SO-AZC-763

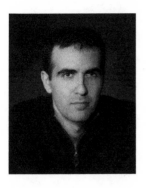

Eliezer J. Sternberg
# NeuroLogic

Eliezer J. Sternberg, M.D., is a resident neurologist at Yale–New Haven Hospital. With a background in neuroscience and philosophy, he studies how brain research can shed light on the mysteries of consciousness and decision making. He is the author of *Are You a Machine?* and *My Brain Made Me Do It.*

Also by Eliezer J. Sternberg

*Are You a Machine?*
*My Brain Made Me Do It*

*Praise for Eliezer J. Sternberg's*

# NeuroLogic

"Each chapter in Sternberg's book reads like a detective novel. His passion for neurology shines through every page. Unlike many brain books, it is encyclopedic in range and scholarly in content, yet highly readable. It is also a valuable antidote to the 'neuron envy' syndrome that many philosophers and psychologists suffer from."
—V. S. Ramachandran, author of *The Tell-Tale Brain*

"The more we learn about the brain the more illogical it seems we are, until you look inside our skulls and examine the brain from an inside perspective, at which point a certain neuro-logic emerges. Eliezer Sternberg's brilliant examination of the human mind reveals the many reasons for our many seemingly unreasonable beliefs and actions. If you want to know why people think and act as they do in such irrational ways, *NeuroLogic* is the first book you should turn to for some rational answers."
—Michael Shermer,
author of *The Believing Brain*

"With his explanation of the hidden logic behind the brain's quirks, Eliezer Sternberg establishes himself as a fresh new voice for neuroscience."
—Sebastian Seung, author of *Connectome*

"In *NeuroLogic*, Sternberg takes us on a fascinating exploration of the impulses and quirks that make us human. An innovative, engaging look inside the black box that is the mind."
—Maria Konnikova, author of
*Mastermind: How to Think Like Sherlock Holmes*

"Dr. Sternberg's enthusiasm for neuroscience bursts out of every page. In clear language he tackles a series of fascinating neurological curiosities that are windows into the wonder of the brain."
—Dr. Sally Satel, coauthor of
*Brainwashed: The Seductive Appeal of Mindless Neuroscience*

"An enchanting journey. . . . The author writes with brio and dash [of] the brain's ability to draw the story of our life, from experience and from thin air."                              —*Kirkus Reviews*

"*NeuroLogic* is an exciting adventure, bringing the most fascinating mysteries of the mind to a very human level. It is a deeply engaging, thought-provoking, and fun read. Sternberg reaches a new level of popular neuroscience literature in the footsteps of Oliver Sacks but with fresh, novel appeal."                    —Hal Blumenfeld, M.D., PhD, author of *Neuroanatomy through Clinical Cases*

# NeuroLogic

# NeuroLogic

*The Brain's Hidden Rationale Behind Our Irrational Behavior*

Eliezer J. Sternberg, M.D.

VINTAGE BOOKS
A Division of Penguin Random House LLC
New York

FIRST VINTAGE BOOKS EDITION, DECEMBER 2016

*Copyright © 2015 by Eliezer J. Sternberg*

All rights reserved. Published in the United States by Vintage Books, a division of Penguin Random House LLC, New York, and distributed in Canada by Random House of Canada, a division of Penguin Random House Canada Limited, Toronto. Originally published in hardcover in the United States by Pantheon Books, a division of Penguin Random House LLC, New York, in 2015.

Vintage and colophon are registered trademarks of Penguin Random House LLC.

The Library of Congress has cataloged the Pantheon edition as follows:
Sternberg, Eliezer J.
NeuroLogic : the brain's hidden rationale behind our irrational behavior /
Eliezer J. Sternberg.
pages ; cm
Includes bibliographical references and index.
1. Cognitive neuroscience.   2. Neuropsychology.   3. Subconsciousness
4. Perception (Philosophy)   I. Title.   II. Title: NeuroLogic.
QP360.5.S74   2016   612.8'233— dc23   2015016491

**Vintage Books Trade Paperback ISBN: 978-0-345-80725-0**
**eBook ISBN: 978-0-307-90878-0**

*Author photograph © Paul Duda*
*Book design by M. Kristen Bearse*

www.vintagebooks.com

Printed in the United States of America
10   9   8   7   6   5   4   3   2   1

For Sharona
and our beautiful children, Alex and Sam

In all chaos there is a cosmos, in all disorder a secret order.

—Carl Jung, *The Archetypes
and the Collective Unconscious*

# Contents

# Introduction

*Our Unconscious Logic*

The mind has its own logic but does not often let others in
on it.

—Bernard DeVoto

Walter had been acting strangely. When friends or family visited, he
ignored them unless they spoke directly to him. Until they uttered a
sound, it was as if they weren't even there. While walking around his
living room, Walter stepped right into his coffee table, then into the
wall. He missed widely when reaching for a cup of coffee and knocked
over a vase instead. At age fifty-five, Walter was having problems with
his vision, yet, inexplicably, he said there was nothing wrong with his
eyesight. But why, Walter's family wondered, would he deny it? Why
wouldn't he seek out help? Confused, they pressed him to go see a neurologist. Walter reluctantly agreed. When he arrived, Walter had the
following exchange with his doctor:

NEUROLOGIST: How are you?
WALTER: Fine.
NEUROLOGIST: Anything wrong with you?
WALTER: No. Everything's perfect.
NEUROLOGIST: Anything wrong with your vision?
WALTER: No. Works fine.
NEUROLOGIST (showing a pen): Then can you tell me what this is?
WALTER: Doc, it's so dark here; nobody can see anything.

With daylight streaming in through the window, the room was plenty bright. Nevertheless, the doctor humored him.

NEUROLOGIST: I put the light on. Can you now see what I have here?

WALTER: Look, I don't want to play games with you.

NEUROLOGIST: Fair enough. But can you describe how I look?

WALTER: Sure. You are a small, fat chap.

The doctor, who was actually tall and thin, understood that Walter wasn't simply denying that he was blind. He actually didn't *realize* it. Was he delirious? Was it early Alzheimer's? Perhaps he needed to speak with a psychiatrist.

The neurologist could infer that there was a connection between Walter's loss of sight and his delusion that everything was fine. Behavioral tests, however, would not be able to identify that connection. He would have to peer inside Walter's brain. A CT scan of his head revealed that Walter had suffered a massive stroke, causing damage to both sides of his occipital lobe, which processes vision. That explained the blindness. But the CT showed something else: damage to the left parietal lobe. Among its many functions, the parietal lobe helps interpret sensory signals, especially visual ones. It compiles the basic visual information sent from the occipital lobe and integrates it to help construct a streamlined picture of the world. The parietal lobe is involved in monitoring how the visual system is working. But what if that monitoring function were impaired?

Walter was diagnosed with Anton's syndrome, a rare disorder in which blind people don't realize they are blind. Patients with Anton's syndrome tend to make excuses for their perceptual mistakes, such as "I'm not wearing my glasses" or "There's a lot of glare from the sun." As one theory goes, this happens because there is a disconnect between the visual system and the brain regions that monitor it. As a result, the brain never gets the message that there's a problem with vision. That's why Walter didn't realize he was blind.

But this story goes deeper still. Not only did Walter fail to admit his blindness, but he came up with an alternative explanation for his symptoms ("It's so dark here"). Walter's brain was faced with a confusing situation. On the one hand, the brain was having trouble perceiving the world. On the other hand, because of the stroke, the brain didn't know that the visual system had been destroyed. What could explain a loss of sight in a person with an intact visual system? It must be dark in here. Faced with contradicting pieces of information, the brain came up with a story to reconcile them. And it was a pretty good one. You might even say that given the circumstances it was perfectly logical.

Deep within our subconscious, there is a system that quietly processes everything we see, hear, feel, and remember. Our brains are constantly bombarded by innumerable sensations streaming in as we interact with our surroundings. Like a movie editor who collects and organizes all the footage and audio to create meaningful stories, the underlying logical system in the brain assembles all of our thoughts and perceptions into a sensible narrative, a narrative that becomes our life experience and sense of self. This book is about that underlying logic and how it creates our conscious experience, whether in those suffering from the weirdest neurological illnesses or during our simplest day-to-day feelings and decisions.

Our objective will be similar to that of other books in the popular science and psychology domain: Can we discover the underlying reasons for the way we think and act? However, we will take a different approach. Many books you might have encountered on the brain rely on behavioral research that, while enlightening in its own right, often doesn't look *inside* the brain to tell us where that behavior comes from. Suppose I give you a machine hidden inside a black box and ask you to figure out how it works. The catch, however, is that I don't let you see what's inside. All the gears and pulleys and levers are concealed within the dark encasing. How would you assess what the machine does? Without the ability to examine the underlying mechanics, all you can do is try using the machine in various ways and look for patterns. From there, you can *infer* how the machine works, but there would still be an element of conjecture. This is a real-world problem in fields like engineering and software development. Consider a software engineer who tries to decipher how a program works without having access to the underlying code. In what is called black box testing, the software designer enters a variety of inputs (such as pushing a button) and records the outputs (seeing what happens) to make educated guesses about how the system works, all without any knowledge of its actual internal structure or mechanics.

That approach is used today to study the human brain. For instance, in a popularized 2010 study, researchers from Harvard, Yale, and MIT had eighty-six volunteer subjects participate in a mock financial negotiation: bargaining down the price of a car with the sticker price of $16,500. One by one, each subject would sit in a chair facing an experimenter who was playing the part of the car salesman. But there was a catch: half the participants were seated in hard, wooden chairs, and the other half were treated to plush, cushioned ones. The result? Those given the hard chairs were the harder bargainers. They were more forceful in their negotiations and bargained the salesman down to a price that was on average $347 lower than that of the comfy chair group. Apparently, the added comfort of the cushioned chairs led the other group to agree to a higher price. Magazines, books, and other commentaries cited the study as yet another breakthrough in the new science of the unconscious. Take, for example, this response from a 2012 article in *Ode* magazine:

> This "hard chair effect" is part of a torrent of new research that is unlocking the mysteries of the human unconscious and show-ing how its enormous powers can be harnessed . . . Over the past decade, neuroscientists and cognitive psychologists have been gradually decoding this unconscious operating system and can now tap into it to induce everything from cleanliness to cleverness in unwitting subjects.

The study tells me that there's an association between chair comfort and the force of negotiation, but it doesn't explain the *cause* of that interaction. What has been "decoded" here? How does the sensation of hardness affect decision making? What system is at work? What model have we discovered that can be applied and connected to other phenomena?

This study is an instance of black box testing. Just like the software designer, the experimenters never gain access to the underlying "code." They observe a trend of inputs and outputs, but the crucial workings of the machine that generate that trend remain hidden.

In this book, we will explore questions about human consciousness by cracking open the black box of the brain and peering at its inner workings. In the process, we'll discover that underlying many of the most mysterious phenomena of human experience, and even the simplest day-to-day decisions, there are distinct neurological circuits, uniting seemingly disconnected facets of our life experience with a single explanation.

The structure of this book is in the form of questions. I have a lot of questions. I am a grown-up version of that kid in the backseat of a minivan who asks his parents a question and then, upon hearing the answer, incessantly responds with "but *why*?" until he drives them to near insanity. In college, this tendency led me to study the art of asking questions: philosophy. Philosophy teaches us to ask questions with precision, to cut through the surface of an issue until you reach the core principle that explains it in all its aspects. As my education moved on from philosophy to neuroscience, to medicine, and eventually to their overlap in medical neurology, I tried to apply that same rigor to a new set of questions: How does decision making work? How do mental illnesses affect the way we think? How do we interact with our brains, and how do they make us who we are?

Our questions will lead us to the mysteries of perception, habit, learning, memory, language, and the very existence of our selfhood and identity. We'll touch on everything from alien abductions, detecting fake smiles, and the real story of schizophrenia to sleepwalking murderers, the brains of sports fans, and the secret of ticklishness. We'll open the black box and, as best we can, use the findings of neuroscience to trace those behaviors to the underlying brain mechanics from which they emerge. With each question we answer, new ones will arise. Every question and answer will build on the previous one as we inch closer to understanding the central questions facing modern neuroscience.

In this book, we will follow the workings of two systems in the brain, the conscious and the unconscious, investigating how they work in parallel and, more important, how they interact in order to create our life experience and preserve our sense of self. My hope is that by the time you finish this book, you'll see that there are discrete patterns in the way that unconscious mechanisms in the brain guide our behavior. There is an underlying *neuro-logic* that drives our experience of the world. You might think of it like a piece of software. Our challenge is to decipher that logical system, not only by observing its inputs and outputs, but also by seeking out the brain systems that generate it. Cracking the code of our internal software has far-reaching implications for neurological and psychiatric research, for the study of human relationships and interactions, and for our understanding of ourselves.

So, where do we begin? In briefly mentioning Walter (note that throughout this book, I have changed the names of people I mention in order to protect the identity and privacy of patients), I said that he failed to detect his blindness because of a broken connection between his visual hardware and the brain systems that were supposed to monitor that hardware. But there may be another explanation as well. Though blind to the external world, patients with Anton's syndrome can still visualize things in their minds. They haven't been blind their entire lives, so they can still *imagine* visual images. Many researchers believe this to be the second reason why people with Anton's syndrome don't feel that they're blind: they mistake their own imagined visual images for actual eyesight. So, when Walter said that his neurologist was a "small, fat chap," it might not have been a simple guess. Perhaps that's how Walter imagined him.

Walter was able to visualize images in his mind because he wasn't always blind, but what if he had been? If a person were born blind, would she have any concept of what it is like to see? How would she "visualize" objects or people in her mind? What do the blind "see" in their dreams?

# NeuroLogic

# 1

# What Do the Blind See When They Dream?

*On Perception, Dreams, and the Creation of the External World*

> What is a television apparatus to man, who has only to shut his eyes to see the most inaccessible regions of the seen and the never seen, who has only to imagine in order to pierce through walls and cause all the planetary Baghdads of his dreams to rise from the dust?
>
> —Salvador Dalí

I'm on the phone with Amelia, a forty-four-year-old insurance agent who has been blind from birth, and I'm scraping the bottom of my mental thesaurus to find descriptive words that will have the same connotation for both of us.

"How do you . . . perceive things?" I ask.

"What do you mean? I just see them."

"You see them?"

"Well, not visually, of course."

"Right." I need a more specific question. "Could you describe the color red?"

"Red is hot," she says. "Red is like fire."

"What about blue?"

"Blue is cold like the ocean."

For most of us, vision is central to the way we navigate the world. It's hard to grasp how members of the blind community are able to function so well without it. When you ask them how they do it, they often respond that the key is using their other senses to compensate for the deficit in vision. Research even confirms that blind individuals have much better hearing than sighted people do.

Most blind people remember what it's like to see. They don't have to construct a mental picture of the world from the ground up. They remember what people, and cars, and sidewalk curbs, and escalators look like. When they tragically go blind, they can build off of what they know.

Amelia never had that luxury. Due to a problem in fetal development, Amelia was born without either of her optic nerves, so she has never seen . . . anything. She has never experienced colors or seen her own reflection. She had to create her mental model of the world from scratch.

"How do you recognize people?" I ask Amelia.

"That depends," she says. "If I've hugged them or felt them, I remember their features. Otherwise, I remember their voices, I guess. I just have a sense of people. I know who they are, who I like, who I don't like."

"Can you describe someone you dislike?"

"Ugh, this woman from work. I can't stand her. She thinks she's *all that*."

"How do you know?" I ask.

"The way she dresses. Her big earrings and long fingernails. Her smelly perfume. Her voice."

What I want to know is what happens in Amelia's mind during the hours she spends unconsciously. Does she have dreams? If so, what are those like?

"I definitely dream," she tells me. "I had a dream last night, quite a vivid one in fact."

"Would you tell me about it?" I pry.

"It's a little embarrassing, but I had a dream that I made love with a man on the beach. He was sexy! Tall, very handsome. He had gorgeous blond hair. The sand was getting everywhere and—"

"Wait, really?" I cut in before the dream becomes too graphic. "You saw him? I mean, did you actually see what he looked like?"

"I saw him," she says. "Definitely. It was real vision. At least I think it was."

During this conversation with Amelia, I couldn't help but grapple with the question of how the dreaming mind and the waking mind compare. In both states, we have some level of consciousness. In both states, we perceive imagery and have experiences. Yet there's something different about dreaming. Something special. But what? And whatever that thing is, is it special enough to lend sight to the blind?

## Filling in the Gaps

Take a look at this image:

Do you see the white triangle? A crisp white triangle appears to cover up the shapes in the background. Technically, though, there is no white triangle. You might have seen this illusion before. The Kanizsa Triangle, as it is known, is a classic illustration of the fact that human vision is not a simple window onto the world. It is an interpretation.

Before we can tackle the issue of whether the blind can see in their dreams, we need to know a little bit about seeing and a little bit about dreaming. Human vision is the brain's highly processed *representation* of what's out there. Why is that? Why couldn't the visual system have been simpler, like a video camera displaying just what's in front of us? It certainly adds intrigue that we can point out the hidden white arrow in the FedEx logo (between the *E* and the *x*), but the reason is more fundamental: our visual system is designed for survival.

From the moment that photons of light become electrochemical signals in the eye, this sensory raw material is passed through an assembly line of processing engines that systematically construct our vision of the world.

It all happens in the well-understood neurological circuit known as the visual pathway. It begins at the rear of the eye, at the retina, where light is translated into electrical signals that zip along the optic nerve through the brain. The signals proceed through the thalamus, the brain's sensory switchboard. From there, the visual information is

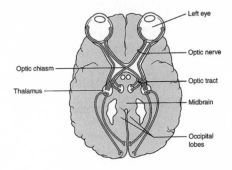

routed straight to the visual cortex, located in the back part of the brain known as the occipital lobe.

To create its interpretation, the visual cortex divides the processing job into components, calculating things like distance, shape, color, size, and speed. An interruption in any of these processes could lead to striking visual distortions. In Riddoch syndrome, for example, patients lose the ability to perceive stationary objects and can only see things in motion. Neurologists first observed the condition in 1916, when a lieutenant colonel was shot in the head while advancing into battle during World War I. The bullet entered his right occipital lobe, destroying much of his visual cortex but sparing the region known as area MT, which is responsible for the perception of motion. The soldier was blind to most visual characteristics of objects, but he could perceive their movements. In his words, "The 'moving things' have no distinct shape, and the nearest approach to color that can be attributed to them is a shadowy grey." You know the blur you see when a ball is thrown past you? Imagine if that's all you could see.

On the flip side, isolated damage to area MT causes a selective loss of motion perception. Imagine standing at a street corner watching a car pass by. Instead of seeing it smoothly cruise along, you perceive sequential snapshots of the car in different places. First it's on your left, then it's on your right, but you never saw it move. That would make crossing the street a terrifying ordeal. It's no wonder that motion is one of the first components of vision to be processed. When an object travels past you, the most prominent thing you see is its motion, while most of the details of its appearance seem glossed over by the brain. Perhaps the reason for this is evolutionary: if a wild beast is running at you, the most important thing to realize is not necessarily the color of its fur or the length of its tail but the fact that it's running at you.

Our visual system doesn't just display patterns of light. It constructs an interpretation based on billions of neuronal calculations. The brain anticipates what things will look like based on what we've seen in the past. It even uses environmental cues to fill in supposed gaps in a scene, as it does with the Kanizsa Triangle. The brain fills in the edges of the nonexistent shape, inferring their location from cues provided by the neighboring shapes. For another example, try reading this:

Dseitpe the fcat taht the ltetres in tehese wrdos are jmbuled, you are sitll albe to raed tehm. Bceasue the frsit and lsat ltertes are in the rghit palce, yuor bairn can use tohse ceus to fgirue out waht I'm syanig.

You might have seen paragraphs like this circulating the Internet, with claims that we read words "all at once" rather than using the individual letters. That's actually not something that research has demonstrated. Rather, what's interesting about our ability to read that paragraph is the way we infer the words from their context, both from the meaning of the sentence and from the fact that the first and last letters are in the correct places. Neuroimaging studies show that the brain processes not only the meaning of words we read but also the patterns of letters and the syntax of the sentences.

The brain often takes shortcuts when we read, skipping certain connector or filler words that aren't crucial to the meaning of a sentence. It makes reading more efficient. At times, however, that anticipatory approach can backfire. For example, here's a question: How many animals of each kind did Moses take on the ark? If you are like most people who were asked this question as part of a study, you would probably say the answer is "two." With a more careful reading, however, it's clear that the correct answer is "zero." It was Noah, not Moses, who built an ark and invited the animals on board. People likely make the error because the question is a close match to one we would expect to hear about Noah. When we hear "How many animals of each kind," we anticipate the end of the question and jump the gun on coming up with the answer.

Neurologists can see this process occurring in the brain using functional magnetic resonance imaging (fMRI). The fMRI technique measures, in real time, the rate at which blood releases oxygen to brain tissue, providing what's called the BOLD (blood oxygen level dependent) signal. The interpretation of the measurement is based on the principle that the neurons that extract the most oxygen are the ones that are most active, so the BOLD signal is a measure of neuronal activity. In a 2013 fMRI study, participants read 160 sentences, half of which were true. Of the other eighty sentences, half were clearly false, while the other half were meant to appear true but had subtle distortions, including the one about Moses and his supposed ark. While an fMRI machine monitored their brain activity, the participants read through the sentences and marked them as true or false.

The results showed that there wasn't much difference in the subjects' brain activity while they read the true and clearly false statements. But what happened when the subjects read the trick statements, like the one about Moses and the ark? Well, that depended on whether they noticed the distortion. For those who failed to detect it, and incorrectly thought the statements were true, the fMRI revealed an activation pattern similar to the one seen while reading the true or clearly false statements. However, for the participants who discovered the distortion and realized that Moses was too busy in Egypt to build a boat, the fMRI revealed that a radically different neurological system was at work. Many more regions of the brain were recruited to interpret the sentence, like the anterior cingulate cortex, involved in error detection, but most notably the prefrontal cortex, which is the center of many higher-level cognitive tasks including, interestingly enough, the power to overcome our tendency to rely on habit.

The brain tries to maximize the efficiency of our thinking by recognizing familiar patterns and anticipating them. Moses's ark and other distorted sentences require the greatest concentration to interpret, because they introduce a conflict between their expected and their actual meaning. As the neuroimaging results imply, the only way to successfully identify the distortion is to use the higher cognitive powers granted by the prefrontal cortex to suppress our tendency to anticipate what's coming and just focus on what's actually there. The self-reflective capacity of consciousness can override the brain's unconscious, automated processes, preventing them from filling in the gaps as they normally would.

When we look out into the world, two systems in the brain mold our perceptions. On the one hand, there is the unconscious system that recognizes patterns, anticipates based on those patterns, and deduces how the perceptual fragments fit together. On the other hand, there is the conscious system that accepts the calculations of the unconscious— questioning them when necessary—and formulates decisions based on the wealth of background knowledge to which it has access. Both systems have their uses. The fact that automated processes help us read words with jumbled letters is just a single instance of the myriad ways that the unconscious anticipates patterns, completing a picture using incomplete information. Yet, as the Moses example reveals, the conscious system is equally crucial in helping us decide when to *trust* the unconscious system's prediction, especially when something in our environment is trying to trick us or outmaneuver us.

A group of psychologists and sports scientists published a 2013 study looking at the brain regions activated as experienced soccer players watch their opponents come at them. The experimenters recruited two groups of players: active professionals and recreational soccer players who competed occasionally. The researchers instructed the athletes to imagine that they were on defense in the midst of a competitive match. They would each watch video clips of offensive players dribbling toward them. The challenge? Determine whether an offensive player's next move will be a normal crossover or a deceptive step-over. All the while, the experimenters used fMRI to watch the subjects' brains at work.

As expected, the professional players were a lot better at reading their opponents. Yet the fMRI results showed that regardless of skill level, whenever players correctly detected the step-overs, they used their prefrontal cortices more than they did when detecting the straightforward crossovers. It was the same region of the brain that the subjects in the reading experiment used to identify the distortion in the sentence about Moses's ark. The soccer players used the higher cognitive faculties of the prefrontal to override pattern recognition of a standard move and instead detect deception. In reading, in sports, and in other situations, it takes the discerning power of the prefrontal cortex to stop your unconscious from jumping to conclusions and possibly falling for a trick. Through conscious analysis, we can distinguish typical patterns from those that are manipulated or distorted.

What would happen to our perceptions if the prefrontal cortex were shut down? We would lose the ability to judge whether our experiences are typical or whether they diverge from the norm. That can occur in instances of brain damage. In 2010, a team of neurologists and psychologists recruited seventeen patients for a study using that same sentence with the Moses for Noah switcheroo (and other sentences with similar formats). The patients had all endured ruptures of a key blood vessel that feeds the prefrontal cortex, causing profound damage there, while the rest of their brains were spared. Just as predicted, the prefrontal lobe patients, compared with healthy controls, were much worse at detecting the distortions in each sentence.

The unconscious system in the brain pieces together fragments of our perceptions, anticipating patterns and filling in gaps when necessary, in order to devise a single, meaningful interpretation. It tells a story. The conscious system experiences that story but can also reflect on it and even question it. However, cases of isolated prefrontal lobe damage create a scenario in which most of the brain is working but the self-reflective capabilities of prefrontal cognition are lacking. In the absence of that supervision, the unconscious, gap-filling processes of the brain are unchecked as they anticipate and piece together our experience, possibly leading to nonsensical interpretations and bizarre stories. But brain damage isn't the only way to bring about that scenario. It can also happen in perfectly healthy people, and it can happen often. It might even have happened to you last night.

## The Stuff That Dreams Are Made Of

In his famous 1944 painting *Dream Caused by the Flight of a Bee Around a Pomegranate,* the Spanish artist Salvador Dalí depicted a vision he imagined his wife dreamed moments before awakening from a nap. In the painting, Dalí reveals some insight into the true nature of dreams. He illustrates their vividness, their emotional intensity, and their propensity for being peculiar or fantastical. This particular painting has inspired a diverse set of interpretations, a prominent one being that it depicts a scene of imminent rape, given the violent imagery and the possible use of the rifle as a phallic symbol. Others take a more straightforward approach, using the title of the painting as a guide.

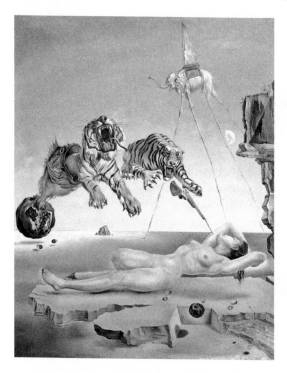

If you look carefully, you'll notice that there is a second, small pomegranate toward the bottom of the painting, with a bee buzzing over it. Perhaps Dalí thought that the buzzing of a real bee around his wife's sleeping figure somehow entered her unconscious and guided the narrative of her dream. Her mind translated a sudden fear of being stung into violent imagery, with the stinger represented by the sharp rifle tip pressing into her arm. But how could such a simple stimulus, a buzzing sound, engender such an elaborate mental mirage?

Dalí painted what most of us already suspected: though they can often be bizarre, dreams may incorporate elements of our daily life and connect them in novel, occasionally nonsensical, or even metaphoric ways to create a narrative. The sleeping brain is a master storyteller, and that power emerges from its unique environment. When we sleep, our eyes are shut, sounds are muted. Essentially closed off from external sensory noise, the mind begins to fill with imagery generated from within.

However, when we dream, we are not *completely* cut off from the outside. Certain stimuli, like a buzzing insect, can make their way into our nocturnal imagery. External sensations infiltrate our dreams all the time. One of the most powerful effects of this kind occurs when you spray a sleeping person with water. Over 40 percent of the time, that stimulus becomes directly integrated into the person's dreams. Awakened subjects describe visions that incorporate things like a rainy day, being squirted by someone, or having to repair a leaky roof.

Still, most of what we dream is a quilt of our memories, thoughts, and emotions. Often our dreams are abstract reflections of things that occur to us in our daily lives, things we contemplate, worry about, and long for. Most dreams incorporate aspects that are familiar to the dreamer. In 2004, researchers in Belgium used positron emission tomography (PET scans, which track brain activity by following a radioactive tracer as it moves to active areas) to monitor the brain activity of subjects as they played a first-person shooter video game. The researchers noted the areas of the brain activated as the subjects moved through the streets of the virtual reality town. In the second part of the experiment, the research group had the participants go to sleep, but not before their scalps were outfitted with EEG (electroencephalogram) electrodes to monitor their brain waves overnight. The next morning, a comparison of the EEG recordings with the PET scans revealed that the same areas of the hippocampus that illuminated during the video game were again stirred as the subjects began to dream.

We know that vision is made possible by the visual pathway and that blindness can result from an interruption anywhere along that circuit. There's also a dream pathway in the brain. Like vision, dreams allow for the perception of imagery, even though the eyes are closed and effectively blinded to the outside world. The fact that we are *still* able to perceive this imagery implies that the dream circuit must be separate from the visual one. If it's true that the blind can see in their dreams, then the dream pathway must be the key. So, the obvious question is, what constitutes that circuit? How does the brain create our dreams?

As you enter REM sleep, while your eyes are shut, the dream system takes over the thalamus and the visual cortex. It controls your internal sensory switchboard, as well as your center of image processing, but it still has to get the images from somewhere.

Neurologists have discovered that, as we dream, the thalamus begins behaving differently: instead of responding to signals arriving from the eyes (of which there are none), the thalamus falls under the control of the brainstem, the central stalk that adjoins the brain to the spinal cord. A major function of the brainstem is to maintain REM sleep, when most dreaming occurs. Many neurologists believe that this link between the thalamus and the brainstem that occurs nightly during REM sleep is the basis of dream imagery.

By watching the brain waves that appear as we dream, neurologists have picked up on unique waves, called PGO (ponto-geniculo-occipital) waves. They have a recognizable shape and size. This same wave is seen in three locations in the brain as we dream: the pons (in the brainstem), the lateral geniculate nucleus (the visual part of the thalamus), and the occipital lobe (where the visual cortex lives). We can infer, therefore, that these regions are working together. Perhaps the brainstem, thalamus, and visual cortex form their own visual pathway, but the eyes are cut out of the process. The dream pathway is similar to the visual pathway except that the brainstem replaces the eyes as the source. The imagery is generated from within.

The renowned dream researcher John Allan Hobson, a psychiatrist at Harvard Medical School, has theorized that dreams occur due to random neuronal firings in the brainstem. From the brainstem, these haphazard signals go to the thalamus, which treats them as it would any visual signal. The thalamus is just a switchboard. It has no idea whether the signals it receives come from the eyes or the brainstem. It just routes them where they need to go: to the visual cortex.

Now imagine what the visual cortex has to deal with. It's 2:00 a.m., and a barrage of signals has just arrived from the thalamus. What's more, the signals are a mess of disorganization. After all, they were randomly generated by the brainstem. But the visual cortex doesn't know that. It assumes that whatever information it receives from the thalamus must have come from the eyes. How does the cortex respond? Just as it would do if we were awake, the visual cortex tries to make sense of the information. Using our store of knowledge and memory, it attempts to connect disparate signal fragments into a single narrative, creating a unified visual spectacle that we experience as dreaming.

The brain does its best to tell a story. The unconscious system in the brain has a knack for finding patterns, anticipating what comes next, and using contextual clues to fill in the gaps when encountering an incomplete picture. These might all come into play as the unconscious stitches together our nightly visions from the tattered signals it receives. The resulting patchwork of thoughts, memories, fears, and wishes can come together as an engrossing, occasionally metaphoric narrative. Usually, however, our dreams are pretty weird.

As weird as dreams can be, we never seem to notice their outlandishness while we're in them. Only when we wake up do we realize how bizarre the imagined scenario was. Why is that? In learning which parts of the brain are involved in dreaming, neuroscientists have also discovered which parts go dormant for the night. Most prominently, the prefrontal cortex, where higher-order decision making takes place, is utterly quiet. The prefrontal cortex, if you recall, is the region involved in discovering the Moses/Noah distortion and spotting deceptive soccer moves. It's involved in self-reflective thinking.

When we dream, we don't actively plan or strategize, nor do we reflect much on our thoughts. Those are abilities mediated by the prefrontal cortex, which is shut down during REM sleep. That's why we can't tell that we're dreaming. It's why dreams can get away with being so bizarre without our thinking, "Wait a minute . . . this doesn't make any sense." If you do happen to realize how weird the dream is, you're likely in the process of waking, and your prefrontal cortex is starting to fire up.

The prefrontal's inactivity may also be the explanation for why we don't feel as if we can control our imagined avatar and make decisions while dreaming. The dream is like a movie that's happening to us. We can't choose our own adventure; at least we usually can't. There is one major exception, known as lucid dreams, in which a person knows he is dreaming and can even willfully explore his imagined internal world.

How are lucid dreams possible? We just got finished saying that the prefrontal cortex is deactivated as we sleep, so how could someone actively control his dreams? In 2012, German sleep researchers asked that same question. They recruited some lucid dreamers to fall asleep in the company of their fMRI machine. As the participants entered REM sleep, the fMRI picked up an interesting pattern of activation. The BOLD signal, in addition to highlighting the regions normally active during dreams, appeared prominently in the prefrontal area. The prefrontal cortex was *active*. For reasons unknown, some people's prefrontal cortices resist the nightly shutdown that the rest of us experience.

Lucid dreamers have access to their capacities for self-reflection, self-control, and decision making, rendering each dream a thrilling exercise in virtual reality. What's more, lucid dreaming is a skill that you can acquire with training and has been used successfully as a treatment for nightmares. With practice, you can just politely ask the ghosts and ax murderers to get lost.

Most dreams are not simple replays of our daily lives; that accounts for just about 1 to 2 percent of dreams. The rest of the time, our unhinged thoughts and visualizations come together in new, often creative ways. Through dreams, the unconscious system in the brain provides us with an alternative way of associating concepts, closed off from all the distractions of waking life. Ideas can dance freely through the mind.

Perhaps that's why we think of great new ideas as we sleep. How often have you awoken from sleep only to frantically seek out a pen and paper to jot down a moment of inspiration? Studies demonstrate that if you give a math problem to two groups of people, one that tries to solve it right away and one that does so after sleeping through the night, the group that sleeps on it is much more likely to discover creative shortcuts.

What is it about the dreaming brain that makes our thoughts and experiences come together in unique ways? One explanation is that sleep protects us from external stimuli, preventing interference and allowing our imagination to flourish. Another possibility is that the prefrontal cortex is largely deactivated, so our more abstract, and even bizarre, thoughts can frolic without being subjected to our usual judgmental analytic rigor. There may be a third, more fundamental explanation for why dreams are so creative. Some neuroscientists theorize that during sleep the brain relaxes preformed synapses (the spaces between neurons through which they communicate), loosening connections between our memories and learned concepts. This is thought to enhance neuronal flexibility, allowing new pathways to form in the brain and fresh, creative ideas to burst forth. In fact, some studies show that the neurons that have worked together most extensively during the day are the most quiet as we sleep. The theory is that relaxing our synapses opens the door for dreaming. It creates the opportunity for novel connections between our thoughts to emerge, allowing the brain to spin its stories.

However they arise, our dreams are wildly different from our waking perceptions, and it's because we have two fundamentally different systems at work in the brain. On the one hand, there is the active, conscious system that we use when we're awake. On the other hand, there's the passive, inner world of dreaming that takes over when the conscious system shuts down. Lucid dreaming would represent some sort of in-between state that recruits brain regions from both systems. Dreams tend to happen as we sleep and end when we wake up; we generally don't dream and make conscious decisions simultaneously. When we awaken, we slip out of our internal fantasy as consciousness overtakes us. The conscious and unconscious systems take turns seizing and ceding control. However, as Dalí's painting and lucid dreams imply, that boundary between dream and reality can be a tenuous one.

## Down the Rabbit Hole

Marcy first went to see her doctor for a severe headache. For most of her life, she had suffered from headaches that seemed to last for ages. Her mom, dad, and sister had migraines, so it came as no surprise to her when her doctor gave her that diagnosis. Like many others with migraines, Marcy experienced an "aura" before each one. Most people describe the aura as a disturbance of perception in which they see spots or lights or zigzagging lines. The experience varies depending on the person, but Marcy's auras were particularly memorable.

"I suddenly get a feeling that my hands are huge," she began, "and I mean huge: ginormous; as though I am wearing triple boxing gloves—this lasts for a while, then I get a funny physical feeling while my hands are staying big that I am shrinking into a tiny, tiny, tiny little girl."

Sometimes, she would feel as if she had suddenly grown into a giant: "I sort of feel as though I am on spongy platform shoes like we used to wear in the '70s. It's really weird; I am only five foot and it's the most peculiar feeling to suddenly feel that you are tall."

Marcy's symptoms are curiously reminiscent of the famous scene from the first chapter of Lewis Carroll's *Alice in Wonderland,* titled "Down the Rabbit-Hole." After entering her fantastical realm, Alice comes upon a bottle labeled "DRINK ME":

So Alice ventured to taste it, and finding it very nice, (it had, in fact, a sort of mixed flavour of cherry-tart, custard, pine-apple, roast turkey, toffee, and hot buttered toast,) she very soon finished it off. "What a curious feeling!" said Alice; "I must be shutting up like a telescope." And so it was indeed: she was now only ten inches high, and her face brightened up at the thought that she was now the right size for going through the little door into that lovely garden.

Whatever ailment Marcy was suffering from, it apparently caused hallucinations much like those which Alice's mysterious cocktail provoked. Marcy was diagnosed with the aptly named Alice in Wonderland syndrome, a neurological condition in which people perceive distortions of the size, position, movement, or color of objects in the environment.

First described in 1952, Alice in Wonderland syndrome can be caused by any number of things, like infections or seizures, but it usually happens in association with migraines. Though it isn't common, Alice in Wonderland syndrome might have influenced the work of prominent artists who, at times, experienced the world as if looking at a circus mirror. For instance, Käthe Kollwitz, a twentieth-century German artist, became known for her drawings inspired by her political impressions of Germany during wartime. Yet at some point in her career, her style appeared to shift from the genre of realism to more abstract representations of people who appeared to have enlarged hands or faces.

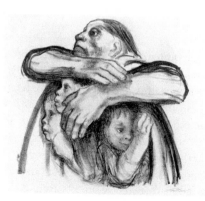

In her diary, Kollwitz lamented being stricken by the following symptoms: "Then there was a horrible state I fell into when objects would
begin to grow smaller. It was bad enough when they grew larger, but
when they grew smaller it was horrifying."

Some scholars have speculated that Lewis Carroll himself had Alice
in Wonderland syndrome, as he was known to have suffered from
migraines. Perhaps he perceived visual metamorphoses similar to those
of his most famous literary character.

Why does Alice in Wonderland syndrome happen? Preliminary
research seems to indicate that the hallucinations arise from a blockage
of visual processing. As we know, the visual cortex constructs our picture of the world by making a series of calculations: distance, size, orientation, shape. If parts of that processing pathway were skipped or
blocked, that would lead to distortions in perception. A 2011 study of
a boy with Alice in Wonderland syndrome used fMRI to monitor his
brain activity while he tried to judge the size and orientation of pictures
presented to him. For example, the experimenters showed him versions
of the Ponzo illusion (below) and asked him to judge whether the two
parallel lines were each the same size.

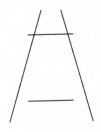

This tricky task requires careful study of the image and, presumably,
thorough processing in the visual cortex. The fMRI results revealed
that compared with healthy control subjects, the boy had *reduced*
activation of parts of his visual cortex. The theory is that this finding
represents incomplete processing of visual signals and, depending on
which stage of processing is missed, that might cause distortions of size,
orientation, or anything else. While far from proven, this hypothesis is
consistent with reports of patients with targeted damage to parts of the
visual cortex who suddenly perceive objects around them as shrunken.

In some cases, Alice in Wonderland syndrome can be a component of a larger hallucinatory disorder. One that comes to mind is Lhermitte's peduncular hallucinosis, a rare cause of vivid hallucinations that occur as a result of damage to the brainstem. People with peduncular hallucinosis can see anything from bright colors, to distortions of size (Alice in Wonderland syndrome can be a subtype of peduncular hallucinosis), to extremely convincing, cinematic hallucinations. It was first reported in 1922 by the neurologist Jean Lhermitte, who told the story of a woman who suffered a stroke in her brainstem and, as a result, began having hallucinations. Whenever it was dark, she would see a parade of brightly dressed little children. A rare disorder, peduncular hallucinosis has not been the subject of a large, controlled study. What we know about the disease comes from a series of individual reports, beginning with Lhermitte's first patient and continuing to the present day.

In 2008, neurologists in Italy described a disturbing case of an eleven-year-old boy who developed striking hallucinations after recovering from a fever. One evening, after an afternoon of watching television, young Bernardo began hysterically crying. His parents ran into the room to find their son trembling in fear. He had just seen Voldemort, the villainous sorcerer from the Harry Potter stories. It might have been dark, but Bernardo insisted that the vision was real. He had not been dreaming.

The next night, Voldemort returned. Bernardo knew that this time he would have to defend himself. He looked down and saw a battle helmet and sword, ready to be brandished. Glaring through the metal eyeholes, Bernardo looked upon his adversary and, sword in hand, hallucinated an epic duel.

A complete neurological work-up revealed that young Bernardo had endured inflammation of his brainstem, which is why he had a fever. When the inflammation went away, so did Voldemort. It was a case of peduncular hallucinosis, but a temporary one. While the brainstem was inflamed, the hallucinations emerged. When the inflammation dissipated, the hallucinations went with it. From this and other reports of the syndrome, it appears that damage to the brainstem is the cause. Most cases of peduncular hallucinosis arise from brainstem injury, or sometimes from damage to the thalamus, and persist as long as that injury goes unrepaired.

Neurologists have noticed two other things that these patients have in common. First, people with peduncular hallucinosis also complain of particularly vivid dreams. Second, people tend to experience the hallucinations when it's dark. When the lights come on, the visions disappear.

Why do the hallucinations surface in darkness? From what we know about the neuroscience of dreaming, it all begins in the brainstem, which contains the on/off switch of dreaming. As we enter REM sleep, tucked away under the blankets with only moonlight brightening our bedrooms, the brainstem initiates the dream pathway. The switch turns on. As morning arrives, and we wake up, the brainstem shuts down the dream pathway as our eyes open and light floods in.

Usually, the switch only turns on during REM sleep, but damage to the brainstem lowers its threshold for initiating dreams. Rather than during sleep, the brainstem prematurely flips the switch when it senses darkness. In peduncular hallucinosis, *people dream while awake.* Simply turning out the lights is enough to rouse the dream machine to fill the darkness with imagery of its own making.

But what if those lights were turned off forever, as they are for the blind? What would we see then?

## A Vision for the Sightless

The neighbors were growing increasingly concerned about Mr. Weiler. An eighty-seven-year-old widower living alone, Mr. Weiler had lost his sight due to long-standing macular degeneration, a common cause of blindness in old age. His neighbors' concern reached new heights when he reported that he had started seeing again . . . seeing things he didn't expect. For the previous six weeks, he saw people in his house whom he didn't recognize and who never spoke to him. The week before, a bear lumbered into his kitchen. Every so often, he saw cattle grazing in his living room. They would stare at him while quietly chewing at the grass that was apparently growing out of his carpet. Mr. Weiler also mentioned seeing a family of bluefish in his house, darting from wall to wall.

The neighbors worried that the kindly old gentleman was developing dementia. Mr. Weiler wasn't particularly concerned, though. He recognized that the visions weren't real, and they didn't bother him much. A complete work-up by a neurologist showed that it wasn't dementia after all. Mr. Weiler's condition was consistent with a diagnosis of Charles Bonnet syndrome.

When we hear the term "hallucinations," the first thing that comes to mind is a psychiatric or neurological disorder (or illicit drugs), but Mr. Weiler didn't have anything wrong with his brain. Charles Bonnet (pronounced "bon*ney*") syndrome is a condition in which people experience rich visual hallucinations not because of a neurological problem but because of a visual one. It happens to people who are blind or partially blind. Hallucinatory episodes can last from a few seconds to most of the day and can occur on and off over a period of years. The content of the hallucinations varies but usually includes things like people, animals, buildings, and patterns of shapes. Many have tried to depict their hallucinations. The artist Cecil Riley, for example, would paint his vision of blue and green eyes surrounding him, glaring at him threateningly.

Here's a sketch by another patient with macular degeneration and Charles Bonnet syndrome (not an artist) who described seeing an "elongated face with disproportionately large teeth and ears."

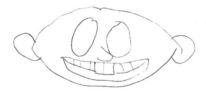

Charles Bonnet syndrome is seen in about 10 percent of people with visual problems, regardless of the underlying cause. Why does this happen? Could it be that the brain is filling in the gap in vision with hallucinations? As the Kanizsa Triangle teaches us, the brain fills in the gaps of what we see, and that which we perceive may not be the same as what's actually in front of us. However, seeing an illusory white triangle is slightly different from seeing cattle grazing in your living room. When we look at optical illusions, we aren't hallucinating. Our brains are extrapolating a scene by processing visual cues. Hallucinations, on the other hand, arise solely from our minds.

It's no coincidence that the hallucinations of Charles Bonnet tend to happen to people who are blind. Visual impairment is the key. A research group in London was able to demonstrate the brain activity that occurs during Charles Bonnet hallucinations. They recruited six people with the diagnosis to tell them whenever a hallucination began and ended. All the while, the researchers recorded their brain activity. All the volunteers were visually impaired, so the fMRI revealed minimal activity in their visual cortices most of the time. However, as soon as one of them signaled that a hallucination had begun, the occipital lobe suddenly ignited with activity. When the hallucination ended, so did the illumination of the visual cortex on the screen.

The fMRI told a lot more about the hallucinations than just the time course. The BOLD signal revealed which visual processors were being utilized to create the visions.

In Charles Bonnet syndrome, the visual cortex activates without any input signal from the eyes. There are two theories as to why this happens. The first is that because of the absence of signals coming in from the damaged eyes, neurons of the visual cortex have nothing to do and begin behaving erratically. The theory is that these bored nerve cells occasionally release spontaneous electrical discharges. The visual cortex is freed from the constraints of being regulated by sensory input and starts generating its own signals—leading to the use of the term "release hallucinations" for the symptom of Charles Bonnet.

These release hallucinations can even be caused by a temporary visual disturbance. On September 3, 2004, a young woman was struck by lightning while mountain climbing in the Alps. After being thrown to the ground by the blast, she blacked out. When she awoke, she was blind. An air rescue team brought her to a hospital where a CT scan showed fluid accumulation around her occipital lobe, interfering with her visual processing. When night came, she began to hallucinate. First she saw an old lady perched on top of the radiator at the edge of the room. The lady started shrinking, getting thinner and thinner until she slid down and vanished through one of the radiator slots. Her visions popped up at random times. At one moment, she would see a cowboy on a horse galloping toward her, firing off his rifle. Later she would see two doctors attempting sexual intercourse in her room, then trying to draw her blood. But as the fluid was drained from the back of her brain and her vision recovered, the hallucinations stopped coming.

Even if the blindness is short-lived, it appears that the absence of visual input causes the brain to generate its own visions. The theory is that the underused visual cortex neurons begin firing for no reason. When these spontaneous discharges are detected, the brain mistakes them for meaningful visual signals because, after all, they are coming from the visual cortex. This is just like what happens in dreaming, only there the random signals originate in the brainstem, earlier in the dream pathway. Here, it is the visual circuitry itself that fills the gap left by patients' blindness with dreamlike imagery. Within moments, the images spit out by the visual cortex reach consciousness and patients experience them as realistic hallucinations, as if seeing them with their own eyes.

There's a second theory for why Charles Bonnet syndrome affects the blind. It involves brain plasticity, the vast, dynamic interconnectedness of our neuronal network. We tend to think of our five senses as being distinct from one another, but that isn't the way the brain treats them. The brain can't tell the difference between visual, auditory, and tactile signals except for the fact that they are transmitted by different pathways. As long as the circuits are hooked up correctly, the information will get to the right place. In the brain, it's all just electrochemical signals; neurons have no idea what the signals they transmit and receive are for. The reason we experience five separate senses—seeing through our eyes and smelling through our nostrils—is that the chains of nerve cells are organized into discrete pathways.

Though each sensory conduit has its own route, there is some crossover between them. Think of these nerve pathways as major highways that intersect. They are isolated most of the time, but there are exit ramps that connect them. There have to be, right? After all, we experience all five senses at once, and they all fit together seamlessly. Picture yourself drinking a cup of coffee. Not only do you simultaneously smell and taste the French roast, but you feel the mug against your lips, see it as you tip it toward yourself, and hear the sound of your sips. Each sensation is perfectly coordinated with the rest, creating the sensory symphony that is your morning caffeine kick. Five completely separate systems couldn't possibly create such a well-orchestrated experience consistently. Somewhere along the line, our senses have to merge.

So, the highway map of the visual cortex has on-ramps and off-ramps that link it to other brain systems. Now imagine a person who becomes blind. The principles of brain plasticity dictate that nerves slink away from areas that are dormant and proliferate in areas that are active. After a person becomes blind, the visual pathway deteriorates as the occipital lobe stops getting visual input from the eyes. The road empties out. Suddenly the on-ramps from other, nonvisual systems are the only source of cars on the road. That once small percentage of the visual cortex that links up to other sensory systems grows, while the rest of the visual system atrophies. This neuronal growth reinforces the connection between the inactive visual pathway and the nonvisual brain systems.

With all this crisscrossing circuitry, some nonvisual signals might enter the occipital cortex and be mistakenly interpreted as visual input from the eyes. Remember, the brain can't tell one signal from another. It's all about the pathways. Therefore, if previously discrete circuits become linked, signals sent by another sensory system might take the ramp toward the visual cortex and be processed as vision. It could be the smell of garden flowers or the sound of a subway car. Whatever the signal is, if it crosses over to the visual circuitry, it may cause visual hallucinations.

Luckily, Charles Bonnet patients are aware of their own blindness, so they tend to realize that what they're seeing isn't real. Unlike during dreams, the prefrontal cortex is working, allowing them to reflect on the peculiarity of their perceptions. But what would happen if they didn't know they were blind? That scenario is called Anton's syndrome, which we discussed in this book's introduction. We heard the story of a gentleman named Walter who denied his own blindness. When asked to describe his tall, thin neurologist, Walter confidently declared that he was a "small, fat chap." In Anton's syndrome, there is a missing link between the visual system and the higher-level sensory regions that monitor it. Without the ability to detect when the visual cortex is compromised, patients with Anton's syndrome falsely think their vision is intact. Therefore, if they were to have a release hallucination, the way Charles Bonnet patients do, their brains might be unable to detect that the vision isn't real. In fact, many people who suffer from Anton's syndrome mistake their own imagination, the images they generate internally, for actual vision. That's probably why Walter fabricated that depiction of his doctor. His brain was unconsciously filling in the gap of his visual perception without realizing it had done so.

If it's true, as all these cases imply, that visual deprivation can lead to hallucinations, shouldn't the same thing happen for our other senses? Shouldn't damage to the circuit that controls our hearing, for example, cause us to have auditory hallucinations?

Consider the case of Mr. Pasche, a fifty-two-year-old man with a long history of ringing in his ears who arrived at a mental health clinic concerned about a peculiar new symptom. Over the previous few weeks, the simple ringing in his ears had become a shrill, repeating beeping noise like an alarm clock. Just like a real alarm, it would wake him up at night. Over time, the alarm sound dissipated but was replaced by music. Sometimes he hallucinated mash-ups of popular songs, including the vocals, while at other times he heard classical symphonies. It was as if his brain were constantly tuned in to an imaginary radio station. He noticed that very loud noises, like a passing subway train, would relieve the hallucinations. Moderately loud noise, on the other hand, would have an additive effect. In fact, if he passed a bongo player on the street, the music in his mind would begin to synchronize with the beat of the drum.

After a neurological and psychiatric work-up found no problems, Mr. Pasche went to see an otolaryngologist, who decided to test his hearing. Apparently, his hearing was poor enough that he met the criteria for deafness. It turns out that musical hallucinations tend to happen in people with hearing loss. This scenario has even been given the term "auditory Charles Bonnet syndrome."

With minimal activity happening in the auditory circuit, Mr. Pasche's brain filled in the void with sounds of its own making. If a sound was loud enough, like that of the subway rushing past, Mr. Pasche was able to hear it, and the hallucinations stopped as the sensory vacancy disappeared. Quieter sounds, however, could not overcome his hearing condition. As his auditory pathway sat idly, the unconscious system in the brain switched on the hallucination radio to fill the silence.

Though Mr. Pasche experienced auditory, rather than visual, hallucinations, it's thought his symptoms developed in the same way that they do in Charles Bonnet, with the same twofold explanation. First, brain tissue deprived of its normal function may begin to act spontaneously, firing off random signals. Depending on whether that happens in the auditory or visual cortex, you get the corresponding type of hallucination. Second, the underused brain region may gradually become a site for growth of nerves from other systems, allowing for novel patterns of interaction. When a sensory highway isn't being used, a formerly trivial on-ramp from one of the other senses becomes a major source of cars on the road. As a result, the brain develops that intersection by adding more lanes until it becomes a significant traffic junction. Before you know it, the auditory cortex is being activated by traffic that originated on a different pathway.

If you prefer computer analogies to transportation ones, just imagine what would happen if you cracked open your friend's laptop's circuit board and started reconnecting wires. After crisscrossing the circuitry, you hand the computer back to your friend, who soon discovers that typing vowels causes his sound system to blast rap music. So too, the brain can acquire new functions as its neural pathways evolve and merge. For the blind or the deaf, those neural changes can help compensate for their deficit in perception. When it comes to crossing our senses, however, the brain needs only to enhance the intersections that are already in place. In fact, our senses are far more connected than we may realize. Just ask Luke Skywalker.

## Luke Skywalker Lives in Your Temporal Lobe

What does the name "Luke Skywalker" mean to you? If you are a *Star Wars* fan, those words don't simply refer to a character from a movie. When you read them, you are momentarily transported into a science fiction universe, a clash between good and evil, and an iconic pop cultural sphere. But what if you had merely heard the name read aloud? What if you saw a picture of Mark Hamill, the actor who portrayed him?

We've seen that the neural pathways of our five senses overlap, perhaps promoting the development of hallucinations if one of our senses is lost. Those intersections exist in all of us, so how do they affect the way our brains perceive and interpret our environment? A team of neurologists asked the following questions: Does the type of sensory system we use affect the way that our brains process information? Does it make any difference to the brain whether information comes from our eyes, ears, nose, or elsewhere?

The researchers used EEG electrodes to record the neuronal activity in the brains of volunteers. The participants looked at a computer screen as a sequence of pictures appeared—pictures of celebrities, famous buildings, nature scenes, or animals. Watching the EEG monitor, the neuroscientists noticed a pattern. The pattern appeared in a region known as the medial temporal lobe, which sits next to the hippocampus, the brain's hub of memory formation. Neurons in the medial temporal lobe showed category-specific responses to the images. Famous people consistently activated one area of the medial temporal lobe, while famous landmarks activated another.

But this pattern went deeper. Using very precise electrodes, the research group tried recording the firing of individual neurons in the medial temporal lobe. Each neuron responded not only to a specific category but to a certain person or place. One neuron would only fire in response to pictures of Jennifer Aniston. The so-called Jennifer Aniston neuron fired after exposure to lots of different photographs of her yet was silent in response to shots of other famous personalities, like Julia Roberts and Kobe Bryant. Another neuron fired exclusively in response to images of Halle Berry, even when she was dressed as Catwoman, the masked superhero whom she played in a 2004 film. The Halle Berry neuron also responded to her written name. This same effect arose with each of the other picture categories. For example, the researchers found a neuron that responded to pictures or words referring to the Sydney Opera House but not to ones of the Eiffel Tower or the Leaning Tower of Pisa.

Finally, the experimenters expanded the range of stimuli to include not only written words and images but also spoken words. A single neuron responded robustly to the concept of Luke Skywalker in many forms: three different pictures of Mark Hamill, the words "Luke Skywalker," and even the character's name as spoken by a male or female voice.

As before, pictures of other famous people, such as Leonardo DiCaprio, did not activate the neuron, nor did the written or spoken names of other celebrities. Interestingly, however, the neuron *did* fire in response to a picture of the *Star Wars* character Yoda.

Evidently, the cell was not responding solely to Luke Skywalker, but also to concepts very closely related to him, like his little green mentor. In many cases, the Luke Skywalker neuron also responded to images of Darth Vader. Similarly, the Jennifer Aniston neuron often fired when subjects were shown photographs of Lisa Kudrow, one of Aniston's co-stars on *Friends*.

Every sensation we have is a stream of information. Regardless of the route by which that information arrives, whether via the visual, auditory, or other pathway, the unconscious system in the brain is tasked with interpreting that information in the context of the situation—as well as our knowledge, emotions, and memory—and synthesizing it into a meaningful representation of the world. Our unconscious processors analyze five simultaneous sensory streams, scrutinizing them for similar features, in order to create the abstract concepts that we consciously experience, such as the relation of the *Star Wars* characters.

The medial temporal lobe is a major intersection for all the sensory highways. Anatomical studies of primate brains support this notion by showing that the various sensory pathways have nerve projections that crisscross in the medial temporal lobe. By allowing our sensory pathways to interact, the brain translates five sets of perceptual data into meaningful ideas and experiences.

For some people, there's so much sensory cross talk in the brain that using one sense can simultaneously activate another. This is best seen in the phenomenon of synesthesia, a syndrome of overly connected sensory pathways. For example, some people have an auditory-visual connection in which hearing certain pitches causes them to see colors. And those associations are consistent: one color associated with one sound. Others have reported having an olfactory-visual connection in which the scent of fresh lemons makes them picture angular shapes while the smell of raspberry or vanilla brings to mind rounded shapes. There are many varieties of synesthesia, because there are many combinations of senses, but they all demonstrate the same insight: our sensory pathways are linked.

We can see evidence of our sensory interconnectedness in everyday life. It's well-known, for example, that losing your sense of smell can dull your sense of taste as well. Vision and hearing are also deeply intertwined. When someone is speaking to you from afar, it's much easier to make out what she's saying if you read her lips at the same time. In fact, those two senses can also interfere with each other. This is best illustrated by a phenomenon known as the McGurk effect.

If you were to listen to a recording uttering the syllables "ba-ba-ba" while watching the lips of someone silently mouthing "ga-ga-ga," you would perceive a distinct third sound: "da-da-da." That's the McGurk effect, discovered by accident in the 1970s when Harry McGurk and his colleague were designing an experiment about language perception in infants. You can also have a reverse McGurk effect, in which hearing certain sounds affects the way you see. When looking at ovals of various sizes and orientations, and asked to describe their shapes, subjects in experiments tend to judge them as taller while hearing the sound "weeeee" and wider while hearing the sound "wooooo."

Our sensory systems are designed for survival. Initially processed through parallel pathways, sensory signals are eventually integrated with each other, interpreted, and organized into a conceptual network. Our senses merge to create a singular, streamlined perception of the world. This collaboration doesn't just enhance our conscious experience; it also creates a backup system in case one of our senses fails. When a person goes blind, the other sensory systems kick into gear, attempting to fill the gap in perception. The brain does its utmost to rebuild our picture of the world, even by re-creating one sense by combining others.

## A Corridor of Sound

"I can figure out what things look like through other means," Amelia tells me. I'm back on the phone with Amelia, the congenitally blind woman we met who claimed to see in her dreams. She's describing the way she creates a mental picture of her environment.

"As I'm walking down a hallway, I can picture it. By the echoes of my heels against the ground, I know that it's a marble corridor. I can tell how long and wide it is. I sense whether the hall is congested with people or if it's empty. I'm aware of all the other footsteps. I feel the slight whoosh of air as someone passes me."

The echo of her heels against the marble changes as she enters the building's main lobby. "I can sense the grandeur of the atrium," she says. "This is clearly a fancy tower." Even in the absence of vision, Amelia can picture her surroundings by integrating her other sensations. Her brain exploits the interconnectedness of its various sensory pathways to reconstitute her vision using nonvisual means. Despite being blind, Amelia can appreciate the dimensions of a hallway, assess how crowded it is, detect the position of people around her, and even sense the elegance of the building she's in. She can navigate her environment using a nonvisual mental map.

I closed my eyes and tried to imagine what it might be like to perceive the world as Amelia does, but visual images kept popping into my mind. I wondered whether her concept of perceiving a corridor of sound was something like the way bats sense their environments using echolocation, their biological sonar that works by detecting the reflections of sounds they emit. Apparently, I'm not the only one who noticed the parallel.

Blind since he was a baby, Daniel Kish founded World Access for the Blind, an organization aiming to help people confront and overcome their blindness by developing their other senses. Kish is particularly known for his ability to use his own form of echolocation. The technique involves rapidly clicking his tongue against the roof of his mouth and listening for how the sound reflects off walls, cars, people, or anything else in his environment.

"It is the same process bats use," Kish says. "If a person is clicking and they're listening to surfaces around them they do get an instantaneous sense of the positioning of these surfaces." By carefully listening for the echo, Kish can discern even subtle differences between materials: "For example, a wooden fence is likely to have thicker structures than a metal fence and when the area is very quiet, wood tends to reflect a warmer, duller sound than metal."

Using fMRI, researchers in Canada were able to peer into the brains of people who use this human echolocation. Two blind individuals who were trained in the technique and two sighted control subjects participated in the study. All four volunteers first sat in a chamber specially designed so that echoes do not occur. The researchers monitored their brain activity while they tried the technique in the anti-echoic chamber. The purpose of this was to determine the baseline brain activation, to map the BOLD signal triggered by the activity of just hearing one's own clicks so as to eventually subtract that from the final results. In the next phase of the experiment, the control subjects were blindfolded, and along with the blind volunteers they tried echolocating outside near trees, cars, or lampposts. All the while, tiny microphones implanted in their ears recorded the sounds they heard. In the final stage of the experiment, the participants entered the fMRI machine one by one, where they listened to the recordings of their own echolocation attempts.

To generate the results, the researchers subtracted out the effects of hearing participants' own clicks from each of their BOLD signals, leaving only the neurological response to the echoes. The brains of the sighted volunteers showed almost no additional activity. As expected, they were just hearing their own clicks. The results for the blind group, on the other hand, were astonishing. As they heard the recordings of their tongues clicking, the fMRI revealed activation in the *visual cortex:*

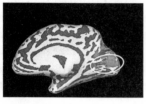
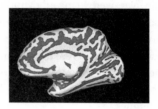

Echolocation expert                Control subject

They weren't just hearing echoes of clicking sounds. Their brains were listening to sounds and translating them into a visuospatial map of the environment.

Despite being unable to see, blind people don't stop using their occipital lobes. The purpose of vision is to navigate our environment. The purpose is survival. Even when visual input is cut off, the occipital lobe keeps trying to be our compass, processing spatial information through other means. The brain constructs our picture of the world by piecing together whatever information it has, even crossing sensory boundaries—and not just those of vision and hearing.

In 2013, neuroscientists in Denmark published a study looking at how the brain allows for navigation when vision is deactivated. The experiment required that the participants find their way through a virtual corridor using only their sense of touch . . . on their tongues. They used a device called the tongue display unit, which created a tactile map by stimulating the tongue whenever the user bumps into a wall of the maze. Subjects could navigate the maze using arrow keys on a computer. The challenge was to use trial and error to find their way through. Participants might first try going straight until they hit a dead end, which they could feel as a buzzing sensation, and then have to figure out which way to turn, all the while constructing a map of the maze in their minds.

The neuroscientists trained two groups of participants to use the tongue display unit: congenitally blind subjects and sighted but blindfolded controls. As neuroscientists tend to do, they watched the participants' brains with fMRI as both the blind and the blindfolded subjects maneuvered through the virtual maze.

The fMRI results looked just like those of the human echolocation study. The blind subjects, who had never perceived a photon of light in their lives, were firing all cylinders of their visual cortices during the tongue stimulation task. Their brains had translated tactile signals into a visuospatial map. The blindfolded subjects exhibited no such activity. Their visual cortices remained quiet. In fact, when the sighted subjects stripped off their blindfolds and navigated the maze with their eyes, their brain activity matched that of the blind subjects navigating with their tongues.

Whether it's from our eyes, ears, or tongue, the brain will accept whatever sensory information it can get to construct a model of the world around us. Though members of the blind community lose the ability to see with their eyes, they can still generate a picture of the world through other means. Imagine how much more prominent these intersections are in the brains of blind people, who depend on sensory cross talk to substitute for their visual deficit. Their unconscious system can reprogram the visual cortex by remodeling the sensory highway system, pixelating the world around them by interweaving their other senses. They keep their sense of navigation and spatial relationships. They can enhance their use of one sense to fill the gaps of another. They retain their ability to imagine and to dream.

## The Dream Machine

In 2003, sleep researchers in Portugal made a bold pronouncement. They argued that people who are blind—and were born blind—can see in their dreams, just as Amelia claimed.

The researchers, led by Professor Helder Bértolo, recruited nineteen people, ten of whom were congenitally blind, for a sleep study. The volunteers slept in their own beds at home with EEG electrodes attached to their scalps. For two consecutive nights, the researchers recorded the participants' brain waves. An alarm clock rang four times each night, and the subjects had to dictate a description of any dreams they experienced into a tape recorder. On the mornings that followed, the blind and sighted subjects were tasked with illustrating their dreams on a sheet of paper. To keep things fair, the sighted group did it with their eyes closed.

Without knowing who contributed which drawing, Bértolo and his colleagues graded the illustrations for their graphic content on a scale from 1 to 5, with a score of 1 being a meaningless scribble and 5 being a detailed scene. Their idea was that the more visual the dream was, the easier it should be to illustrate. Of course, the degree of artistic talent among the participants could have skewed the results. To control for that, the researchers had both groups, with their eyes closed, draw a human figure as best as they could. Here's what they came up with:

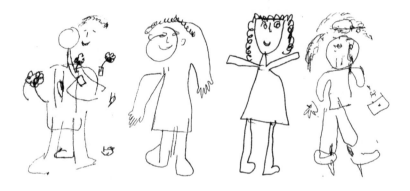

Can you tell who drew which ones? The two pictures on the left were drawn by members of the sighted group. The two on the right were drawn by people in the blind group. Did you guess correctly? It's very hard for us to tell, and the sleep researchers agreed: after grading the full set of drawings, they found no difference on average between the artistic talents of the two groups.

So how did the dream illustrations look? Again, Bértolo found no statistical difference between the average scores. The drawings of the blind and sighted subjects were *equally visual*. For example, take a look at the scene at the top of the next page. The drawing depicts a dream about a day at the beach. We can easily visualize the real-life scene that it represents. The sun is shining, the birds are flying overhead. You and a companion relax under a palm tree as a sailboat cruises past. As you

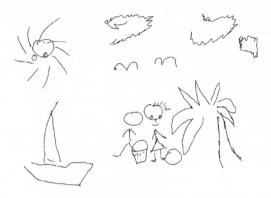

imagine this snapshot in your mind, it seems impossible to take the "visual" part out of it while still experiencing it. Yet this illustration was made by someone who has never seen sunlight or birds flying overhead. She's never seen a palm tree or a sailboat.

Does that mean that the blind see in their dreams? Not so fast. Being able to illustrate a dream doesn't necessarily mean that it's visual. Suppose that I hand you a puzzle piece. With your eyes closed, you feel its corners, its curves, and its protrusions. Don't you think you'd be able to draw it, even though you never saw it with your eyes?

So, perhaps the drawings, as impressive as they are, don't prove anything. But remember that the sleep researchers did more than just a behavioral test. They had the EEG recordings. What they were looking for among the brain waves is a phenomenon known as alpha blocking. Alpha waves are seen on an EEG when a person is relaxed, with eyes closed, and not actively visualizing anything. When you "clear your mind," your EEG will show a predominance of alpha waves. They are seen, for instance, in the brains of people who are meditating. On the other hand, alpha blocking is the disappearance of these waves, which is thought to occur when a person is experiencing mental imagery. That includes not only the visual imagery of actively looking around but also the internal imagery that we call upon when we picture things in our minds. Studies show that if you ask someone to answer a question that doesn't require visual imagery, such as "What's the capital of Massachusetts?" an EEG will not show alpha blocking. However, if you ask something like "What does the inside of your house look like?"

the EEG will show the alpha blockade in the visual cortex, presumably because the person answering is harnessing visual imagery in his mind. This correlation seems to hold up during sleep, with alpha blocking peaking during REM sleep, when dreaming is most movielike.

With that in mind, what did the blind participants' EEG results reveal about the visual content of their dreams? Just as we would expect to see in a sighted person, the blind participants showed a clear correlation between alpha blocking and visual dream content. The more illustrative their drawings were, the fewer alpha waves the EEG detected in the visual cortex (more alpha blockade), implying that their brains were processing more visual imagery. They had never seen anything in their lives, yet Bértolo's experiment suggested that they were visualizing in their dreams.

How could this be? How could someone who has been blind his entire life be able to *see* in his dreams? It's difficult to fathom how that could be possible. As we might expect, Bértolo's result is highly controversial. George William Domhoff, a psychologist and dream researcher at the University of California, Santa Cruz, responded with a direct critique of Bértolo's study. For one thing, it is well documented that congenitally blind people can perform just as well as sighted people on visual imagery tasks like drawing. As we have seen, their brains compensate for their deficit exquisitely well, so perhaps it's no surprise that they can sketch a person's body or illustrate a beach scene. Like the puzzle piece example, this finding doesn't necessarily mean that the blind can actually see in their dreams.

But what about the EEG results? Interpreting brain waves is always difficult, because you can never be completely sure of what they represent. You are simply correlating what you see to what has been noticed in the past. Alpha waves represent a relaxed, low-activity state. So, when we detect the disappearance of alpha waves in the visual cortex, the implication is that the person is experiencing visual imagery; at least that's the correlation that's been noticed in sighted people in the past. We know, however, that the visual cortex of a blind person does not sit idly. Over time, it becomes integrated with all the other senses and maintains its role as a center of spatial perception and navigation. Therefore, when we see the alpha blockade in congenitally blind individuals, it's possible—even likely—that the waveforms don't represent true visualization, as sighted people experience. Rather, they represent the blind person's *version* of visualization: a depiction of a scene that vividly integrates different senses, an internal experience reminiscent of Amelia's "corridor of sound."

The unconscious mind is a powerful storyteller. In dreams, it connects the random firings of the brainstem during REM sleep and weaves them into a striking narrative. In the blind, it can reconstruct spatial perception using other senses, even creating a kind of echolocation. But most people born blind don't think that they see in their dreams. In fact, polls reveal that those who go blind before the age of five do not report experiencing any true visual imagery, whether during the day or in their dreams. However, when they go blind later in life, especially if after age seven, people remember what it was like to see and can usually imagine and dream visual scenes. People who go blind after age seven *do* see in their dreams.

Those who were born blind have a different internal experience. Of all the congenitally blind people I spoke to, only Amelia claimed to have had a visual dream. I suspect that what she felt was something like that corridor of sound. She had a sensual dream (sex on the beach) that interwove her emotions and intimate physical sensations into a singular fantasy.

As we have seen, one crucial ingredient that sets dreams apart from reality is the deactivation of the prefrontal cortex. Free from the prefrontal lobe's constant reality checking, the brain's dream circuitry is unfettered. It can conjure up a fantasy so vivid, so immersive, and so wildly detailed that it might, for the briefest of moments, appear to someone as if she has experienced something beyond the bounds of her usual sensory perception. Only when she awakens might she begin to doubt it, as was the case with Amelia.

Compared with the conscious system, the unconscious abides by a different set of rules. Within each of these systems, different processes are at work that allow for deliberate, conscious reflection during the day and unbounded sensory explorations at night. Yet we have barely seen a glimpse of how these systems function and interact. The hallucinations of Charles Bonnet, Alice in Wonderland syndrome, and peduncular hallucinosis are ways in which they overlap, by allowing dreams—generated by our unconscious circuitry—to invade our waking consciousness. But those are cases of circuit breakdown. Our two systems in the brain are not merely separated by sleep and wakefulness, and they interact far more often than during hallucinations.

Modeling the brain as containing two systems of behavioral control—the conscious and the unconscious—goes a long way in explaining not only the subtleties of our everyday thoughts and decisions but also the various ways in which human experience can be disturbed and distorted. There is an underlying logic to the way these two systems interact as well as how they attempt to compensate, for better or worse, when gaps or defects in processing arise. In blindness, the brain may fill the void in perception by generating visual hallucinations or attempting to reconstruct vision using our other senses. In dreams, the unconscious brain collects the random bursts of activity from the brainstem and, as logically as possible, connects them into a single narrative, an all-encompassing fantasy that permeates our minds as we sleep.

# 2

# Can Zombies Drive to Work?

*On Habit, Self-Control, and the Possibility of Human Automatism*

> For if habit is a second nature, it prevents us from knowing
> our first, whose cruelties it lacks as well as its enchantments.
>
> —Marcel Proust

Local officials in Huntsville, Alabama, were dumbfounded. In a two-week period, a slew of eight car accidents had occurred, and all of them at the same place: the intersection of Adventist Boulevard and Wynn Drive. Equally puzzling, each accident occurred in exactly the same way. Cars driving along Adventist took a left onto Wynn, directly into oncoming traffic. This seemingly ordinary intersection, a common route for morning commuters, had never had such a problem. Now, all of a sudden, the wreckage and injuries were piling up. What was causing this disturbing pattern? Huntsville officials put local traffic engineers on the case.

It turned out that the string of car accidents began after a slight change was made to the traffic light at the intersection. Previously, the only way you could turn left from Adventist onto Wynn was with a green arrow. To help reduce congestion on Adventist, traffic engineers added another setting to the light, allowing drivers to turn left on a green light in addition to the green arrow. Just like at countless other intersections, if you made the green arrow, you could turn left immediately, but at the green light you'd have to wait for traffic to clear before turning. Apparently, drivers were so used to only having the green arrow that they turned at the light instinctively without checking for traffic. They were in the habit of just turning left at the sight of green and therefore didn't notice the change. As one traffic engineer put it, "When you drive by habit, you drive quite dangerously."

How many times have you arrived at work in the morning after having driven for thirty minutes or so, only to have no memory of the actual driving experience? You get lost in your own thoughts, especially if there's something specific on your mind, such as a presentation you have to give at nine o'clock. The actual driving experience of your commute does not register in your conscious mind. Suppose that on a certain day you have to drive to a meeting across town instead of your office. It's possible that you could drive to your office out of habit, neglecting to remember your meeting. You might not even realize your mistake until you arrive. It's almost as if you drove your car unconsciously, while your mind was occupied with other endeavors.

What's startling about this scenario is that driving is an incredibly complex task. You use your foot to switch back and forth between the accelerator and the brake, both of which respond to subtle differences in the degree of pressure you apply to them. You coordinate the movement of your foot with that of your hands operating the steering wheel, guiding the momentum of your two-thousand-pound vehicle. As you drive, you abide by the rules of the road. You consider right-of-way, pedestrian crosswalks, and speed limits. There are stop signs, yield signs, and traffic lights to follow. There are countless other cars on the road that can sometimes behave erratically. Every time you switch lanes, speed up, or slow down, you have to account for their position, speed, and intentions to move, as suggested by the patterns of illuminating brake lights and turn signals they exhibit. Yet despite all of these challenges, experienced drivers on a familiar route can do it without paying much attention at all, to the point at which they feel that they do it automatically.

In Huntsville, that automatic driving had dire consequences. Motorists didn't notice the new signal in the traffic light. They made the turn automatically, careening into cars coming the other way.

If a preoccupied driver is not consciously aware of traffic signals or any driving-related activities, and has no memory of having driven at all, then who (or what) was driving the car? If we can commute to work without using our conscious faculties, then there must be *another system* in the brain capable of driving a car—a system that isn't dependent on consciousness. If this unconscious mechanism can do something as complex as driving a car, perhaps it can do much more than that. How much does it contribute to the world of our experience without our knowledge?

## Zombies Among Us

Imagine that a family of zombies arises from a long-forgotten crypt. When they reach the surface, pedestrians shriek in horror as they see the undead trudging along the sidewalk. Much offended by these judgmental reactions, the zombies head over to a plastic surgery center in the city and get full-body makeovers. The surgeon is world renowned, and these zombies are her masterpiece. After the procedure, the zombies look completely alive and well. In place of the rotting flesh is soft, moist skin. Where there were once exposed ribs, there are now pudgy love handles. The surgeon did so well that the zombies plan to blend into society as model citizens, and no one will be the wiser. There's still one problem, though. The zombies aren't conscious.

Both human beings and thermostats detect temperature, but only human beings experience warmth or coldness. The post-op zombies are like thermostats, but with respect to all experiences. The philosopher David Chalmers writes that these creatures are "physically identical to [us], but [have] no conscious experience—all is dark inside." Chalmers and others pose the question of whether human beings could behave the way we behave without awareness, feelings, or imagination. Is consciousness necessary for human behavior, or could we potentially be just as successful without it?

An airline pilot can leave the cockpit, and the plane will fly just as well on autopilot. Without him, nobody is making the conscious decisions to steer the plane or change its altitude. The plane's computer system takes care of those things automatically.

A zombie is like a plane on autopilot: the functionality is the same, but there's nobody having the experience inside. Could human beings, like planes, operate on autopilot? Or, put another way, could the post-op zombies successfully blend in with human society and do everything humans do, despite not having human minds?

Let's start with perception. Much of conscious experience consists of the way the brain interprets the information it receives from our five senses. As we saw in the previous chapter, the brain goes to great lengths to rebuild our experience of the world when vision is lost. The most crucial element of vision appears to be not the visual detection granted by the eyes but rather the conscious experience associated with that detection. What is perception without consciousness? Our sensory detection and the conscious experiences associated with that detection are intimately connected. But could we disconnect them? For example, could we see something without consciously knowing that we saw it?

## Vision Without Seeing

The preoccupied driver doesn't remember having the conscious experience of driving. He doesn't remember making the decision to stop at a red light or activate his turn signal. He has been running on autopilot. Consider a situation in which the driver nearly gets into an accident and is suddenly jolted out of his daydream as he slams on the brakes and his car comes to a screeching halt, inches from a U.S. postal truck. After settling his nerves, the driver reflects on what just happened. He doesn't feel as if he had merely tuned out for a while. His momentary loss of awareness seems to have been much more severe. He feels as though his conscious mind had been completely withdrawn from the process of driving. It's as if, during his period of spacing out, he had been effectively blind.

Research on cell phone use during driving seems to confirm the feelings of the preoccupied driver. In one study, participants used a driving simulator while speaking on the phone with a headset. The simulator was programmed with a three-dimensional map of a small suburban city with residential, business, and downtown districts that spanned over eighty blocks. Billboards scattered throughout the city displayed bold advertisements and were in clear view of the participants. After practicing with the simulator for a while, the volunteers followed the normal rules of the road as they drove along a predetermined route. During the drive, they spoke on the phone, using the headset. At the end of the drive, the volunteers took a multiple-choice quiz to identify the billboards that were placed along their route. The accuracy of their answers was compared with those of participants who drove the same route but weren't on the phone. As you might expect, those participants whose attention was occupied by the cell phone conversation did poorly on the quiz compared with those who were solely focused on driving. Though the billboards towered over the road, the cell phone group didn't even notice them.

How could the participants fail to see the billboards? Did they just happen to not look at them? To find the answer, researchers fitted the drivers with eye trackers while they drove their simulated cars. Using this device, the research group discovered that when drivers become deeply involved in a cell phone conversation, there is no decline in their shifts of gaze to targets on the road. Their eyes still move appropriately to focus on all relevant objects, including street signs, other cars on the road, and, yes, even billboards. Strange. Drivers on cell phones look at all the same things that drivers without cell phones do, yet they can't seem to remember the things they looked at. How could that be? The theory is that even though the eyes are looking at the targets, the drivers' conscious vision is partially deactivated while they are engrossed in conversation.

If objects on the road as big and obtrusive as billboards can be missed just because of a cell phone conversation, why aren't accidents more frequent? People have conversations while driving all the time, whether on the phone or with other people in the car. How can we possibly drive safely while conversing if doing so impairs our vision? It seems obvious that continuous conscious vision is crucial to keep a safe distance from other cars, stay in your lane, make turns, and whatever else you have to do to get home without totaling your car. Yet the research on distracted driving shows that, though your eyes might dart between targets on the road, you often don't consciously process what you're looking at.

If the conscious experience of vision is turned off, who is controlling the movements of the eyes? The brain takes care of that *unconsciously*. The unconscious system in the brain is able to generate the necessary eye movements to cars and street signs to keep the driver and passengers out of harm's way. That's why accidents are not more frequent and why preoccupied drivers can usually drive safely. Even though conscious vision is limited, the brain's unconscious processes take over the visual system and guide us to our destination.

That's an example of how consciousness and vision can be disconnected. The visual system is working, because the car isn't spinning out of control, but the driver doesn't have the conscious experience of seeing.

Certain neurological disorders further expose the fact that visual detection and the experience of seeing are separate processes. For example, patients with neglect syndrome have perfect vision, yet they are only conscious of one-half of their visual field and seemingly ignore the other half. To test for neglect syndrome, neurologists ask patients to copy drawings. Here's what happens:

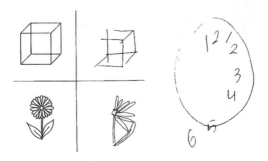

The drawings on the right were done by patients who had no problems with their vision yet inexplicably failed to draw the left side of the images they were copying. Neglect syndrome is caused by damage to the right parietal lobe (located at the top of the brain), which is involved in focusing our attention. Even though vision is appropriately processed, the brain fails to pay attention to the left half of any given scene, and it never enters consciousness, but that's not to say the brain doesn't see it *unconsciously*.

In another test of neglect syndrome, called the target cancellation task, the neurologist hands a patient a whiteboard with short lines drawn all over it. The challenge for the patient is to cross out each line on the board, transforming each one into an *X*. As the photographs in the figure (parts B and C) on the next page show, a person with neglect syndrome will cross out the lines on the right half of the page while ignoring those on the left. In a modified version of this test, however, the patient has to erase the lines rather than cross them out (parts D and E of the figure). When the test is done this way, patients with

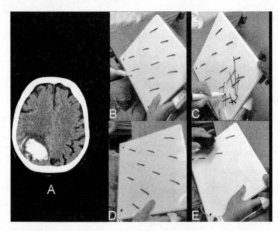

Target cancellation tasks. (A) CT scan of the brain showing a hemorrhage in the right parietal lobe. (B, C) In the target cancellation task, the patient crosses out the lines on the right, neglecting those on the left. (D, E) In the modified version, the patient is much better able to erase the lines as attention progressively moves toward the left.

neglect syndrome are able to erase all the lines. Neurologists theorize that when patients erase the lines on the right part of the board, their attention shifts leftward, because there's nothing to see there anymore. Shifting attention leftward reveals another column of lines to erase. This trend continues until the patient has cleared the board.

Even though patients can't see the left side of the page, the visual information must still make it into the brain. The visual system is working fine, so there's nothing preventing the brain from detecting what's out there. Only conscious awareness is left out of the loop.

In neglect syndrome, the conscious system can't see the left half of the world, but the unconscious system can. Similarly, the preoccupied driver isn't consciously aware of the road, but since his car doesn't crash, we learn that unconscious processes watch the road. So is it true, then, that the unconscious can really see without our knowledge?

It's true: our brains see things that we don't know we're seeing. For the most striking medical example of this, we turn to the mysterious phenomenon known as blindsight.

Consider Darren, a thirty-four-year-old man who suffered from debilitating headaches for twenty years. After imaging of his brain revealed a malformation of the blood vessels in his right occipital lobe, he realized his symptoms were not going to improve without surgery. A neurosurgeon cut out the malformation in his brain but, in doing so, also removed a large chunk of Darren's right occipital lobe.

In the weeks after his surgery, Darren happily reported that his headaches had improved but that he was still adjusting to the unfortunate side effect of the procedure: he was blind to everything on the left side of his body. The right occipital lobe controls vision in the left half of the visual field, so Darren's partial blindness was to be expected. However, there was one aspect of Darren's visual symptoms that was quite *un*expected.

In a dimly lit room, Darren was asked to sit in a chair and place his head on a chin rest. With Darren's eyes looking straight ahead, experimenters flashed a spot of light in the blind part of his visual field. Despite being blind to everything in that area, Darren was able to detect that the light had been flashed, and he moved his eyes to focus on the source. The research group asked Darren if he could see the light. He insisted that he couldn't. The experimenters shined the light again at the blind field and asked Darren to point at the source—just to take his best guess. Shrugging his shoulders, Darren stuck his finger out. He pointed right at it. His "guess" happened to be correct, but perhaps he got lucky. The neuroscientists repeated the test again . . . and again. Each time they shined the dot of light in a different position in his blind field, and each time Darren got it right.

Scratching their heads, the experimenters took things a step further. In another experiment, they flashed horizontal or vertical lines at Darren's blind side and asked him to guess which one they were showing. Trial after trial, Darren answered correctly. In a third experiment, he was even able to identify the color of lights in his blind field. Darren's ability has come to be known as blindsight.

Research on blindsight shows that patients with isolated damage to the primary visual cortex can correctly identify the location of a target, its color, and even whether it is moving or stationary. Accuracies of up to 100 percent have been reported. What's more, analysis of eye movements in these patients reveals that they properly move their eyes to focus on the locations of the targets. They are blind, yet they follow objects with their eyes and can accurately describe them.

A 2008 study focused on a blind gentleman named Tad, who lost his sight after having two strokes in a row that obliterated his visual cortex. Usually, Tad walked with a cane, but on this day he was asked

not to bring it. An experimenter led Tad to the entrance of a long hallway that was set up like an obstacle course. Littering the corridor were
a variety of objects: two trash bins, a tripod, a stack of paper, a tray,
and a box. However, the experimenter told Tad that the hallway was
completely clear and asked him to walk through it. Tad began to do so.
As he approached the first trash bin, he turned sideways to avoid it . . .
then did the same with the next trash bin. Next, he turned to avoid the
tripod, sidestepped between the stack of paper and the tray, and deftly
snuck right by the box. When asked how he had so skillfully avoided
all the obstacles, Tad had no idea how he had done it. He was blind, yet
somehow he could navigate his way through a complex environment.

Clearly, Tad and Darren have some form of visual detection, even if
it isn't conscious. Their brains both process light and have intact visual
circuits to process the information their eyes receive. Because the damage in blindsight is at the end of the pathway rather than at the eyes, the
brain still detects the patterns of light, but consciousness is cut out of
the loop. What's left is blindsight, a form of unconscious vision. Visual
information travels from receptors in the eyes along the arcing chains
of neuronal fibers until it arrives at the occipital lobe for analysis. It's
then sent to the relevant motor areas to coordinate eye movements and
generate a programmed behavioral response, all without ever reaching
conscious awareness.

Something similar is happening with the preoccupied driver. The
brain processes perceptual information about road conditions from the
eyes and ears and guides the movements of the steering wheel, the accelerator, and the brake. The driver's conscious mind doesn't contribute to
the driving decisions, because it is occupied with other thoughts. The
brain is using blindsight to navigate. That's how the drivers in Huntsville failed to notice the change in the traffic light. Blindsight may be
able to navigate to work for you, but it isn't sophisticated enough to
detect changes as subtle as a green light in place of a green arrow.

In the instance of preoccupied drivers, the effect occurs when traveling a familiar route. If you were driving through an unfamiliar neigh-
borhood to an address you've never been to before, you'd be very aware
of the road as you struggle to find your way. You would pay close attention to every traffic signal. After you had made the trip twenty or thirty
times, the drive would become second nature, and your mind would be
more likely to wander. What's changed? The drive has become *habit*.
Maintaining a habit doesn't seem to require the same level of mental

effort that is needed when attempting a task for the first time. Not only does "practice make perfect," it seems to make our actions automatic. This is a pervasive effect that we all experience, and possibly take for granted, but it isn't uniquely human.

## Mice in a Plus-Maze

Let's return to that fateful intersection in Huntsville, Alabama. Imagine that your commute to work involved navigating only those two streets: drive straight on Adventist and make a left on Wynn. After making the trip a number of times, you would probably be able to drive without paying much attention. It would become a habit, but how would this transition occur in the brain? How does practice cause our behaviors, such as driving to work, to become automated? Neuroscientists have studied this question by designing an experiment that re-creates the process of navigation but for mice. The map is the same: two interacting streets in the shape of a plus sign. The mouse is placed in the south arm of the map, and a reward (food of some sort) is placed in the west arm, as shown below.

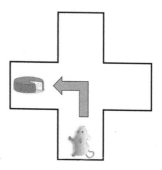

When initially placed in the maze, the mouse cautiously inches forward until it reaches the intersection. At this point, it turns its head back and forth as it attempts to decide which way to go, often venturing the wrong way. Eventually, it discovers the reward in the west arm of the maze. When placed in the maze for a second or third time, the mouse still pauses at the intersection but is more likely to make the correct turn to the left on its way to the goal. Neuroscientists repeated this procedure over and over again, each time placing the mouse in the south arm and the reward in the west. Eventually, the mouse's behavior changes: it no longer pauses at the intersection. It runs forward and makes the left turn without hesitation. The behavior has become habit, just as it does for someone who has taken the same route to work for years.

When the traffic light in Huntsville was modified, the expectation was that drivers would notice the change and immediately adjust their behavior. But that isn't what happened. Many drivers failed to notice the change because, after years of turning at that intersection, they made the turn out of habit. A similar effect occurs in a driver who suddenly has to take a different route to work. What would happen if the mouse suddenly had to adjust to new circumstances, such as to travel a different route?

After allowing the mouse much practice navigating up from the south arm of the maze to the west, the experimenters made a change: they had the mouse start from the *north* arm. They didn't move the food pellet: it was still in the west arm. However, from the mouse's perspective, navigating to its goal now required a new route: a right turn rather than a left. The mouse could have approached this situation in two ways. If its habit system had truly taken over its navigation, it would still make that same left turn, only to find that it had reached a dead end with nothing to munch on. It would take the route it was habituated to taking, just like the preoccupied driver. On the other hand, if the mouse was not operating based on habit, it should have paused at the intersection, evaluated its options, and then turned right, toward the reward. The setup looked like this:

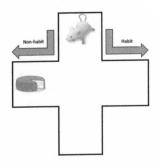

When placed in the north arm of the maze, after having much practice starting from the south, the mouse proceeded forward to the intersection and made a left, leading it toward the dead end. It made the same mistake as the preoccupied driver because its navigation was being controlled by the habit system. It was accustomed to making a left turn without thinking, and that's what happened.

The researchers then tried the experiment with a mouse that had not been trained to navigate from the south arm. In theory, without the extensive practice navigating from the south arm, this mouse shouldn't develop the habit of turning left. The untrained mouse scurried down from the tip of the north arm to the intersection, paused as it peered in both directions, and correctly made a *right* turn, westward toward the food pellet.

It seems as if the mice in these experiments behave one way if habit is in control and another way if it's not. But how can we be sure of whether the mouse is acting out of habit?

Neuroscientists have traced the habit system to a region located in the deepest recesses of the brain known as the striatum. The more practice the mouse gets, the stronger the activity in the outer striatum. Simultaneously, as the mouse continues to undergo its training, the activity level decreases in the inner striatum and the hippocampus (memory formation), both of which scientists believe to contribute to non-habit behavior. If we know the precise location in the brain that generates our habits, then theoretically we can shut down that region and prevent those habits from being formed.

There is a technique in neuroscience research known as lesioning in which one can temporarily shut off an area of the brain by infusing a deactivating chemical or zapping it with a well-aimed electrical current. What would happen if scientists lesioned the mouse's outer striatum, thereby deactivating the habit system, before putting it into the north arm? The answer: the mouse made a *right* turn! With its habit system out of commission, the mouse was no longer able to navigate the maze on autopilot and make the automatic left toward the dead end. Instead, it had to pause at the intersection, look both ways, and travel west to score itself a snack.

The habit system works faster than the non-habit system. The mouse doesn't pause at the intersection; it makes the left turn automatically. Driving to work is quicker when you don't have to focus on the navigation. However, this system is prone to make errors, as it does when the mouse begins from the north arm or when your presentation is moved to a new location. In contrast, the non-habit system allows the mouse to reflect on its new circumstances and adjust its behavior accordingly.

Together, these parallel systems split the job of controlling our actions, and we can see the differences in our behavior depending on which one is at work. In theory, both could also operate at the same time. While the habit system is automatically guiding us through traffic on our way to the office, the non-habit system can talk on the phone.

## Focusing by Being Unfocused

When we try to do two things at once, like drive while talking on a cell phone, what if only one system splits its attention between the tasks, rather than two systems that take one each? That would imply that the quality of our performance in each task would depend on how much attention we decide to devote to it. The more we focus our attention, the better our performance. However, that model doesn't fit with our experience of habit behavior. When we've practiced something a lot, to the point at which we can do it out of habit, it's often better if we *don't* pay much attention and just let our body do it automatically.

On February 10, 2011, Ray Allen, then a member of the Boston Celtics, hit the 2,561st three-pointer of his career to break the all-time record for three-pointers, previously held by Reggie Miller. Throughout his years in the NBA, Allen was known for his work ethic. He often arrived on the gym floor three hours before the start of a game to practice his shooting form. In an interview, Allen was asked how he was able to achieve his success and what went through his mind as he shot the ball. He said, "If you're aiming, if you start aiming, that's when you miss to the left or the right. All these things go into play. You just try to get to a point where you are comfortable enough to where you *don't* aim . . . you just take one step in the air, flick of the wrist and the ball's in the hoop."

For Ray Allen, shooting is a habit, which is probably what athletes are referring to when they talk about muscle memory. The way Allen focuses when he has to make a big shot is by *not focusing on it*. When he thinks too hard about his shooting, his performance suffers. He plays his best when he lets his habit system do what he has trained it to do.

The same goes for other athletes. In a study of skilled golfers, participants had to swing their clubs in two different conditions. In the first condition, they focused intently on the mechanics of their swing, carefully monitoring how hard they hit the ball, where they were aiming, and how good their form was on the release. In the second condition, the golfers didn't think about their swing at all. As they set up in front of the ball, they were distracted by a second task: to listen to a recording of sounds until they heard a certain beep. At the beep, they announced, out loud, that they heard it. The experimenters compared the performance of the golfers in the two conditions. On average, the ball was hit closer to the hole when the golfers were not thinking about their stroke mechanics than when they were. Just as in Ray Allen's experience, the golfers performed better when they didn't think about their craft.

The fact that an athlete's performance changes depending on whether habit or consciousness is at the helm lends support to the notion that there are two parallel systems in the brain that control behavior. When we practice a behavior enough, we can automate it, allowing the habit system to take over. This frees up the conscious, non-habit system to focus on something else.

The division of labor between our two brain systems doesn't stop with basketball or golf. Our most subtle behaviors can be controlled by habit or explicit conscious direction, and depending on which system is in command, we can detect the differences.

## How to Identify a Fake Smile

What is it about fake smiles that make them feel so ungenuine? Why is it so difficult to fake a smile? In 1862, the French neurologist Guillaume Duchenne published his finding that real and fake smiles are actually accomplished using different muscles. All smiles require that we flex muscles around the mouth, but the difference is the way we involve the muscles around our eyes, called the orbicularis oculi. In a genuine smile, we contract those muscles, pulling in the skin next to our eyes, as you can see in the picture of this handsome fellow:

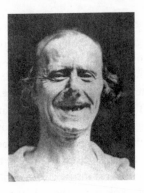

Teeth or no teeth, doesn't he look genuinely happy to see you (and not at all creepy)? Look at the contraction of the muscles around his eyes. That only happens with smiles that reflect true, happy emotions. On the other hand, a fake smile doesn't use those muscles. When forcing a smile, we use a muscle in each cheek, called the risorius, to pull our lips into the right shape, but the eye muscles don't contract. To demonstrate this, Duchenne electrically stimulated the risorius muscles of his toothless friend. Here's what that smile looked like:

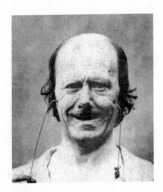

There are creases on his cheeks but not around his eyes. The orbicularis oculi muscles are not contracted. The skin around the eyes is not pulled in tightly as it is in the first picture. That is the mark of a fake smile.

The differences in muscle contraction in genuine versus fake smiles illustrate the separation between the habit and the non-habit systems in the brain. When a smile comes naturally to us, one set of muscles is activated. When we use our conscious powers to feign a smile, we alter the pattern of muscle activation, and people around us can tell.

One more example. Recently, I noticed a colleague in the hall of the hospital where I work who was visibly distracted by his smart phone as he walked. As he passed by me, I asked, "Hey, how's the patient doing?" He replied, "I'm good. How are you?" The automated response was evidently a response to "Hey, how are you?" which is not what I asked. With his mind preoccupied by his phone, the doctor replied out of habit. When I asked him about the incident later, he had no recollection of the unfitting remark. I then did a little experiment by asking distracted people similar questions and found that this kind of thing happened a lot (and I know I've done it too). Interestingly, most people I asked about it, like my colleague, also did not remember giving me an inappropriate response.

Our dual control systems involve different regions of our brains and have distinctive effects on behavior, whether in sports or in the way we interact socially. But the incident with my colleague implies that they differ in yet another way: they are associated with separate forms of memory.

## Why We Forget to Pick Up a Gallon of Milk

As I am preparing to leave work on a late Tuesday afternoon, my wife calls and asks me to pick up a gallon of milk on the way home. No problem. I make a mental note of it as I step into the elevator and head to the parking lot. As I get in my car, I remind myself once more as I adjust the mirrors and turn the ignition key. I drive home as I usually do, along my normal route. It is not until I arrive home, as I am walking toward the door, that I suddenly realize I forgot to pick up the milk . . . again. However, I'm not worried about it—not only because my wife is very understanding, but also because there is strong neurobiological evidence to suggest that I had a good excuse for not remembering the errand in the first place.

A number of distinctions are used to describe the way we store and retrieve information in the brain. One such distinction is between the categories of procedural and episodic memory. Procedural memory is memory for how we do things, like ride a bike, tie a knot, type on a keyboard, or drive a car. This memory becomes stronger the more we practice that procedure. In contrast, episodic memory is for autobiographical events, such as past experiences, feelings, places, and ideas, such as the idea that one must pick up a gallon of milk on the way home. It's how we remember the episodes that have taken place in our lives.

Not only do these forms of memory store different types of information, but they also arise from different regions of the brain. Episodic memory is stored in the hippocampus, located deep within the brain and next to the temporal lobe. It tends to be active during non-habit behavior and, as we saw with the mouse in the plus-maze, quiet during habit behavior. On the other hand, procedural memory comes from the outer section of the striatum, the same area responsible for generating habits. This is no coincidence.

When an electrical current is fired at the mouse's hippocampus, temporarily turning it off, an untrained mouse can't make its way through the maze at all. It can't remember where it is, where it wants to go, and what it's been placed in the maze to do. Without the hippocampus to store and retrieve these memories, the disoriented mouse runs around in a random pattern. However, if the hippocampus is shut off *after* the mouse has been successfully trained, the mouse will run straight and make a left as usual. That's because the outer striatum is in charge of habit. The hippocampus is not involved in habit behavior, so deactivating it has no effect on a mouse that is navigating on autopilot.

So what does all of this have to do with my forgetting to pick up a gallon of milk? Recall that when the preoccupied driver arrives at work, he doesn't remember having driven there. That's because he drove out of habit. Habit occurs exclusively by retrieving and storing procedural memory. He doesn't remember the drive to work because whenever something is done using the habit system, the memory of that activity is not recorded in the hippocampus using *episodic* memory. If a segment of our lives doesn't get recorded into episodic memory, we can't recall the imagery (like billboards), sounds, or feelings associated with it. It will quietly strengthen the habit of the procedure, and that's all.

Not only is habit unable to record information into episodic memory; it can't *retrieve* information from it either. It just doesn't have access. This is the trouble I face as I drive home with my wife's instructions in the back of my mind. Because I'm spacing out, procedural memory takes over as I drive home. As a result, I lose access to episodic memory and therefore can't retrieve the important fact that I wanted to remember. My habit system doesn't know anything about gallons of milk, and by allowing it to take over the drive, I put myself in a position that made it difficult to remember my task. So, I guess I wasn't totally blameless because, thinking back on it, I probably could have tried harder to overcome my tendency to let habit take over.

## Why Do We Eat When We're Not Hungry?

When the habit system takes control, our ability to retrieve information stored in episodic memory is compromised. Episodic memory stores the contextual knowledge that helps inform decision making, be it an awareness of our location or the thought that we must run an errand. That knowledge also includes all the reasons for refraining from eating when we are not hungry. Among those reasons might be the worry that we will gain weight, concern about our state of health, or just the simple feeling of fullness that makes eating unnecessary. Yet it's all too common for us to eat when we aren't hungry, a behavior that most would agree is just a "bad habit," but nobody means that literally or scientifically. However, research shows that eating when we're full may be controlled by the habit system after all.

Thirty-two healthy volunteers were asked to sit in front of a computer screen and press a button whenever an image appeared on the screen signaling them to do so. When they pressed the button, a machine next to them released either a Fritos corn chip or an M&M. They ate whichever snack the machine ejected. Half of the subjects did this task for only two sessions of eight minutes each, while the other half did *twelve* eight-minute sessions. The second group had six times as much practice with the task as the first group and was more likely to eventually start pressing the button out of habit. To ensure that the first group did not develop habits and the second group did, the experimenters monitored the brain activity of both groups. Because the striatum is where habits develop in the brain, the experimenters could confirm that the second group (the group that received more practice) developed habits because they exhibited a dramatic increase in activation of the striatum by the end of their training. With this in mind, we'll call this group the habit group and the first group the non-habit group.

To determine how the development of habits affects our eating behavior, the researchers were interested in the activity of a certain brain region known as the ventromedial prefrontal cortex, located in the mid-lower section of the frontal lobe. A major function of this region is to anticipate the value of an expected event. This is important in the brain's reward pathway, which manages positive and negative reinforcement of behavior. For example, when we are sitting hungrily at a restaurant and the waiter approaches the table with plates of food, neuronal fireworks go on in the brain in anticipation of the meal. The ventromedial prefrontal cortex is one of the primary regions that contribute to this excitement. It revs up whenever it anticipates that a certain experience will yield a high reward. This allows for positive reinforcement as it encourages us to keep doing the behavior in question. So, when we are eagerly awaiting the plate of food to be set in front of us, the ventromedial prefrontal cortex is firing away because it detects high reward. Once we are full, however, the response is vastly diminished. If the waiter were to bring another plate of food, the ventromedial prefrontal cortex would barely respond at all. The low response *devalues* the experience of eating, discouraging us from continuing to chow down. Scientists believe further that neighboring regions in the prefrontal cortex inhibit the feeling of being hungry generated in the hypothalamus. So, the ventromedial prefrontal cortex participates in a feedback loop. It positively reinforces eating when we are hungry, but that act of eating eventually causes the ventromedial prefrontal cortex to *discourage* us from eating and to recognize that we are full.

The researchers wanted to compare the responses of the ventromedial prefrontal cortex in the habit group and the non-habit group. In the non-habit group, the ventromedial prefrontal cortex was activated before each press of the button in anticipation of the snack, encouraging them to eat. But that was while the subjects were hungry. What would happen once they were full? The researchers had the members of the non-habit group eat a full meal until they were no longer hungry.

Then they returned to the task. This time, as the subjects pressed the button on the machine, the activation of the ventromedial prefrontal cortex was diminished. The participants were not hungry, so the projected reward of eating an M&M or a corn chip was minimal. The ventromedial prefrontal cortex downgraded the reward value of the snack food to discourage further consumption.

The habit group was tested next. In the first condition, when they were hungry, their ventromedial prefrontal cortices exhibited the anticipatory signal as they pressed the button, indicating that their brains assigned high reward to the food. Next, the subjects ate a large meal. Once they were satiated, the habit group returned to the task. They proceeded to press the button once again as the experimenters continued to monitor their brain activity. This time, the fMRI results revealed that the ventromedial prefrontal cortex activity was just as strong as it was when the subjects still had their appetites. The anticipated reward value of the snack was *not* downgraded, even though they were full. The feedback loop was broken. Apparently, because the subjects were pressing the button and eating the snack out of habit, their brains failed to discourage them from continuing to eat. In fact, by maintaining the reward signal, the ventromedial prefrontal cortex was positively *reinforcing* the behavior of eating without being hungry. The development of habit changed the act of eating from something dependent on the need for nourishment and transformed it into something automated.

This may explain why we often eat despite not being hungry. We let our habit system take over, and our eating becomes automatic. But how do we permit the habit system to seize command? Can we control it? Think of it this way: There are two systems for directing our behavior, the procedural habit system and the thoughtful conscious system. Each system can work in isolation or they can operate simultaneously, but neither system can do two things at once. The conscious system can drive, and it can reflect on the events of the day, but it can't do both at the same time. If the conscious system is preoccupied, the habit system is assigned the driving duties. By passively allowing thoughts to flood our minds (what we might call spacing out), we take our conscious system out of commission. We lose the ability to access episodic memory and reflect on more pressing tasks. The habit system takes over whatever routine activity we are doing.

This often occurs when we are distracted by something, such as television. Doctors strongly recommend that people avoid eating in front of the TV because it can lead to overeating. When we passively watch TV, we allow the television to monopolize our conscious system. Therefore, if we are doing something routine while watching, such as eating potato chips, the habit system will control that behavior. Just as the preoccupied driver may navigate on autopilot, the preoccupied diner may thoughtlessly consume five bags of chips while his mind is distracted by a rerun of *Seinfeld*. Unfortunately, because it doesn't have access to episodic memory, the habit system doesn't know anything about stomachaches, weight gain, heart disease, or even the simple concept of setting limits.

When our minds are preoccupied, our ability to consciously control our behavior is suspended, and our behavior seems to follow a preprogrammed course. What would happen if we lost that capacity for self-control indefinitely? A permanent loss of self-monitoring can be seen in cases of damage to the frontal lobe, which includes the ventromedial prefrontal cortex. When the brain loses the ability to centrally monitor our conduct, we lose our ability to make thoughtful decisions. Our brains switch into habit mode, and a pattern of automaticity arises in our behavior.

## Executive Dysfunction

In cognitive neuroscience, the term "executive function" is used to describe the highest-order functions of the brain, including planning, decision making, the control of attention, and self-monitoring. Executive function is to the brain as a CEO is to a company. It endows us with the ability to broadly control the way we think and act.

When people suffer injury to the frontal lobe and executive functioning is compromised, they can lose the ability to plan, make sound decisions, and even control their own behavior so as to maintain social decorum. What's more, they tend to act in ways that resemble habit behavior. A young Russian engineering student in his twenties named Vladimir suffered frontal lobe damage after being hit by a train when he ventured onto the tracks to retrieve his soccer ball. Tragically, he lost his ability to engage in decision making and higher-level thinking. He usually sat motionless, staring off into space. When nurses would try to get him to talk, he would ignore them or start cursing. He even had trouble following basic instructions. When given a sheet of paper and asked to draw a circle, he looked vacantly at the examiner and did nothing. The examiner intervened by taking his hand and helping him draw the circle. Vladimir finally did successfully draw the circle on his own, but he didn't stop there. He continued drawing circles again and again until the examiner had to pull his hand away from the page. Evidently, Vladimir's procedural memory allowed him to effectively draw circles. Yet because of damage to his frontal lobe, he was unable to stop himself from doing so.

Another, even more vivid example of frontal lobe dysfunction is a condition known as alien hand syndrome, in which a patient's hand might spontaneously grab a nearby object. The patient does not intentionally move the hand; it happens automatically. Sometimes the patient is even powerless to make the hand release the object and may have to use the other hand to remove it. Reports of this syndrome include a patient who found that he could make his "alien" limb let go by screaming at it as well as another patient who said that her alien hand tried to strangle her. Alien limbs tend to rebel against what the rest of the body is doing, like unbuttoning your shirt while your normal hand is trying to button it. Patients also report that their alien hands grab objects from their other hands and generally behave mischievously. Frontal lobe dysfunction in these patients leads to strikingly automatic movements of their limbs.

The French neurologist François Lhermitte became known for his work on how patients with frontal lobe damage may automatically start using tools or objects in their surroundings, even if doing so is socially inappropriate. In one experiment, Lhermitte invited a patient with frontal lobe damage to his room. On a table by the door, Lhermitte placed a framed picture beside a hammer and nail. When the patient arrived, he saw the picture and the tools on the table, and without hesitation he banged the nail into the wall and hung the picture on it. He was, of course, not asked to do that. Evidently, he noticed the hammer and nail and instinctively did what he habitually does with hammers and nails, much like the preoccupied driver who drives to work even when he isn't supposed to, simply out of habit. If better judgment does not intervene, through the exercising of executive function, the habit system will take over and do what it is accustomed to doing.

In another experiment, two patients with frontal lobe damage, a mother of several children and a working single man, were led to a room that contained an unmade bed. The mother entered first. When she stepped into the room, she walked over to the bed, tucked in the sheets, fluffed the pillow, and laid the blanket down with care. Next, the bed was unmade by one of the experimenters and the man was asked to enter the room. He immediately walked up to the bed, plopped himself onto it, and took a nap. As in the first experiment, the deficit in executive function led both patients to automatically behave in the ways in which they were habituated, in this case falling in line with gender stereotypes.

Lhermitte demonstrated that this effect, which he called "utilization behavior," is only seen if the person in question is accustomed to using the object in the experiment. When he tried the test by placing a cigarette and lighter in front of a smoker and a nonsmoker (both of whom had frontal lobe damage), only the smoker lit himself a cigarette. The nonsmoker did nothing. Because he didn't have a smoking habit, he did not exhibit the same automated response.

Is this automatism in cases of frontal lobe damage precisely the same as the habit response? Not exactly. Frontal lobe injury can have a wide range of effects, and no two cases are exactly alike. There is an element of habit behavior observable in the way that frontal lobe patients conduct themselves. The striatum, the region responsible for habit behavior, is spared in cases of isolated frontal lobe disturbance. When executive function is out of order, the brain depends more on the habit system, and more automated, stereotyped behaviors arise.

In the absence of executive function, whether from injury or because the person is preoccupied with other thoughts, the brain falls back on its other means of generating behavior, and this leads to automatism. For short periods, we can operate on autopilot and do so without having any conscious awareness of our actions—just like zombies. The question is, if the automatic processes in the brain can drive for us, hang up picture frames, and make the bed, what else could they accomplish?

## Murder on Autopilot

Kenneth Parks, twenty-three years old and living in Toronto, Ontario, had a steady job in the electronics business. He had been married for about two years and had a lovely five-month-old daughter. Parks also had a very close and warm relationship with his in-laws, feeling even closer to them than to his own parents. His mother-in-law affectionately called him "her gentle giant."

In the spring of 1987, Parks found himself overwhelmed by the consequences of some poor life decisions. He had become a heavy gambler, frequenting horse races and placing hefty wagers on long shots, the horses with the worst odds but highest potential payoff. After a number of failed bets, Parks began embezzling money from his job to conceal the losses from his wife. Going to work became a nightmare as he tried covering up evidence of the stolen funds. When his theft was inevitably discovered, Parks was fired from his job, and charges were brought against him. It became increasingly difficult to explain his gambling to his wife, especially once they were forced to put their house up for sale.

The weight of the debt Parks had accumulated often kept him up for entire nights. When he did manage to fall asleep, he often awoke in the middle of the night with pangs of anxiety in his chest. After attending a meeting of Gamblers Anonymous, Parks decided that the time had come to openly discuss his financial difficulties with his family and in-laws. The night before the meeting, he did not get a moment's sleep. Exhausted the next morning, he told his wife to push off the family meeting until the following day. At 1:30 a.m. on Saturday, May 23, Parks finally fell asleep on the couch.

The next thing Parks was able to recall was looking down at the terror on his mother-in-law's face as she collapsed on the floor in front of him. He then ran to his car, and as he reached for the steering wheel, he realized that he was holding a knife and it was dripping with blood. He threw it to the floor and drove straight to the police station, where he told the officers, "I think I have killed some people."

After many separate rounds of questioning, Parks's story was remarkably consistent. He remembered nothing from the time he fell asleep until the moment he saw his mother-in-law's face. But during this period that he could not recall, investigators learned, Parks had accomplished quite a bit. He had gotten off the couch, put on his shoes and jacket, walked outside, driven his car twenty-three kilometers (more than fourteen miles), stopping at up to three traffic lights, entered the home of his in-laws, fought with and strangled his father-in-law, and stabbed his mother-in-law to death. Yet he remembered none of it.

After a medical evaluation found no signs of physical illness or drug abuse, a team of four psychiatrists gathered to help shed light on the case. It was clear that Parks was horrified by what had happened, and there were no signs of premeditation. There was no clear motive, because he had nothing to gain from the murder. Parks also did not have any problem controlling aggression. He was of average intelligence and didn't suffer from delusions, hallucinations, or psychosis of any kind. Astonished by the absence of medical findings, the psychiatric evaluators had no answers.

Finally, with the help of a neurologist, it was suggested that a sleep disorder could have had something to do with it. Parks had a history of fragmented sleep as well as sleepwalking, as did many members of his family. His own sleepwalking traced back to when he was a child. Once his brothers had even caught him climbing out of a window while fast asleep, and together they had to drag him back to bed. He also had a history of nocturnal bed-wetting, night terrors, and talking while asleep, all of which are associated with sleepwalking. The neurologist called for a full sleep evaluation using a polysomnogram, a device that simultaneously measures brain waves, eye movements, heart rate, respiratory rate, and muscular movements during sleep. The readings demonstrated that Parks had unusually high levels of slow-wave sleep, a finding typical of chronic sleepwalkers. When all the evidence was finally compiled and brought to trial, the court concluded that Parks had assaulted his father-in-law and killed his mother-in-law while sleepwalking. He was found not guilty on both counts. As a judge stated on the ruling,

Although the word "automatism" made its way but lately to the legal stage, it is a basic principle that absence of volition in respect of the act involved is always a defense to a crime. A defense that the act is involuntary entitles the accused to a complete and unqualified acquittal ... At common law, a person who engaged in what would otherwise have been criminal conduct was not guilty of a crime if he did so in a state of unconsciousness or semi-consciousness. Nor was he responsible if he was, by reason of disease of the mind or defect of reason, unable to appreciate the nature and quality of an act or that its commission was wrong. The fundamental precept of our criminal law is that a man is responsible only for his conscious, intentional acts.

To better understand what might have been going on in Kenneth Parks's brain on that terrible night, we need to think about the four stages of sleep. In stage 1, you are just barely falling asleep. It's pretty easy to wake up at this stage, and when you do, you might not even realize you've been sleeping. In stage 2, your muscles relax, though at times there may be spontaneous contractions. Your heart rate slows and body temperature cools as the body readies itself to enter deep sleep. Stage 3 is known as slow-wave sleep and is the deepest period of sleep in the cycle. It is during slow-wave sleep that people can have night terrors or nocturnal urination. It is also the part of the cycle in which people sleepwalk. Finally, during REM (rapid eye movement) sleep, your muscles are completely paralyzed. This is the stage in which we experience our most vivid dreams. The muscle paralysis prevents us from acting out those dreams in reality. However, the same cannot be said for slow-wave sleep, which is, as I mentioned, the stage found to be unusually long in Kenneth Parks's case.

Sleepwalking is a mysterious example of how a person's behavior can be overtaken by automatic processes he can't control, and as we have just seen, it can lead to terrifying consequences. The American Academy of Sleep Medicine has determined that incidents of sleepwalking share the following characteristics:

1. Difficulty to arouse the person during the episode
2. Mental confusion when awakened
3. Complete or partial amnesia for the episode
4. Potentially dangerous behaviors

Reports of sleepwalking have included everything from throwing heavy objects, jumping out of bedroom windows, and even sexual acts during sleep. Sexuality during sleep has even been given a name in scientific literature: "sexsomnia." It is just another frightening example of the complex behaviors people are capable of while fast asleep.

People who sleepwalk, and potentially commit dangerous acts, most often can't remember doing so. People tend to find out that they were sleepwalking when someone else, such as their spouse, tells them so. Some people figure it out by suddenly waking up and realizing that they are not situated in the same place in which they went to sleep. Why are sleepwalkers consistently unable to remember having sleep-walked? One might think that it's because their brains are not active and lack the ability to process what's going on around them. After all, they are *sleeping*. In fact, however, the mind is quite active during slow-wave sleep. People have simple dreams during slow-wave sleep, and because their muscles are not yet paralyzed, the brain can even activate muscle contractions and complex movements.

Alternatively, perhaps the reason people don't remember sleepwalking is that the brain does not record these incidents in episodic memory. Sleepwalkers would therefore have something in common with the preoccupied driver. The preoccupied driver can't remember driving his route to work, because his mind is immersed in other thoughts, such as those about an upcoming presentation. The driver remembers those thoughts about the presentation but not the complex task of driving. So, what might be occupying the thoughts of sleepwalkers? Their dreams.

Sometimes we remember our dreams, but it seems that equally often we don't. Research shows that it depends on the stage of sleep we are in. If the dream occurs during REM sleep, we remember it about 75 percent of the time. In contrast, if the dream takes place during slow-wave sleep, the stage in which sleepwalking occurs, we remember it just under 60 percent of the time. The reasons for this difference are unknown. During slow-wave sleep, our dreams are shorter than those during REM sleep and are usually described as being more like interrelated thoughts than actual dreams. If normal slow-wave sleep presents short, choppy dreams that we recall little more than half the time, how does sleepwalking affect our dreams and how we remember them? A 2009 study of sleepwalkers investigated this very question.

The forty-six participants in the study, who had been followed by sleep specialists for at least two years, were asked to describe any thoughts or dreams they could remember having during their episodes of sleepwalking. The research team then compiled the data on whether the subjects remembered dreaming and, if so, what they dreamed about. What they found was that 71 percent of them remembered at least part of the dreams that were linked to their episodes of sleepwalking. Of those who could remember their dreams, most of them (84 percent) described them as being frightening or similarly unpleasant. The table below shows some of the dreams they reported, as well as what they did while sleepwalking.

| Content of dream | Behavior, as observed by bed partner or reported by dreamer |
|---|---|
| A truck was bearing down on her and she was about to get run over. | She jumped out of bed and out of the mezzanine. |
| Her baby was in danger. | She grabbed her baby and ran out of the room. |
| Spiders were crawling toward her and she wanted to drown them. | She started spitting on the bed. |
| People were following him. | He climbed onto the roof of his house. |
| His girlfriend was in danger and he had to save her. | He grabbed his girlfriend and pulled her out of bed. |

People often remember the dreams they had around the time they were sleepwalking but don't remember the sleepwalking itself or the things they did during the episode. All they can do is piece together what happened after the fact. When conscious analysis is not applied to our behavior, whether because it is damaged or simply preoccupied with other endeavors, our automated system takes over. Looking at the table above, there is a clear parallel between dream content and sleepwalking behavior. During the episodes of sleepwalking, with the mind engrossed in an internal fantasy, the body runs on autopilot. It's as if sleepwalkers are automatons acting out their dreams.

Kenneth Parks did not sleep well. He was under incredible pressure, at his psychological breaking point, as he prepared to face his in-laws and come clean about the lies and recklessness that had brought his family to ruin. In his fragile mental state, it's possible that a fantasy crept into his mind during that night. Perhaps he dreamed of a way to avoid the confrontation. If only his in-laws were dead before he had to meet with them. Parks would never have committed murder, it seems, if he were awake and consciously reflecting on his own behavior. But in dreams, a person can imagine anything.

There's a good chance that Kenneth Parks's mind was preoccupied by a terrible dream that night. Without his conscious faculties to monitor his actions, his automated system took over. He became a most deadly preoccupied driver as he traveled more than fourteen miles in his car and committed murder—all on autopilot. Evidently, zombies *do* exist, and they're capable of committing atrocious acts.

We are wired with an automatic system that can control our behavior. The fact that this system is capable of acting against our best interest, whether by leading a mouse down the wrong arm of a maze or by causing a man to commit murder, raises an obvious question: Why does this system exist? Presumably, natural selection kept it around because it has some usefulness. So, what advantage do we gain from having such a system?

## Two Systems for Multitasking

In his classic song "Piano Man," originally released in 1973, Billy Joel played two instruments at once, the piano and the harmonica. It's difficult enough to coordinate two hands on the piano while maintaining the flow of the piece, but playing another instrument simultaneously is a feat that few can accomplish. How does he do it? It's tempting to say that Billy Joel has unlocked certain abilities that the rest of us cannot access. Yet he himself disagrees. When Alec Baldwin interviewed him in 2012, Joel had this to say about his skills on the piano:

> BILLY JOEL: I know what good piano playing is and I'm not good. My left hand is lame. I am a two-fingered left-hand piano player.
> ALEC BALDWIN: As opposed to?
> BILLY JOEL: As opposed to somebody who knows what they're doing with their left hand. I never practiced enough to use all my fingers on my left hand, so I just play octaves, bass notes. My right hand tries to compensate for my left hand being so gimpy, so I overplay on my right hand. My technique is horrible.

Despite his humility, Joel seems honest when he says that he struggles with playing complex bass lines with his left hand because he *hasn't practiced that enough*. So how does he manage to play the harmonica at the same time? He plays simple octaves or single notes on the piano— patterns that are easy enough for him to automate. With his fingers mindlessly playing simple combinations, Joel is able to focus on playing the melody on a second instrument.

In the interview, Joel also admitted that he struggles with reading music notes:

> ALEC BALDWIN: If I took a piece of music that you didn't know, if I got a score and put it in front of you and I said, "Play this—"
> BILLY JOEL: It would be Chinese.

Imagine that Joel attempted to play the piano part from a piece of sheet music while playing the harmonica. That wouldn't work. Billy Joel's secret to playing two instruments at once is that he makes one of the parts simple enough that he can play it automatically.

When driving a route, playing a song, or even walking up a staircase becomes habit, we can do those things faster and without thinking. It might even produce better results. The real advantage of being able to automate certain parts of our behavior may be that it allows for multi-tasking. The preoccupied driver is able to focus on thoughts to improve the upcoming presentation because the habit system has taken over the drive. Billy Joel is able to play the harmonica and piano simultaneously because he plays the piano without thinking. Even walking is an automated behavior that at some point required practice. The reason we can speak on a cell phone while walking and not fall over is that we don't have to focus any conscious attention on each swing of our legs or placement of our feet.

How could we prove that this kind of multitasking is occurring? We would have to demonstrate that a person who extensively practices a task (until it becomes habit) is able to take on a second, brand-new task and execute it simultaneously with little or no loss of efficiency or performance. A research group at the University of Illinois conducted exactly this kind of experiment. They taught thirty-nine volunteers how to play a computer game called *Space Fortress,* in which players navigate a spaceship using a joystick. The objective was to destroy the space fortress at the center of the screen by launching missiles at it using a trigger button on the joystick. This had to be done while avoiding damage to the ship from mines that were located throughout the virtual environment. Points were awarded for accurate missile hits against the fortress and taken away whenever the ship bumped into a mine.

The setup of this game was complex and might be compared to the task of a driver who must avoid other cars along his route as he navigates to his destination.

Playing *Space Fortress* was task 1. Task 2 was a listening activity. Participants were to listen to a sequence of sounds and identify which of the sounds was different from all the others. This could get tricky if the tones were close in frequency and therefore required that the subjects pay close attention.

Once the volunteers were shown how to approach both tasks, the experiment could begin. When performing the listening task alone, subjects correctly identified 97 percent of the mismatched tones. Then they were instructed to do the task again, but this time while simultaneously playing *Space Fortress*. This did not go so well. Without practice, *Space Fortress* scores were in the negative range, indicating that there were more collisions with mines than successful attacks on the fortress. In addition, because they now had to split their attention, the participants achieved only an average of 82 percent on the listening task.

In the next phase of the experiment, subjects were asked to just play *Space Fortress*. They played it again and again for a total of twenty hours. Now well trained at the game, the subjects were asked to play it again while concurrently attempting the listening task. This time, the subjects were just as proficient at firing missiles accurately at the fortress, and their score on the listening task rose to 91 percent. The interpretation? Without practice, conscious attention had to be split between the two tasks, and the resulting interference caused the subjects' overall performance to suffer. In contrast, practicing the video game allowed them to play it more or less automatically. This gave them the ability to allocate more of their conscious attention to the listening task, and as a result they were able to accomplish it with only a small loss of proficiency. If your boss ever catches you, this is how you can justify playing *Minesweeper* at work.

The investigators also monitored the subjects' brain activity using an EEG. They wanted to know whether the distribution of neuronal activity in the brain before and after the training would shed light on how the brain allocates resources to tasks performed together. Every time the subjects successfully struck the fortress with a missile, a distinct waveform appeared in the EEG recording. Similarly, each time the subjects heard a tone, an equivalent increase in neuronal activity was detected. Before the training, the size of these EEG waves was about the same for the missile hits and the auditory tones. However, after the twenty hours of training, the EEG activity for the missile hits was significantly muted, implying that fewer neuronal resources were committed to the task. On the other hand, neuronal activity during the auditory tones was significantly *increased*. With the video game task more or less on autopilot, the subjects' brains were able to focus more of their processing power to succeed at the listening test. Both the behavioral and the electrophysiological results revealed that automating the first task allowed for more mental resources to be devoted to the second. It allowed for the emergence of multitasking.

Allocation of resources for several complex tasks is a difficult endeavor, but the brain does this for us. We are endowed with two parallel systems in the brain that can be used to control behavior. These systems have different strengths and access to different forms of memory. The habit system is procedural, programmable, and fast. It enables us to carry out jobs that are routine, such as driving a familiar route to work or simply turning left in a maze, in a way that is efficient. The automaticity of this system affords us the ability to use our second system simultaneously. This system is that of deliberate, conscious analysis. It may be slower than the habit system, but it is more flexible. It can account for differences in context, such as when construction on the road closes off a familiar driving route and an alternative one must be found. The brain uses its logic to find tasks it can automate, as a computer might free up RAM, so we can focus our conscious efforts on any other undertaking we choose.

The key to multitasking is being able to accomplish one of the tasks by habit. Peeling an orange, for example, is something we can easily do while engrossed by our favorite TV show or while speaking to a friend on the phone. However, it would be incredibly difficult to interpret a physics textbook chapter while doing those things. That is not a process that can be automated; it requires conscious attention. But we could read that chapter while peeling an orange because the conscious system can read the chapter and the habit system can peel the orange. This is how we benefit from having dual systems of behavioral control.

Just ask Barack Obama. In an interview with *Vanity Fair* near the end of his first term, President Obama described the way he tries to automate his more trivial daily decisions so as to focus his conscious energies on the important ones. "You'll see I wear only gray or blue suits," he said. "I'm trying to pare down decisions. I don't want to make decisions about what I'm eating or wearing. Because I have too many other decisions to make. You need to focus your decision-making energy. You need to routinize yourself. You can't be going through the day distracted by trivia."

The brain's internal logic creates the infrastructure for multitasking. That's something that zombies don't have. Because they can only operate on autopilot, without consciousness, zombies have only one system to control their behavior. Zombies may be able to drive to work, but, sadly for them, they can't multitask, at least not in the way that we can. For our part, it is only when one system is damaged, as in executive dysfunction, or when we misuse the system, as in daydreaming or sleepwalking, that we lose the advantage our brains provide.

With what we know about how the brain can automate certain behaviors with enough training, it seems that we have found a neurological basis for why practice is so crucial. The more practice we have, the more automated an act can become, and the better we are able to multitask. However, the Kenneth Parks case still leaves us with certain questions. He never practiced strangling or stabbing anyone. He had no experience with murder whatsoever. Yet he was able to commit such a heinous crime in his sleep. He did it completely on autopilot. Maybe *physical* repetition is not the only way to accumulate experience. Perhaps there is another way to train the brain, using only the mind.

# 3

# Can Your Imagination Make You a Better Athlete?

*On Motor Control, Learning, and the Power of Mental Simulation*

Golf is a game that is played on a five-inch course—the distance between your ears.

—Bobby Jones

"Tiger's favorite thing has always been getting ready, preparing for a major," Earl Woods once said of his son. "He is an analytical, systems-oriented person, and that's how he likes to manage his golf."

Since he was young, Tiger Woods has been known for his meticulous preparation. His daily routine includes nearly eight hours of golf plus an hour and a half of weight lifting and another hour of cardio. Yet when discussing Tiger's preparation for a major tournament, his father fondly recalls a different aspect of his routine, which doesn't appear anywhere on the training schedule. "Every year he would take the week before his major to mentally and physically fine-tune," he says. "We'd drive to the site and play practice rounds, and after we got home, I'd find him lying on his bed with his eyes closed. He told me he was playing the shots he was going to need in his head."

For athletes to succeed at the highest levels of professional sports, mental readiness is a prerequisite. Physical fitness alone isn't enough. To Woods, that readiness meant more than just psyching himself up for the big match. He was practicing the golf strokes in his mind.

As the winner of fourteen major tournaments so far, Tiger Woods is second in wins only to one player: Jack Nicklaus, who won eighteen majors between 1962 and 1986. A legend in the golf world, Nicklaus preached a similar mental strategy in his book *Play Better Golf:*

Before every shot I go to the movies inside my head. Here is what I see. First, I see the ball where I want it to finish, nice and white and sitting up high on the bright green grass. Then I see the ball going there; its path and trajectory and even its behavior on landing. The next scene shows me making the kind of swing that will turn the previous image into reality. These home movies are a key to my concentration and to my positive approach to every shot.

When two all-time great golfers claim to use mental rehearsal to improve their performance, the golfing community will take notice.

Mental practice in sports doesn't end with golf. Consider the British javelin thrower Steve Backley, who won bronze in the 1992 Olympics in Barcelona. Three and a half years after Barcelona, just months before the 1996 games in Atlanta, Backley sprained his ankle. Unable to walk, he would need crutches for six weeks and was not allowed to train—at least not physically. Refusing to give up hope that he would compete in Atlanta, Backley began a grueling workout in his mind. With his crutches leaning against the wall, Backley sat down in a chair and closed his eyes. He imagined the javelin in his hand, feeling his fingers curl around the cool metal shaft. He pictured using perfect throwing form, tensing his muscles as he released the javelin on a high-arching path. He watched as it sailed into the distance, looking like a pin as it reached its peak, and came careening down as gravity thrust the spear into the earth.

When Backley recovered from his ankle injury, after over one thousand imaginary throws, he was surprised to find that he hadn't lost any ground in his preparation. His throws were just as good as they were before he hurt his ankle. Backley won silver at the Atlanta Olympics.

It's hard to believe that imagining yourself playing sports could actually make you better, yet some of the greatest athletes in history, like Michael Jordan and Roger Federer, have claimed to employ the technique. Then again, athletes engage in plenty of rituals before and during matches that probably don't affect the outcome. For instance, Brian Urlacher, former linebacker for the Chicago Bears, would eat two Girl Scout cookies before every game, and no other type of cookie would do. Cristiano Ronaldo, the 2008 World Soccer Player of the Year, always gets a haircut before a match. When playing in a tennis tournament, Serena Williams likes to wear the same pair of socks through every round.

In the world of pregame rituals among athletes, where does mental imagery fall? Does practicing a sport in your mind really improve your performance, or is it about as effective as wearing dirty socks?

## The Internal Simulator

Imagine that you are sitting comfortably on your couch watching television when you decide that you'd like to grab some food from the refrigerator. How long would it take you to get there? Picture yourself standing up, walking out of the living room, past your napping cat, and around the kitchen countertop, until you finally reach the fridge and the bowl of leftover chili within it. So, in your mind, how long does that trip to the fridge take?

When you imagine that voyage, you are using mental imagery to create a simulation of your walk to the fridge. Believe it or not, that simulation is really accurate. Experiments have compared the time it takes for people to walk between two points with the time it takes them to *imagine* making the same trek. Trial after trial, the results showed that the mental and the physical trips take almost exactly the same amount of time. For short walks, the times are within one second of each other. This close correlation occurs when imagining not just walking but any kind of movement. It takes the same amount of time, for example, to imagine yourself drawing a triangle as it does to actually draw it.

It's a surprising discovery. We generally don't think of imagination as something realistic. The things we think about are . . . imaginary. They are fictional. Yet it cannot be coincidence that the timing of imagining ourselves doing certain actions so perfectly mirrors the time it takes to actually perform them. Imagination and movement must somehow be connected in the brain, allowing our internal imagery to be not just an exercise in fantasy but a reliable simulation of exercise.

Neurologists in California ran an experiment to compare the brain activity of people while they engage in real versus imagined movements. Faced with a set of four numbered buttons, the participants practiced pressing them according to a sequence: 4, 2, 3, 1, 3, 4, 2. Their brain activity appeared on the fMRI as their fingers pushed the buttons. Next, with their hands on their laps, the participants closed their eyes and just *imagined* pressing the buttons in that same order. How would the fMRI results compare? The activation patterns overlapped, most notably in the area of the motor cortex that controls finger movements. Mentally picturing finger movements triggered an fMRI signal that was nearly indistinguishable from the signal observed during actual finger movements.

Evidently, mental imagery and physical performance activate the same parts of the brain. When we imagine ourselves doing a task, the brain runs a simulation modeled after our past experience with physically performing that task. The more experience we have, the more accurate the brain's internal model. Since we have lots of experience with walking to the fridge and sketching triangles, the brain is excellent at simulating those movements. People who practice other forms of movement like rowing, canoeing, and ice-skating show similarly accurate mental simulations.

Simulation alone, however, will not make you a better athlete. The question is, does imagining yourself playing golf or tennis or any other sport actually make you better, the same way physically practicing your swing or your serve might?

## Flexing Mental Muscle

A group of neuroscientists in France gathered forty volunteers for a study of whether mentally executing a motor task has any impact on the physical performance of that task. The subjects were each seated in front of two shelves supported by a pole that displayed numbered cards. The setup looked something like this:

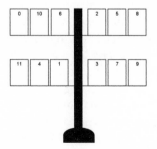

The task was to point at the numbered targets in numerical order, from 0 to 11, and to do it as quickly as possible. The participants were not allowed to just move a finger. Rather, they were asked to move their entire extended arm to point at each card, creating a wide, complex pattern of arm movements that could get faster with practice.

The researchers divided the subjects into three groups. The first group practiced the arm exercise exactly as instructed. Their goal was to do it as quickly and accurately as possible. The second group had the same goal but wasn't allowed to flex a single muscle. Over and over again, they mentally pictured themselves moving their arms in the correct pattern, intently imagining the stretch in their shoulders and outstretched fingertips. The third group was the control group and didn't move their arms or imagine doing so. They simply moved their eyes from one number to the next.

All three groups tried the pointing task once, then did their respective training regimens, and then tried the pointing task again so that the researchers could gauge their improvement. The results showed that the physical practice group completed the arm movement significantly faster after their training. The control group (in which participants just moved their eyes) showed no improvement at all. So, what about the mental imagery group? They improved nearly as much as the physical practice group.

Not only can mental rehearsal improve physical performance, but it also enhances actual muscle strength. In one study, led by Dr. Guang Yue of the Cleveland Clinic, participants imagined flexing one of their elbows and pinkie fingers for fifteen minutes a day, five days a week. After twelve weeks, the experimenters found that the strength of their muscle contractions had increased by 13.5 percent in the elbow and 35 percent in their little fingers. For comparison, physical practice for that same time period enhanced muscle strength by about 50 percent, and participants who didn't practice at all showed no improvement.

Yue's study demonstrated that mental practice not only improves your performance but also strengthens the muscles that you imagine yourself using. How could your imagination make you physically *stronger*?

Using EEG monitoring, Yue observed the brain waves that appeared in the motor cortex (which controls muscle) before, during, and after the practice sessions. The amplitude (height) of brain waves represents their electrical voltage, the strength of the signal sent from brain to muscle. Yue hypothesized that mentally rehearsing a motor act would amplify the signal voltage that reaches muscle cells, causing them to contract more intensely.

As expected, the control group showed no difference in the amplitude of the waves. Also as we would expect, physical practice increased the amplitude. And mental practice? It, too, heightened the brain waves and did so just as much as physical repetition. This finding lends support to the idea that using mental imagery enhances the brain's stimulation of muscle, making our movements faster and stronger. So, even if you don't see or feel your muscles moving, the nerves in their vicinity are causing them to tighten.

Our thoughts are not inert, not trapped in the vacuum of the mind. Underlying each instant of imaginary exploration is a current of electrical information that trains and molds the neuronal cells that carry it. Mental simulation is a means by which the conscious system can change the unconscious system. By mentally rehearsing one simple movement, we can enhance the functioning of the habit-driven, neuromuscular circuitry that underlies it. But what about more complex movements? What can imagination do for Steve Backley's throwing form or Tiger Woods's slice?

## PETTLEP

In 2001, the sports scientists Paul Holmes and David Collins proposed a seven-point mental imagery program for athletes, represented by the acronym PETTLEP. Here's what it stands for, along with a blurb of how an athlete, say a baseball player, might use it to improve his swing:

Physical—Mentally simulate every movement necessary to swing the bat perfectly.
Environment—Imagine the lights illuminating the field, the roar of the crowd.
Task—Imagine not only the swing but what you're swinging at. Feel the ball coming.
Timing—Simulate the time it would take to complete the swing in real life.

Learning—Adjust the imagery as you improve to reflect your progress.

Emotion—Feel the big moment: the pangs of nervousness, your heart racing.

Perspective—Experience the mental imagery in the first person.

Each component of the program is intended to make an athlete's mental imagery more precise so that it more closely resembles the physical experience. Holmes and Collins believed that the more accurate the simulation an athlete conceives, the better the resulting brain activity will map onto the brain regions used for the real thing.

The PETTLEP method, or variations of it, is the standard for motor imagery regimens in sports. So, the obvious question is, does it work?

In a study of thirty-four golfers with at least ten years of experience, researchers tested the PETTLEP method to see whether it could improve performance. The challenge was to hit the golf ball out of a bunker (a sandy pit on the golf course) and onto the green, as close as possible to a pin. The researchers awarded a score between 0 and 10 based on how close the ball landed to the pin:

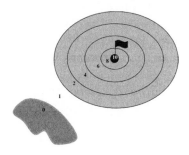

The golfers' total score was derived from the average of fifteen shots. After obtaining an initial score, the participants were assigned to one of four groups: physical practice, mental practice, both mental and physical practice, and a control group that didn't practice, but instead read sections of Jack Nicklaus's biography. The physical group trained by taking fifteen bunker shots twice a week for six weeks. The mental group, on the other hand, prepared by using the PETTLEP method to *imagine* those same fifteen shots twice a week for six weeks. To help fulfill the "environment" criterion of the PETTLEP guidelines, they ran those mental simulations while standing on clumps of dirt or sand in their gardens.

After the six weeks of practice, the golfers returned to the course. Again, they took fifteen shots from the bunker, the average of which became their overall score. The researchers could then compare the average change in score of all four groups:

| Practice group | Percent change in score |
| --- | --- |
| Physical practice | +13.27 |
| PETTLEP | +7.79 |
| PETTLEP + physical practice | +22.38 |
| Control group | −1.94 |

Mental imagery does work, not as much as physical practice, but it makes a significant difference. What's more, when combined with physical practice, it complements the overall training, having an additive effect on improving results.

The beneficial effects of mental imagery have been similarly demonstrated in other sports. A recent study of experienced tennis players found that using mental imagery improved the accuracy and velocity of their serves. It even led to higher scores in actual tennis matches. It helps soccer players make more precise passes. In basketball, it improves shooting percentage. It's even been shown to work in archery, gymnastics, weight lifting, high jump, and swimming.

The success of mental imagery in sports has led to research on other possible applications. For example, consider a pianist on a train on her way to a concert. What if she wanted to get a little extra practice in? She could do it in her mind. Mentally rehearsing the finger movements of the piece will improve her actual piano performance. Studies show that the results of mental practice by musicians are just as good as those that athletes have achieved. Pianists involved in mental imagery studies played their pieces faster, smoother, and more accurately after imagining their fingers gliding across the keys and playing the melodies to perfection.

We've seen myriad examples of how conscious rehearsal affects the performance of unconscious mechanisms. Whether in sports, musical performance, or otherwise, mentally simulating a behavior enhances our ability to accomplish it and can physically change the brain regions underlying it. Nevertheless, the power of mental rehearsal has limits— limits that exist precisely *because* of that inextricable link between imagination and the brain regions involved in doing the real thing.

## Insights from Stroke

In 1996, Jill Taylor suffered a catastrophic stroke, leaving her disabled to the point at which she felt like an "infant in a woman's body." In an instant, she lost the ability to walk or speak, read or write. Over the next eight years, with intensive training and a commitment to rehabilitation, she regained all the functions that had been taken from her.

In Taylor's wonderful book, *My Stroke of Insight,* she details one technique that she believes was instrumental in her recovery:

> Imagery has been an effective tool for regaining physical functions. I am convinced that focusing on how it feels to perform specific tasks has helped me to recover them more quickly. I had dreamed of skipping up steps every day since the stroke. I held the memory of what it felt like to race up the steps with abandon. By replaying this scene over and over in my mind, I kept that circuitry alive until I could get my body and mind coordinated enough to make it a reality.

The success of mental imagery in enhancing motor function has led to high hopes for its application to a variety of medical conditions, including stroke. Taylor believes that the technique helped her, but does it actually work?

Strokes are the sudden onset of oxygen deprivation in the brain, whether because of a blockage or bleed, leading to rapid, inexorable destruction. Without immediate treatment, the affected brain tissue dies. Paralysis results whenever the stroke occurs in the motor cortex. Fortunately, with intensive physical therapy, brain plasticity allows neurons to grow into the affected area and reestablish its functioning.

Mental imagery is already a successful form of rehabilitation for sports injuries. Athletic trainers often use it to help injured athletes get back into shape. It's even been shown to increase athletes' recovery rates. So couldn't we apply the same technique to stroke victims? Because we know that imagining a physical movement activates the same region of the brain used to actually attempt that movement, mental imagery should theoretically be able to stimulate and even revive damaged brain tissue.

Experimental results, however, have been mixed. Some small studies have claimed that mental rehearsal helps in motor recovery after stroke. However, a large study of 121 stroke patients published in 2011 concluded that mental imagery didn't make any difference.

The data don't support Jill Taylor's contention that mental imagery helps with recovery after a stroke. Why doesn't it work? Both injured athletes and stroke victims can experience muscular weakness, so why does mental rehearsal work for sports injuries but not for strokes? Well, consider how mental imagery affects the motor system: by rousing the same regions of the brain that physical movement does. For the technique to be successful, the nerve pathways from the motor cortex to muscle have to be intact. If the brain region that you are targeting is destroyed, mental imagery loses its potency.

On the other hand, in a sports injury the problem is with the actual muscle or tendon or ligament. It's a musculoskeletal problem. The brain is *spared*. Therefore, the recuperative effects of mental imagery can take place unimpeded.

If the stroke were to spare some functional tissue, then there might be a role for using motor imagery, as some small studies have claimed. Perhaps that was the case with Jill Taylor. If her imagination really did speed up her recovery, it's probably because her stroke left behind enough viable brain tissue for her mental rehearsal to activate. However, if an entire motor region of the brain is *dead,* mental imagery would be powerless to motivate it.

Using mental rehearsal to improve your golf game is an example of how consciousness can affect the mostly automated physical process of swinging the club, but that interaction goes both ways. The motor system can affect our imagination in return. Studies show that mental imagery exercises can be disrupted if you try to simultaneously undertake a physical task. It's very hard to imagine moving your arm in one direction while physically moving it in another. Mental and physical maneuvers use the same area of the brain, so trying to do both at once causes a battle for neuronal resources. Most fundamentally, if that area of the brain is destroyed, as in stroke, both the physical and the imagined movements will be compromised.

Strokes not only render mental rehearsal an ineffective treatment but also impair our ability to use imagination in the first place. A group of neurologists in China recently asked eleven patients who had suffered strokes of the left hemisphere and eleven control subjects to participate in a study of mental imagery. Each volunteer sat in front of a computer screen and watched as pictures of a left or right hand were displayed. The hand appeared in a random orientation: right side up, upside down, or at any degree of rotation. The challenge for the participants was to press a button indicating whether they thought the image depicted a right hand or a left hand. This task tested mental imagery skill by forcing the subjects to rotate the pictures in their minds. The neurologists figured that the participants who were more adept at mentally manipulating the images would come up with accurate responses more often, and would generate those answers more quickly, than those who struggled with the task.

The results were clear-cut: the stroke patients did not perform as well as the controls. They took longer to come up with their answers, and when they finally made a selection, their answers were more often wrong. Evidently, the neuronal devastation left by the strokes harmed not only the patients' physical mobility but also their capacity to imagine movements. To support this interpretation, the neurologists had members of both groups undergo EEG monitoring while they took the mental imagery test. Just as hypothesized, the stroke patients exhibited weaker activation of the left brain (the side damaged by their strokes) compared with the controls. Despite their best efforts, their imagination could mobilize only a fraction of the brain regions that the healthy volunteers could.

Our ability to imagine the movements of the body depends on the integrity of the corresponding motor regions of the brain. When a stroke destroys those regions, our capacity for mental imagery may be crippled. That, unfortunately, is why mental rehearsal is likely inept at helping with motor recovery after a stroke. In Jill Taylor's case, it might have been a placebo effect or a source of motivation. Or, perhaps she was one of the lucky few for whom the technique worked, because she had just enough viable neurons for her imagination to arouse.

As long as they remain intact, the conscious and unconscious systems communicate and change each other. By combining physical practice with mental simulation, we can maximize this interaction. Because of injury to the brain, mental rehearsal may not enhance the recovery of motor function after stroke, but that's not to say it doesn't have any medical applications. If the motor impairment is outside the nervous system, such as an injury to the limbs, the mind can overcome the limitations of the body.

## How Do You Scratch a Phantom Itch?

Patients who undergo limb amputations often suffer from the well-known phenomenon of phantom limb syndrome, in which an amputee continues to feel the presence of an appendage even after it is cut off. Suppose a person has his hand removed. He may still feel his wrist, his palm, and his individual fingers. He can sense the invisible hand's position in space and even feel it moving. The problem, however, is that a lot of patients develop uncomfortable sensations in the air where their limb used to be. It's common to feel things like heat, pressure, or tingling. Worse, most patients experience phantom pain, which can be severe. It's even possible to have a phantom itch.

The reason that phantom limb syndrome occurs is not completely clear. The best explanation we have is that even though the limb is gone, the neuronal infrastructure that interprets sensation from that limb is still there. Though the amputee may consciously realize he's missing a hand, his unconscious system hasn't come to terms with it yet. Accustomed to receiving sensory signals from the now-missing appendage, the brain erroneously ascribes certain sensations to it, though they actually arise somewhere else along the nerve pathway.

In 1978, the *Journal of the American Medical Association* reported a case of an elderly gentleman who tragically had both feet amputated because of circulation problems. After the procedure, he had unbearable itching of his phantom feet. He tried furiously scratching the stumps of both legs, but that didn't help. What was he to do? How do you scratch a phantom itch in a nonexistent limb?

We know that this itching sensation was being misattributed to parts of the body that were no longer there. Though the man was consciously aware that he didn't have any feet, his unconscious brain hadn't quite realized that. How could he bridge the gap? By appealing to the principle that the brain regions used to imagine an action are the same as those used to physically execute that action. If you can't actually scratch the irritated skin, then just imagine it as realistically as you can. And that's what the man did. He curled his fingers and raked his nails through the air where he imagined his feet would be.

It worked. Using his imagination, he was able to overcome the phantom sensation by stimulating the same regions of the brain that he would have used to scratch an itch on real feet. Years later, drawing on these same principles, the neurologist Vilayanur Ramachandran would introduce his "mirror box" therapy for phantom limb pain. The box has two mirrors in the center, one facing each way, and a hole on each side to insert arms or legs. Suppose a person has had his left hand amputated and is experiencing phantom pain. To relieve the pain, he places his right hand into one side, and the stump into the other. He then looks at the side of the mirror with his right hand (the good side) and begins moving his hand. Because he sees the reflected image of the right hand moving, it appears as if his left hand were intact and moving simultaneously. This maneuver effectively relieves phantom aches and pains.

Our subjective sensations mirror the functioning of the neuronal circuits that underlie them. By consciously simulating the movement of scratching a missing limb, amputees can trick their circuitry into alleviating their discomfort. The mental simulations we generate internally are not just accurate depictions of real-life events but active contributors to brain functioning, changing the way our neural architecture interprets the world. Mental simulation is a way that the conscious system can manipulate the unconscious. One wonders, however, whether that interaction might also work the other way around. Can the unconscious system trigger mental simulations that affect the conscious system?

In 2009, Ramachandran did a small experiment with four amputees (all of whom lost one of their arms starting at the elbow) who had vivid phantom sensations. One at a time, he had them sit at a table next to one of his assistants. Ramachandran asked his assistant to place her hand on a table in front of the first volunteer. She placed her hand so that it was close to where the volunteer's phantom hand would be, though she was careful not to actually touch his arm. Ramachandran then used his finger to stroke his assistant's hand.

The patient was never touched. He simply watched Ramachandran's finger graze his assistant's hand. Yet to the patient's surprise, he felt as if Ramachandran were stroking his own phantom hand. "It's spooky," the patient said. "Well, I learn something new about my phantom every day." All four of the participants had the same experience. Watching Ramachandran touch his assistant's hand caused them to feel as if their phantom hands were being touched. This happened in sixty-one out of sixty-four total trials, and the effect has been successfully replicated in larger studies.

The amputees knew, consciously and with complete certainty, that no one had touched them. Yet their unconscious systems were somehow tricked into believing it and generated the conscious sensation of touch in an invisible hand. For the amputees, the mere observation of someone's having a sensory experience led to a vicarious sensory experience of their own. How could this be?

## Neuronal Mirrors

Back in the 1990s, an Italian neuroscientist named Giacomo Rizzolatti was studying the motor system in the brain of the macaque monkey when he noticed something interesting. The same neurons that fired while the monkey grabbed a slice of apple from a box also fired when the monkey watched one of the experimenters do so. Specific neuronal groups lit up while the macaque watched others engage in activities like grasping, tearing, and holding. In each case, the active neuronal groups were identical to those that fired while the monkey was doing those same things itself. The same neurons responded to both executing a motor act and observing someone else undertake that same act. It was as if the monkeys were mentally simulating whatever they saw. Brain cells that respond to both the execution and the observation of an action are now famously known as mirror neurons.

Neuroscientists have since discovered the existence of mirror neurons in human brains as well. Just as physically executing a movement and imagining a movement utilize the same brain regions, so too does *observing* a movement. For example, watching someone move her fingers activates the same region of the brain that you would use to move your own fingers. In addition, just as imagination and action compete for brain resources (it's difficult to imagine one movement while performing another), observing movement can interfere with our own motor control. For instance, studies show that subjects are worse at performing vertical or horizontal arm movements if they do so while watching arm movements in a different direction. Can you imagine trying to perform a dance routine while the choreographer at the front of the class suddenly decides to try out some new moves? Your own attempt to dance and the conflicting moves you observe will both call upon the same neuronal groups, making it difficult to stay true to your routine.

Mirror neurons are located in a network in the brain that includes the motor areas as well as the frontal and parietal lobes. When we observe human behavior, this network mobilizes, creating simulations in our minds of what it would be like for us to engage in that same behavior. It automatically triggers our mental imagery. Given what we know about mental imagery and sports, the obvious question is: Does watching skilled athletes make you better at sports?

That question is still under investigation, but early results are starting to emerge. In a 2011 study, twenty expert archers with at least ten years of experience watched close-up videos of an archer using proper shooting posture. As the participants watched the video, fMRI monitoring revealed a surge of activity in the premotor cortex (located next to the motor cortex). In contrast, when a group of control subjects (who were not archers) watched the video, their brains did not exhibit that motor activation pattern. Why the difference? Because the first group had experience in archery, their brains had developed an infrastructure for the complex set of movements involved in shooting an arrow. Therefore, while the first group watched the archery video, their observations could easily map onto that neuronal infrastructure and initiate an accurate simulation. On the other hand, the control subjects had no experience with archery, so the video didn't trigger any sort of built-in archery circuitry.

Among the archers, however, the effect on the brain of watching the video did parallel that of mental imagery, so it's possible that it could improve performance in the same way. Perhaps watching a great athlete's perfect technique trains the brain just as mentally rehearsing that technique, so long as you have some experience in that sport. However, that remains to be seen. Studies have not yet proven (or disproven) that observing a motor task improves a person's performance, but it is certainly a possible application of mirror neurons that warrants research.

That's not to say that mirror neurons need any more hype. They represent one of the most publicized findings of modern neuroscience. That's because mirror neurons, if they do as much as some scientists believe they do, may have implications not only for physical movement or sensory perception but for many of our basest, most intimate human reactions—and some of our most mundane.

## Why Is Yawning Contagious?

Contagious yawning isn't a myth. It's a real, scientifically demonstrable phenomenon. We yawn when we see someone else yawn. The sound of yawning makes us yawn. The yawning contagion can even spread between species. Studies show that chimpanzees start yawning when they watch videos of other primates yawning. Dogs exhibit contagious yawning, even in response to human yawns. You might be yawning right now, as you read this, and it's probably not because you're sleepy and certainly not because you're bored (heaven forbid). So, why then? Why is yawning contagious?

In 2013, scientists in Zurich, Switzerland, had eleven healthy volunteers watch a set of videos while plugged into an fMRI. The videos displayed human faces yawning, laughing, or with neutral expressions. As expected, the subjects yawned in response to the yawning videos more than half the time, which is the typical percentage. Also as expected, the participants did not react to the laughing or neutral faces. The fMRI results, however, were profound. As the subjects experienced contagious yawning, the BOLD signal lit up the inferior frontal gyrus, an area known to be part of the mirror neuron network. In contrast, the mirror system was quiet while the subjects saw the neutral or laughing faces.

Scientists theorize that when we watch someone yawn, mirror neurons simulate the action in our minds. Those simulations can change our behavior. Try to use mental imagery to simulate a yawn in your mind. Really focus on it, using the PETTLEP principles that athletes use. You can probably make yourself yawn that way. Similarly, by simulating an observed yawn, mirror neurons cause us to yawn, imitating what we see.

It might seem silly that yawning has become the target of serious scientific inquiry. At least scientists can have a sense of humor about it, as evidenced by this title of an article from the journal *Frontiers of Neurology and Neuroscience:* "Yawn, Yawn, Yawn, Yawn; Yawn, Yawn, Yawn! The Social, Evolutionary, and Neuroscientific Facets of Contagious Yawning." Nevertheless, the research is not devoid of insight. It has actually revealed a number of potential connections between this seemingly meaningless behavior and the basic components of human nature.

A chain reaction of yawning doesn't happen in every instance of observing a yawn. It happens in some circumstances more than others. For example, consider the following study. Neuroscientists in Italy spent four months studying a group of twenty-one baboons living in a large alcove in the zoo. Over those four months, the researchers observed the baboons from 6:00 a.m. to 10:00 p.m. daily and recorded each yawn that they witnessed, the precise monkey that yawned, and the time at which the yawn occurred. They also noted many of the other behaviors the animals exhibited, including sleeping, walking, feeding, and grooming. The neuroscientists' question was how the interaction between the baboons affected their yawning patterns.

It turned out that the incidence of contagious yawning correlated best with the time the baboons spent grooming one another. This trend persisted even after the experimenters controlled for the effect of proximity among the animals. So, it wasn't simply being around one another that led to yawn spreading but the act of mutual grooming. That's significant because primate grooming is more than just practical; it's a demonstration of affectionate social relationships. Baboons groom each other when they feel close. The more they groom, the closer they feel. The closer they feel, the more infectious their yawns become. If the results of this study are true, emotional closeness correlates with the degree of yawn contagiousness. What does this mean?

Mirror neurons are thought to be involved in the spread of yawning. If that's true, and social closeness makes yawning more contagious, then it would follow that social closeness is associated with mirror neuron activity. Many neuroscientists today believe that the ability to simulate what someone else is doing, using mirror neurons, helps you experience what that person is experiencing. It helps you "put yourself in his or her shoes" as we tend to say when we understand someone around us. In short, the association between primate social relationships and yawning contributes to a body of research that claims that mirror neurons create the basis for empathy.


## Empathy, Pornography, and the Autism Spectrum

Empathy is the capacity to sense another person's emotions. Phrases like "I feel for you" and "I feel your pain" are expressions of empathy. By mirror neuron theory, they are also quite appropriate ones. They imply that we feel empathy by experiencing internally what we observe others to be experiencing, and that's precisely what mirror neurons are thought to do. Though the theory has not been proven, there is emerging evidence that mirror neurons are active as we feel for our fellow man.

Studies show, for example, that when we see someone in pain, the parts of the brain that activate overlap extensively with those that would be active if we ourselves were in pain. Fortunately, this excludes the regions for actual pain sensations, so we don't literally feel each other's pain. Nevertheless, in subtle ways, our bodies behave as if we do. As we watch someone endure an instant of pain, our muscles tense up as if we were the ones going through it. In one cringe-inducing experiment, subjects watched videos of a needle penetrating a human hand. For comparison, the subjects watched two other videos: a cotton swab touching a human hand and a needle puncturing a tomato. As the participants watched the three videos, the neuroscientists stimulated the part of the motor cortex that controls the muscles of the hand using what's called transcranial magnetic stimulation (TMS).

Here's how it works: if your hand is at rest, a jolt of TMS aimed at your brain could activate the muscles of your hand. It's an artificially induced brain signal. However, your muscles can respond to only one set of signals at a time. If you are already using that hand for something, the artificial signal will fall flat. The nerves and muscles will be preoccupied because they are already in use. An artificial TMS signal would be rendered too feeble to stimulate your hand muscles in the presence of the more prominent self-generated signaling.

In the experiment, the subjects' hand muscles all showed normal resting activity while the subjects watched the needle prick the tomato and the cotton swab caress the hand. They responded normally to the zap of TMS. However, when the volunteers saw the needle stab the hand, the activity of their hand muscles suddenly changed. The signal induced by the scientists' stimulus dropped in strength. It was as if the muscle were ignoring the artificial stimulus and instead responding to another signal generated from within. This activity pattern might be seen in a muscle when someone reflexively moves his hand away from something painful, like a hot stove or an exposed nail. Apparently, by merely observing a hand being pricked, the subjects unconsciously activated their own system for withdrawal from pain. The unconscious system in the brain initiated a mental simulation of pain that caused the body to respond as if to an actual needle prick. Extrapolating from this and similar cases, neuroscientists theorize that these unconsciously initiated simulations affect our conscious minds, molding the way we think by setting the foundation for empathy.

As you witness someone in pain, your brain ever so subtly activates the muscles that would be triggered if you yourself were suffering. Similarly, as you watch a friend's face react with emotion, the brain activates the same muscles in your own face. This happens even if you aren't consciously aware of the expression your friend is making. Psychologists flashed pictures of happy, angry, or neutral faces at subjects and used a technique called electromyography (EMG) to measure the muscle activation in the subjects' faces. The images were flashed so quickly that the subjects couldn't tell what they were, yet the muscle activation detected by the EMG matched the expression in the unseen face.

What's more, it seems that our ability to recognize emotions is compromised if we cannot simulate them. If a subject is asked to clench a pencil between her teeth, and is therefore prevented from imitating emotional expressions she observes, she will be less likely to recognize what emotion a person's face is expressing. In fact, there is a rare congenital neurological disorder known as Moebius syndrome, in which people are born with facial paralysis. They therefore can't form any facial expressions. Studies of people with Moebius syndrome show that they are unable to recognize other people's emotions.

However, the ability to recognize emotions is not quite the same as empathy. It's necessary for empathy but not sufficient. To directly study empathy, scientists have used psychological questionnaires to give subjects an empathy score. Using such a scale, psychologists have shown that people with higher empathy scores are more likely to imitate the movements and expressions of those around them. Looking into the brain, fMRI studies reveal that while evaluating people's emotional expressions, people with high empathy scores exhibit greater activation of the motor neuron system than those with low empathy scores. Insofar as the scales can quantify empathy, it appears that the more empathic a person is, the more active his mirror neuron system.

Mirror neurons appear to be active as we witness people undergoing pain, so what about pleasure? Consider pornography, a multibillion-dollar industry that allows subscribers to watch other people have sex. What can explain that level of popularity? The viewer isn't experiencing the pleasure, just observing someone else experience it, yet some estimates have claimed that the porn industry earns more as a whole than Hollywood. What makes pornography so effective?

Neuroscientists in France ran a study in which they recruited a group of heterosexual men to undergo fMRI monitoring while watching pornography (probably the fastest ever recruitment for a study). The erotic videos consisted of scenes of intercourse or fellatio. In addition to using fMRI, the researchers used a technique called volumetric penile plethysmography to monitor the participants' degree of erection while watching the video clips. To serve as a control scenario, the volunteers also watched humorous videos that were free from any sexual innuendo.

So, what does the brain on porn look like? As the participants watched the erotic videos (but not the humorous ones), the BOLD signal on the fMRI lit up specific parts of the frontal and parietal lobes known to be parts of the mirror neuron system. What's more, the degree of mirror neuron activation corresponded to the magnitude of erectile response: the more active the mirror neuron system, the greater the erection.

Why is pornography so effective? Because a person's brain internally simulates sex as he watches it. His body responds as if he were the one having sex. Though it may not seem as if this has anything to do with empathy, it does. The mirror neuron theory of empathy is that it arises because we internally simulate the experiences of others, whether they be pain or pleasure or even extreme pleasure. The fact that the mirror neuron system is active while a person watches sex is, surprising as it seems, consistent with the neuroscientific view of empathy.

More indirect evidence for the role of mirror neurons in empathy and social behavior comes from cases of people whose social functioning is impaired. It's well-known, for example, that people with autism exhibit impairments in social interaction, communication skills, and emotional expression. These parallels have led neuroscientists to wonder whether mirror neuron dysfunction plays a role in autism, leading to the so-called broken mirror theory of autism. What drives the theory is that autistic individuals' difficulty with self-expression extends beyond their own emotions. They can struggle recognizing other people's emotions and simply acknowledging other people's existence.

When he first described the condition of autism in 1943, the psychiatrist Leo Kanner gave examples of children he had seen in his practice. One of the children he discussed was a four-and-a-half-year-old boy named Charles. As an infant, Charles would just lie in his crib staring at the ceiling, seldom interacting with people the way one would expect of a happy baby. According to his mother, things didn't get better as he got older: "He would pay no attention to me and show no recognition of me if I enter the room."

In his clinic, Kanner observed the way Charles interacted with his environment. At one point during the meeting, Charles's mother took an issue of *Reader's Digest* away from her son, placed it on the floor, and stepped on it so that Charles would not fiddle with it. Kanner observed that Charles "tried to remove the foot as if it were another detached and interfering object, again with no concern for the *person* to whom the foot belonged."

The theory is that people on the autism spectrum may have trouble empathizing. On psychological tests of empathy, they score significantly lower than control subjects do. But what about physiological tests? Recall the earlier experiment in which subjects watched a needle pierce a human hand or a tomato while neuroscientists zapped their motor cortices with transcranial magnetic stimulation. In the average person, the results showed that the TMS was ineffective while the subjects watched the needle prick the hand. This occurs because the hand muscles are already in use, unconsciously withdrawing from the needle in the video. When we observe someone in pain, we tend to shrink away as if we were the ones in pain.

When that same experiment was conducted with people on the autism spectrum, the needle-into-hand video had no effect on the subjects' hand muscle activity. The TMS signal was equally strong whether the subjects watched a hand caressed by a cotton swab, a tomato pierced, or a hand stabbed. They didn't attempt to withdraw their hands. They did not shrink away. Their brains did not mentally simulate the experience of pain, and that changed the way their bodies reacted.

It appears that the same thing happens with pleasure. In one study, psychologists measured the heart rate and skin conductance response (a classic experimental measure of arousal) as people with Asperger's syndrome (part of the autism spectrum) looked at erotic pictures. A typical reaction to pornography would be a rise in skin conductance as well as a faster heartbeat. However, the psychologists showed that people with Asperger's don't respond that way. Erotica has a minimal impact on their nervous systems compared with those of control subjects.

The ability to become aroused by pornography, recognize emotion, and express empathy and the phenomenon of contagious yawning are all attributed to the activity of mirror neurons, and we know the first three are diminished in autism. So, what about contagious yawning? It seems to arise from the same mechanism as empathy and emotional recognition, so shouldn't it exhibit the same impairment? A group of psychologists actually attempted to answer this question. In their study, fifty-six children, half of whom had an autism spectrum disorder, sat around a table facing one of the experimenters. "First, I'm going to read you a story," she said, "and then I'll ask you some questions about it." After reading the story for a while, the examiner paused and let out a loud yawn. She did this four times during the story. Because the session was videotaped, the research team could look back at the footage and determine how many of the children in each group yawned within ninety seconds of one of the storyteller's yawns.

The results were clear: 43 percent of the control participants exhibited contagious yawning, but only 11 percent of the autistic kids did. Therefore it appears that the last piece of the puzzle fits: people with autism are less susceptible to contagious yawning.

Some researchers suspect, however, that the yawning deficit exists because autistic children have poor eye contact and tend not to pay attention to people's faces. Perhaps it's just another manifestation of the classic symptoms of autism. The debate extends throughout the literature on autism and mirror neurons. The broken mirror theory is highly controversial. Answers have to come from neurological studies, looking at whether mirror neurons in the autistic brain operate any differently from those in a typical brain. Research is ongoing, with studies finding evidence on both sides. A 2010 fMRI study of autistic individuals, published in the journal *Brain Research,* revealed abnormal activation of the mirror neuron system as compared with controls. Yet that same year a study in the journal *Neuron* said just the opposite: the mirror neuron system is perfectly normal in autism, with activity patterns precisely *matching* those of controls. At this point, there isn't enough neurological evidence to prove that mirror neuron dysfunction has a role in autism.

It may still be only a theory, but it sheds light on just how powerful unconscious mental simulation might be in influencing the way we think, act, and feel. Whether or not they are involved in autism, mirror neurons do help create our sense of empathy, an attribute that we hold dear as part of human nature. By instinctively simulating the experiences of others, we acquire essential information about them, as well as ourselves, and it shapes our own conscious development. Like the mental imagery a golfer might initiate before a tournament, these internal simulations change us. But there's one crucial difference: mirror neurons do their work unconsciously.

Mental simulation is a bridge between the conscious and the unconscious systems. It can be used by either system to affect the other. When used consciously as a form of practice, as in sports, it hones the functioning of the unconscious, fine-tuning the habit-driven mechanisms for motor control. When initiated by the unconscious, through mirror neurons, mental simulation shapes our conscious behavior, mediating our social behavior and helping us internalize the experiences of others.

Without our knowledge or consent, the unconscious system quietly simulates what we observe. We simply feel the effects of those simulations, perhaps as a passing thought or emotion. We might never know the extent to which we are influenced by these ephemeral feelings, or where they come from, other than that they arise somewhere deeply from within.

## Gut Feelings

Suppose that I have a friend who has a serious drinking habit and I am trying to decide whether to stage an intervention. How do I make the decision? As I deliberate, I consider the range of possible approaches I could take and attempt to anticipate the consequences of choosing each one. If I were to confront him alone, he would probably act stubbornly. He might resist my suggestions and perhaps even resent my intruding into his chosen lifestyle. What if the intervention involved a large group of all his friends? Perhaps that approach would more powerfully demonstrate the concern we have about the direction in which his life is heading. Or would he feel cornered and become closed off? If I decide not to confront him, his problem could get worse. He could be arrested after driving drunk or injured while engaged in an angry brawl at a bar. His supervisor at work has already noticed signs of his alcoholism. My friend could potentially lose his job if the situation doesn't improve.

These scenarios rapidly flash through my mind, too quickly to precisely define the details, yet each one strikes me in a certain way. As I mentally run the simulations, one choice doesn't feel right. My gut tells me that a second choice is better. I have certain impressions of which choices are better or worse, even before I actually try to sort out the pros and cons of each. Where do these scenarios, gut feelings, and impressions come from?

The neurologist Antonio Damasio asserts that they come from various emotions we have had in the past and that the effects of these emotions linger in the nervous system until they play a role in decision making. Every time we have an experience, Damasio says, some feelings or bodily states are associated with it. These feelings are impressed upon the nervous system and remain connected to the memories of the events as bodily markers. Our emotions leave behind biological remnants, physical changes in the nervous system. Damasio calls these emotional remnants somatic markers (*soma* is Greek for "body"). So, for example, if a prospective student takes a college tour while it is muggy and rainy, she might unconsciously develop a negative association with that school. Or take the case of someone who has an aversion to a certain food, say Brussels sprouts. It's common for such aversions to be traced back to a bad experience eating that food, often in childhood, such as eating a bad batch of Brussels sprout soup in the school cafeteria.

Just as mirror neurons simulate the experiences of others, somatic markers simulate our own past experiences. Emotional responses that were originally felt in conjunction with a certain food, place, or experience are suddenly retriggered as we encounter similar circumstances or are faced with a relevant decision. As we begin our deliberation, somatic markers have already begun exerting their effects, simulating how each scenario could play out. They influence how we choose and even what choices we are considering in the first place. Before we have a chance to reflect on the merits of each choice, somatic markers have already eliminated choices from the pool of possibilities, and we might be completely unaware of their influence. The simulations are initiated unconsciously.

The somatic-marker system lives in an area of the frontal lobe, right between the eyes, known as the orbitofrontal cortex. Patients who have endured damage there suffer the effects on their emotional and decision-making capacities. The most famous of these is Phineas Gage, a railroad construction foreman who had his orbitofrontal cortex obliterated when a violent explosion caused a metal rod to fire into his head, between his eyes, force its way through the front of his brain, and burst out the other side, landing over a hundred feet behind him. Miraculously, Gage survived the accident, but he was not the same. Without his ability to generate reliable gut feelings through somatic markers, he lost his ability to plan ahead and to make sensible judgments about how to act. Gage lost his ability to make good decisions, and it was not long before he was fired from his job at the railroad. As his friends soon realized, Gage was "no longer Gage."

Damasio recalls a similar story with one of his patients, whom he calls Elliot, who required surgery to remove a brain tumor. As part of the surgery, the surgeons removed a large chunk of Elliot's orbitofrontal cortex. Once Elliot had recovered, it was evident that there had been a profound change in his personality. Once a good husband and father with a successful business, he suddenly couldn't be trusted to get anything done. He couldn't abide by a schedule or properly complete his assignments, and he soon lost his job. He made bad decision after bad decision until he fell into bankruptcy and underwent multiple divorces. It was as if he couldn't appreciate the consequences of his decisions.

Damasio wondered if the explanation had something to do with somatic markers, and he designed a test to help him find out. The test, called the "gambling task," was designed to mimic the uncertainty and possibilities of reward and punishment that people face in real life. He gave Elliot $2,000 of play money and seated him at a table on which four decks of cards were placed, labeled A through D. Elliot was instructed to draw one card at a time from a deck of his own choosing. Written on each card was an amount of money that Elliot would either gain or lose. One card might have said that he gains $50, while another said that he loses $100. Elliot was told to accumulate as much money as possible by the end of the experiment.

What he wasn't told, however, is that the decks were designed in a very specific way. Decks A and B were stacked so that the cards that added money did so $100 at a time, while decks C and D gave $50 at a time. However, each deck also had cards that took money away. In decks C and D, those cards deducted only $100 or less when picked. In contrast, decks A and B took away up to $1,250. The potential for loss in decks A and B far outweighed the potential for gain. The expected, prudent tactic, therefore, was to pick only cards from decks C and D.

Healthy volunteers initially exhibited a preference for decks A and B because of the higher gain. However, after taking huge losses, control participants quickly realized decks A and B were too risky. They changed their card-drawing strategy to focus solely on the good decks.

Elliot had described himself as a conservative person, someone who makes his choices cautiously and seldom takes risks. He described himself this way even *after* the operation on his brain. Yet his choices during the gambling task were anything but cautious. He kept drawing from the bad decks, even after repeatedly losing enormous amounts of money.

It's not as if he didn't know how to play. He was aware of the objective and clearly understood the concepts of gain and loss. He was even able to correctly point out which decks were the good ones and which decks were the bad ones. Nevertheless, every time he was given the gambling task, he kept making the worst choices, seemingly unaffected by the losses he sustained as a result of them. The lessons of each bad consequence didn't sink in.

If Elliot had had an intact somatic-marker system, the frustration and anger that one would normally experience from a significant financial loss would have been imprinted on his nervous system. As he looked at the decks the next time, he would have been able to appreciate the consequences of his choices by recalling those feelings. He would have been able to simulate the results of choosing one deck versus another just as you or I might simulate the consequences of confronting a troubled friend. Unfortunately, the damage in Elliot's brain prevented his unconscious system from using experience to guide his future choices, and Elliot continued to dig himself into a deeper and deeper hole, both in the gambling task and in life.

Somatic markers are a type of emotional memory, re-instantiations of information that the brain has acquired in the past. But we just experience them as "gut feelings." Stored and activated unconsciously, these memories emerge at relevant moments in our lives to help guide our decisions. In this chapter, we have seen the ways in which we can train the unconscious system in the brain. Physical practice, mental rehearsal, and observing others are forms of learning that build up neuronal connections through repetitive use. Once we establish this infrastructure, the unconscious brain gives back. In sports, it improves our performance without our having to think about it, strengthening muscle and perfecting technique. Through mirror neurons, it simulates what we see so we can learn about one another, express empathy, and understand pain and pleasure. Finally, through somatic markers, it uses our past experiences to guide future decisions.

Through the recollection and rehearsal of past experience, the unconscious simulates old information to help us learn and grow. It draws from our vast store of memories to empower decision making. Memory, however, is not always a dependable source of information. Yet the unconscious depends on it to construct its simulations. So, what happens when that information is incomplete or misleading?

We have seen different ways in which the brain fills in the gaps. When we fall asleep and perception goes dark, the brain narrates our dreams. When we lose our sight or endure neurological injury, the brain reconstructs our world through other means, even by concocting hallucinations. When recalling memories to guide decision making, the brain is equally vigilant in trying to create a complete narrative. The logic of our unconscious system dictates that gaps in information be filled by drawing from context or from memory. But what if the gaps were not in perception but in memory itself? How could the unconscious fill a hole in the very store of information it depends on to create its simulations? As it turns out, the brain can make up its own story.

# 4

# Can We Remember Things That Never Happened?

*On Memory, Emotion, and the Egocentric Brain*

He was still too young to know that the heart's memory eliminates the bad and magnifies the good, and that thanks to this artifice we manage to endure the burden of the past.

—Gabriel García Márquez

When I first met Billy, he was sitting motionless in a wheelchair, gnawing on a bedsheet dangling from the side of his mouth. He did not reply to questions. When I asked him something, he would just stare at me with an ear-to-ear smile, as if he secretly knew something no one else did. His muscles were stiff. Occasionally, he would glance from side to side, chew on the sheet, or pick at his arms with his fingernails, but other than that he didn't move. Billy was in a state of catatonia, immobile and stuporous. Yet to the chagrin of those of us responsible for his care, we had no idea how a perfectly healthy guy could become like this in the span of just a few weeks. A CT scan and an MRI were inconclusive. A drug screen came back clean for illicit substances. Blood tests were negative. Billy was a mystery.

Two weeks prior, Billy had gone to the emergency department of another hospital with wet shoes on the wrong feet, saying, "I need to talk . . . about brain damage." His family said that Billy had been completely normal his entire life. With silky black hair, a winning smile, and a cocky, sarcastic edge to his humor, he had enough charm to fill any room and made friends easily. In his early thirties, Billy held a master's degree in chemistry and worked for years in a commercial laboratory. He was moving up in his career and had a steady girlfriend.

But suddenly something changed. He became distant from his

friends and family. He was laid off from his job and broke up with his girlfriend. He lost the ability to pay his bills, maintain his car and apartment, and feed himself. His mother went to look for him in his apartment, where she discovered towering stacks of empty pizza boxes. She found full, untouched containers of home-cooked food that she had prepared for him lying all over the house, spoiled and attracting flies. Billy's car was found abandoned in an off-limits area of a distant public park. No one was sure how he found his way to a hospital. The answers would have to come from Billy himself, but he was mute.

After being transferred to our hospital, Billy began treatment with electroconvulsive therapy (ECT), which involved inducing thirty-second-long seizures by firing electrical pulses at his brain under general anesthesia. It's the best-known treatment for catatonia. After several sessions, the catatonia began to regress, and Billy's personality started to reemerge. He began talking again, and a lot, though much of what he said was initially incomprehensible. He started flirting with female nurses and doctors, giving them an occasional wink or asking them out on dates. His sense of humor returned, and after a few weeks of treatment Billy was able to walk without a wheelchair. One thing, however, did not return to normal: his memory.

Billy could not remember basic information about himself or his past. He could not recall who the president was, who his doctor was, or even that he was in a hospital. Yet he always pretended he knew the right answers. He fabricated bogus replies and said them with confidence, repeating those same answers day after day. Each morning, I would interview Billy, asking any and all questions that came to my mind as I tried to uncover clues that might hint at what caused his sudden transformation. I would write down his answers so I could see how they evolved over time. Here are some snippets of conversations we had over the course of two weeks.

DAY 1

ME: Billy, can you tell me today's date?

BILLY: Sure thing. It's February 20, 2012, but more specifically it's September 3, 1998.

ME: Do you know your name?

BILLY: Yeah, man, of course.

ME: What is it?

BILLY: I don't really think it's appropriate, at this juncture, considering our current rapport, with everything going on here, to reveal that information to you now. But, hey, man, I certainly appreciate the gesture on your part. If you play your cards right, you might just get what you're looking for.

DAY 4

ME: Do you know why you're here in the hospital?

BILLY: Yeah, because of my knee.

ME: What's wrong with your leg?

BILLY: It's been hurting me for weeks. That's why I got surgery on it yesterday.

ME: You got surgery yesterday?

BILLY: Yeah. It was a torn ligament. Surgery went well, though. You guys have been great at taking care of me. I can walk a lot better now. No wheelchair or anything. And my knee doesn't hurt anymore.

ME: Billy, I haven't seen notes from the surgeons in your record about that. Are you sure you had surgery yesterday?

BILLY: Oh yeah. They wanted to keep it hush-hush. Nobody would think a guy like me would need knee surgery.

Billy didn't know the date. He didn't know where he was. He initially didn't even know his own name. He wouldn't admit to not knowing these things. Rather, he would trot out an endless list of excuses, as if to cover up his ignorance, or, more often, he would invent an answer and stick to it no matter how often that answer was called into question by the medical staff. But here's the really mysterious part: Billy wasn't lying. He wasn't *intentionally* misleading anyone or trying to cover himself. He truly believed every answer he gave. He was completely certain, for example, that he was recovering from knee surgery. He had memories of things that never happened.

What happened to Billy's memory?

## A Web of Snapshots

To understand what went wrong in Billy's brain, it helps to have a sense of how memory works. There is a common misconception that memory is a video capture of our past, a simple record of our life experience. However, video recordings emphasize every aspect of a scene equally. They don't pick and choose what's most important to focus on. Video recordings are exact records. Memory makes mistakes and changes over time.

Deep within the brain, in the hippocampus and neighboring regions, the memory machine churns, seated in a meshwork of interconnected neurons. The axons and dendrites, the spiderlike appendages of brain cells, send and receive the electrochemical signals called neurotransmitters. These signals traverse the no-man's-land between axons and dendrites known as the synaptic cleft until they arrive at the receptors on the target neuron. The pattern of these connections evolves throughout our lives. As we accumulate new experiences and reflect on the past, the strength of synaptic connections is enhanced or blunted.

This was first discovered in the 1960s when neuroscientists found that when they shot the same pulse at a neuron more than once, the neuronal response intensified. It was as if the neuron *remembered* receiving that exact signal before. When the experimenters activated two or more neurons simultaneously, the neurons appeared to form an association, a stronger working relationship. If a future signal activated that neuronal group in the same pattern, it elicited an amplified response. The theory is that when neurons are frequently incited as a group, they recruit additional receptors, creating new and stronger synapses. This bolstering of synaptic connections, known as long-term potentiation, is the basis of memory formation.

Long-term potentiation allows not only for memories to be encoded as recognizable patterns of neuronal firing but also for links to form between memories. One of the fundamental principles of neuroscience is that "neurons that fire together, wire together." When groups of neurons are activated simultaneously, especially if this happens often, the pattern of synaptic connections gradually changes, connecting those groups of neurons. Once they're connected, future activation of one group will nudge the other group to rally as well. Memory formation is a dynamic, evolving process that lasts throughout our lives. Our experiences are stored as a pattern of interwoven connections. When you reimagine an experience, or undergo something similar, the pattern is reactivated. The more you think about it, the more entrenched it becomes and the more it can form links to other thoughts and memories.

Think of memory as a collection of disparate moments in time that the brain has to organize to tell a continuous story. When, at a dinner with friends, someone mentions her high school graduation, you instantly think of yours. Thoughts of graduation remind you of your high school crush, whom you haven't seen in years. Your mind wanders to pictures of your past relationships, your wedding, the drunken best man who knocked over the cake, the day you persuaded him to go to Alcoholics Anonymous, the moment he cried and hugged you when he finally became sober.

But those snapshots can be rearranged. The psychologist Elizabeth Loftus designed an experiment to demonstrate how our memory can be manipulated by experiences we have later in life. She told a group of volunteers that an older relative of theirs would remind them of four events from their past. Unbeknownst to the participants, the older relatives were actually in cahoots with Loftus, helping her with the experiment. Loftus instructed the older relatives to remind their younger counterparts of four events that happened to them as children: three of them true and one false. In each case, the false event was about a time the participant got lost in the mall as a child. The participants, however, were told that they truly had all four experiences. Loftus wanted to know whether a trusted family member's reference to a made-up incident could lead to the implantation of that story in a person's mind as a false memory. She chose getting lost at the mall because it made for a good example of a scary event that could reasonably have happened a long time ago. One subject, Chris, was told the following story by his older brother, Jim:

> It was 1981 or 1982. I remember that Chris was 5. We had gone shopping at the University City shopping mall in Spokane. After some panic, we found Chris being led down the mall by a tall, oldish man (I think he was wearing a flannel shirt). Chris was crying and holding the man's hand. The man explained that he had found Chris walking around crying his eyes out just a few moments before and was trying to help him find his parents.

In the days that followed, Chris began to remember details about the supposed incident. He recalled how scared he was and how his mother told him never to do that again. He even remembered the old man's flannel shirt. Two weeks later, Chris's false memory had become even more vivid:

> I was with you guys for a second and I think I went over to look at the toy store, the Kay Bee Toys, and uh, we got lost and I was looking around and I thought, "Uh-oh. I'm in trouble now." You know. And then I . . . I thought I was never going to see my family again. I was really scared you know. And then this old man, I think he was wearing a blue flannel, came up to me . . . he was kind of old. He was kind of bald on top . . . he had like a ring of gray hair . . . and he had glasses.

After Chris was finally informed that one of the stories his brother related was false, he attempted to guess which story was made up, and he guessed wrong. His visualization of getting lost at the mall had become so clear that he was more convinced that it had occurred than one of the true memories. Of the twenty-four subjects who underwent Loftus's experiment, seven (29 percent) of them developed a false memory of being lost at the mall. Loftus concluded that our thoughts truly can alter how our memories are stored.

The interconnected nature of memory is what allows it to change over time. Just as the brain links memories that have similar features and emphasizes the moments that we consider most significant, it can reorganize those connections later based on new thoughts and experiences. No memory is made in a vacuum, and no memory is fixed. Like any well-written story, memory has a direction and a point of view and is subject to revision.

A research group in Israel once filmed a young woman, with no history of memory problems, for two days straight. They were ordinary days in her life, save for the cameras, of course. At various intervals over the next few years, she filled out a questionnaire that tested her memory of those days. While she did so, the researchers monitored her brain activity using fMRI. The longer the interval, the more distorted her memory became for the details. What was interesting, however, was how her brain activity changed over time while filling out the recall questionnaires. As the months and years passed and the memory errors accumulated, her memory appeared less and less reliant on the activity of the hippocampus. The fMRI revealed reduced activation there as her recollection became more distant. Other regions of the brain, including the medial prefrontal cortex and associated regions, became more and more active. Bordering the frontal lobe, the medial prefrontal cortex is associated with self-centered thinking. The young woman's memory was accessing not simply a record from a neurological file folder but a representation stored across multiple systems. As time passed, her memory drifted away from accurately recording the details of that time period and instead became more focused on her.

To a large extent, our memories define us. Our personal history forges our self-image and assembles our store of knowledge. When the unconscious system in the brain encodes our memories, it is shaping who we are. It doesn't record our experiences impartially as a video camera would, because it focuses on our role in the story, on the aspects that we care about. At any given moment, there is a context of how we are feeling, our emotions at that instant, what we are expecting or dreading, and what that moment *means* to us. It is on that basis that the brain begins to compose its first draft.

## The Brains of Rival Sports Fans

College basketball games are a surprisingly ideal setting for studying the way self-centered thinking and emotion affect memory formation. Whenever one team scores, say on a ferocious dunk or a game-changing three-pointer, the two halves of the audience are simultaneously experiencing fervent, perhaps even fanatical, emotions on opposite sides of the spectrum. The fans identify with their team's players and, from tip-off to the final buzzer, are locked in on every play, screaming for their favorites and booing the opposition.

Few rivalries in sports are more impassioned than that between the Duke University Blue Devils and the University of North Carolina (UNC) Tar Heels. In 2010, a group of neuroscientists at Duke University (we'll assume they were unbiased) recruited hard-core basketball fans, twelve from Duke and eleven from UNC, to participate in a study on emotional memory. Over the course of the week, the fans watched a dramatic Duke-UNC basketball game together three times on a big-screen TV. One day after the third viewing, the experimenters presented each fan with sixty-four video clips of the game through liquid crystal display goggles that made them feel as if they were right in the action, surrounded by the roar of the crowd. Half the clips depicted plays that turned out well for Duke, while the other half exhibited sequences that were good for UNC. All of the clips portrayed the action leading up to an emotional play, and the fans rated each one for its level of emotional intensity. But the clips were incomplete. Each twelve-second highlight would cut off just as a player was releasing the basketball. The challenge for the fans was to try to remember whether the player made the shot.

When the behavioral data were gathered, the experimenters found that fans' memories were better for plays that helped their team than for those that hurt it. Apparently, positive emotional memories tend to be more accurate than negative ones.

As the fans watched the action unfold, the experimenters monitored their brain activity using fMRI. The neuroimaging results revealed activation in brain regions we would expect, like the hippocampus (episodic memory) and the amygdala (emotion). But the fMRI data also showed something else: several other regions of the brain seemed to be participating in recalling the plays. One such area was the medial prefrontal cortex, which we said earlier is associated with self-centered thinking. That doesn't mean simply selfish thoughts, like wanting a more expensive car. Whenever we see something that we feel is intimately connected to our identity, the medial prefrontal cortex goes to work. In one study at the University of Toronto, subjects were shown various adjectives, such as the word "stubborn," and asked two questions:

1. Does the word "stubborn" describe you?
2. Does the word "stubborn" describe [the former Canadian prime minister] Brian Mulroney?

On the fMRI, the medial prefrontal cortex lit up while they answered question 1 but not question 2. The medial prefrontal was called upon when the question involved the self but not when it referenced someone else, even though the topic was restricted to the concept of stubbornness.

Why would a region of the brain that specializes in self-referential thinking be involved in recalling emotional plays of a basketball game? It's because these fans are so invested in the performance of their team that they personally identify with the players, so much so that their self-centered thinking shows up on an fMRI while they watch the game. As they think about the players, they think about themselves.

There's more to this neurological story. The neuroimaging results showed that the parahippocampal area (the area bordering the hippocampus) was also active while the subjects recalled the basketball plays. This region is known to be involved with social cognition, such as when we detect sarcasm in a conversation. In one study, volunteers watched videos of conversations between two people. In each case, one of the actors would say a neutral phrase like "I'd be happy to do it. I've got plenty of time." In some of the videos the character said the phrase sincerely, while in others he or she said it bitterly, drenched in sarcasm: "I'd be *happy* to do it. I've got *pleeenty* of time." When patients correctly detected the sarcasm in a character's recital of the phrase, the parahippocampal area fired. When people with damage to their hippocampal area tried the task, they were far worse at comprehending sarcasm than healthy subjects were.

Though the parahippocampal cortex is historically known for its role in processing spatial relationships, the sarcasm study implies that it has a role in social cognition as well. In the context of a basketball game, this makes perfect sense. After all, the fans go to the arena with their friends, or watch the game on TV with a group, as in the study we discussed. Those scenes are rife with social cues: reactions of the other fans, competitions, subtle taunts, or explicit trash-talking. As the events of the game unfold, the brain processes them in the context of the viewer's life at that instant. The emotional intensity of the moment is derived not solely from the game but from *what the game means to the fan*. The fan identifies with the players, so the self-referential processing of the medial temporal lobe is activated. The fan is experiencing the emotional highs and lows of the game with his friends (and adversaries) around him, so the social cognition ability of the parahippocampal area fires up as well.

When the brain encodes a memory, it does so in the context of a vast array of circumstances and emotions, such as the social construct of the game and the excitement or disappointment of the fan. The regions of the brain that mobilize while the fans watch the game become permanently associated with the memories of the game and the memories of each play. As fans recall the plays, they do so together with the personal and social implications, contributed by the medial prefrontal cortex and parahippocampal area. They come to mind all together, bound both conceptually and neurologically.

Though the basketball players may be the stars of the game, the fans are the stars of their own recollections. Whether they realize it or not, the fans remember what the game meant to them and perhaps even reflect on their participation in the experience. When we want to share a moment from our past, we don't simply describe a still moment in time; we tell a story with a beginning, middle, and end. And we each see ourselves as the protagonist.

## Why Do We Remember Where We Were on 9/11?

Do you remember where you were on the Sunday morning of November 18, 2001? Neither do I. I can barely remember what I did two Sundays ago. Yet we remember September 11, 2001, extremely well—not just the tragic events that occurred, but also precisely where we were and what we were doing at the moment the news broke. Whenever people recall the events of 9/11, the first memory that everyone shares is not of the events themselves but something to the effect of "I remember it perfectly. I was at Starbucks getting a cappuccino when I heard the news on the radio," or "I was in class when the professor came in and made the announcement." Strange, isn't it? September 11 was a national tragedy that affected us all, an event that changed the course of history, but the first memory we all share (except for those directly affected) is whatever insignificant activity we were doing on that day.

Our recollection of 9/11 is known as a flashbulb memory, a highly detailed vision of a powerful, intensely emotional event. In a study of flashbulb memories, 168 participants were interviewed in September 2001 and asked to recall the circumstances in which they learned of the attacks on the World Trade Center and the Pentagon. The experimenters repeated the interview two years later to determine whether the memories were consistent. For comparison, a control group of 185 volunteers was told they would be entered into a prize drawing. Each of them was then alerted via text message that they had *not* won the prize. The experimenters asked the participants to describe where they were and what they were doing when they received the unfortunate text message that no prize was coming their way. They conducted this interview twice as well, once in the days following the text message and once a year later.

The results revealed that even though two years had passed since 9/11 compared with one year since the text message, the subjects' accounts of what they were doing on September 11 were more consistent with their original testimony than were the descriptions of the day of the text message. Though the accounts were not perfectly consistent, the participants recalling 9/11 remembered more details than the control group did, and those details better matched the original ones provided.

This conclusion may not seem that startling, but what if we were to compare the memories of different people for events of equal caliber or for the same event? How does the emotional intensity of our reaction affect our memory of that episode? Consider the experience of most people who witnessed the falling of the Twin Towers firsthand compared with the rest of us who saw it on the news.

## Brains in Midtown and Downtown

Three years after 9/11, two groups of New York City residents were enrolled in an experiment to learn how their emotions at the time of the attacks might have affected their memory. The first group consisted of people who were in downtown Manhattan, close to the World Trade Center, and personally witnessed the events on that day. The second group consisted of people who were in midtown, several miles away. As subjects described their memories, the researchers monitored the participants' brain activity using fMRI. The subjects then graded their memories for their degree of vividness and emotional arousal, as well as the level of confidence they had in the accuracy of those memories. As expected, the downtown group rated their memories as being more vivid, more complete, and more emotionally intense than the midtown group did. They also had more confidence in the accuracy of their memories. However, the neurological results told a different story.

The hippocampus is the area classically involved in episodic memory, of which recalling 9/11 is an example. But, depending on the type of memory being accessed, other areas of the brain may be recruited to varying extents. For example, the amygdala may be activated when the memory is of an emotional nature, and the posterior parahippocampal cortex (the region of the brain adjacent to and behind the hippocampus) will become involved when the brain attempts to access the more meticulous spatial details surrounding the event. Members of the midtown group showed activation of the posterior parahippocampal cortex as they recalled the details of 9/11 but only trivial amygdala activity. It was just the opposite case for the downtown group. They exhibited striking activity in the amygdala but not in the posterior parahippocampal cortex. The neuroimaging implies that the downtown group recalled the events of the day for their emotional impact at the expense of remembering peripheral details. In fact, studies reveal that the more emotionally affected people are in recalling 9/11, the better they are at consistently describing the central events of what happened to them that day (such as where they were), but the worse they are at providing reliable descriptions of the emotionally neutral details (what shoes they were wearing).

We remember moments that bring out our emotions. The fact that someone was getting a cappuccino when he heard about the attacks of September 11 is an insignificant fact to nearly everyone in the world except for him. In the narrative of his life, that's where he was and what he was doing when he received world-changing news. The Starbucks trip was a central component of his life experience that day, whereas a fact like the precise time at which the towers were hit was not.

Our experience on September 11 was integral to our personal narrative. It was a transformative moment in history, and we lived to witness the horror and tragedy, whether in person or from afar. We cared so much about how we received the news that the first thing we mention when recounting 9/11 is what we ourselves were doing as the events unfolded.

When organizing the snapshots of our experiences, the unconscious system in the brain takes a self-centered, *egocentric* approach. We consciously remember the aspects of our experience that matter to our own personal story. In a 2013 study, a group of psychologists asked forty undergraduates to imagine that they were stranded in the grasslands, without food or water and with the knowledge that deadly predators stalked the landscape. They showed the students a list of thirty words and asked them to rate how relevant each word was to their survival in the imagined precarious situation. The participants then repeated this task with a different set of thirty words while imagining that some unknown person was stranded in the grasslands instead of them. Finally, they repeated the task with a third set of words but without an imagined scenario; they just rated whether the words were things found in cities or in nature.

After the undergrads completed these three tasks, the psychologists announced that there would be a surprise quiz. They showed the students a set of 180 words; half of them were words the students saw in the preceding tasks, while the other half were new words. The challenge was to indicate which of the words were in the experiment and which were new additions.

The psychologists found that students demonstrated the greatest accuracy for identifying words that they saw while imagining themselves in the grasslands. They did worst with the words in the scenario with no story, and their performance in the scenario involving a third party in the grasslands fell in the middle. The participants' memory was most accurate when it came to details pertaining to their own survival story, even an imagined one. When constructing our memories, the brain homes in on the features that matter most to us, often at the expense of details that, at the time, appear relatively mundane.

Here's just one more example. In 1967, a strange and frightening incident occurred during the fourth inning of a baseball game between the Boston Red Sox and the California Angels. Tony Conigliaro, star hitter for the Red Sox, was up to bat. The Angels pitcher Jack Hamilton fired at him with a fastball that struck Conigliaro in the head. The impact fractured his cheekbone, dislocated his jaw, and caused lasting blurring of his vision. Years later, when interviewed about the pitch that nearly killed Conigliaro, Hamilton said,

I know in my heart I wasn't trying to hit him . . . it was like the sixth inning when it happened. I think the score was 2–1, and he was the eighth hitter in their batting order . . . I had no reason to throw at him . . . I tried to go see him in the hospital late that afternoon or early that evening but they were just letting his family in.

Even though this was a significant event in Hamilton's life, records reveal that parts of his account were false. He was wrong about the inning (it was the fourth) and the batting order (Conigliaro was sixth). Also, Conigliaro was an excellent hitter, and therefore there *was* reason to hit him and force a walk to first base. Most significantly, the game took place in the evening, not the afternoon. Hamilton did not visit the hospital until the next day.

Hamilton had a clear memory for the event, or so it seemed to him. He probably remembered the look on Conigliaro's face when the ball hit him. He probably remembered how he felt at the moment it happened. He likely could have told you all about the visit with Conigliaro at the hospital. Yet circumstantial details like what inning it was, the batting order, and even the time of day fell by the wayside. Hamilton conveniently forgot that Conigliaro was a great hitter and, therefore, that there was good reason to hit him with the ball and force him to walk to first base rather than risk him hitting it out of the park. Maybe Hamilton did think about hitting Conigliaro with the ball but just didn't want to admit it. But there's another possibility: perhaps his brain unconsciously left that detail out of memory because Hamilton didn't *want* to remember it. Hamilton might have seen himself as an ethical player who wouldn't engage in that sort of gamesmanship. Had he believed that he recklessly threw the ball or intentionally hurt Conigliaro, it could have haunted him for the rest of his life. Such a thought could have ruined his self-perception. Perhaps, unconsciously, his brain was protecting him.

## Ignorance Is Bliss

On September 22, 1969, an eight-year-old girl named Susan Nason disappeared after a visit to a friend's house in Foster City, California. With the help of the police, her parents initiated a search that went on for months without success. Then, in December 1969, an employee of the San Francisco Water Department, while on a routine patrol, discovered the remains of a child's body in a ravine near the Crystal Springs Reservoir. Investigators examining the scene noted that there was a crushed silver ring on one hand and that the dress on the body had been pulled up above the waist. Dental records identified the body as Susan Nason. Pathology reports indicated that Nason died from blunt-force trauma to the head, and injuries to her wrist bones were evidence of a struggle near the time of death. But who was the killer? That question remained unresolved for the next twenty years.

In January 1989, twenty-eight-year-old Eileen Franklin-Lipsker was watching her daughter play on the floor when, at one point, her daughter looked up at her. Peering into the child's eyes, Eileen was suddenly struck by a terrifying vision. She recalled being eight years old and sitting in the back of a van with her best friend, Susie. The van came to a halt near a reservoir. Her father, George Franklin, came to the back of the van, straddled Susie's lap, and began grinding his pelvis against her. Susie struggled to fight him off. Eileen was stricken with fear. The vision skipped to another scene. Susie was outside the van, on the ground, crying. Eileen saw her father approach her friend and smash her head with a rock. Susie's hand was bloody, and the ring on her hand was crushed. Clumps of Susie's hair were on the ground.

After initially discussing the memory with her therapist, Eileen told her husband, who immediately called the police, claiming that his wife could identify Susan Nason's killer. Believing that the story had legitimacy, the police ventured to George Franklin's house. Franklin opened the door.

"We are investigating an old homicide case," one officer began, "involving a subject by the name of Susan—Susan Nason."

Franklin stared at the officer for a moment before he replied, "Have you talked to my daughter?"

When Franklin's case went to trial, several expert witnesses testified regarding the concept of memory repression. For the prosecution, Dr. Lenore Terr, a psychiatrist and professor at the University of California at San Francisco, referenced the fact that Eileen had herself been a victim of physical and sexual abuse as a child. Terr asserted that "a particularly hideous, violent act occurring in a childhood filled with repeated acts of both physical and sexual abuse starting at an early age, involving multiple persons, including a parental figure ... would very likely— would probably most likely be repressed." For the defense, Dr. Elizabeth Loftus, a psychology professor at the University of Washington, raised the possibility that repeated retellings of a story can convince a person that it is true, when indeed it is not, like someone coming to falsely believe he had been lost in the mall as a child. What's more, the longer it has been since an event supposedly happened, the more time there is for information acquired after that event to seep into a person's subconscious and alter the way that event is recalled, a phenomenon she referred to as "memory contamination."

The defense argued that the details of Eileen's testimony were derived from news reports that she had seen around the time of the incident. They claimed that "absolutely everything" Eileen claimed to remember was information available to the public. Perhaps she was just remembering descriptions from the investigation that she had read. The defense council also pointed out that Eileen had been inconsistent in her recall of the event. There were subtle variations of the story in each of her retellings. For example, at the trial, Eileen said that her sister, Janice, was in a nearby field when Eileen and her father picked up Susan. However, before the trial, Eileen had claimed that Janice was in the van next to her and that their father told Janice to get out of the car before they picked up Susan. Janice testified that she remembered the day that Susan disappeared but did not remember seeing either her sister or her father at all on that day.

Despite this and other inconsistencies, the jury was convinced by the degree of detail in Eileen's testimony and the confidence with which she remembered the incident. George Franklin was found guilty of murder in the first degree.

Did Eileen truly witness her father murder her best friend twenty years earlier? Or was she simply connecting visions of news reports she had read and images she had seen into a memorylike sequence?

We won't be able to resolve the debate over whether repressed memories are true memories or distorted ones here. The best answer we can provide is that they are a little bit of both. When George Franklin was approached by the police, he immediately referenced his daughter. So, it's quite likely that the central aspects of Eileen's story were true. The fact that she misremembered some of the peripheral details is consistent with the studies of memory we have seen. Eileen did witness her father's crime, but her memory was repressed for two decades.

Memory repression typically occurs in the context of trauma. Children who are victims of physical or sexual abuse, for example, sometimes don't remember what happened to them until many years later, when something triggers those memories to flood back. Emotional trauma like sexual abuse can destroy a person's psychological functioning, injuring his or her sense of self-worth and personhood. The predominant theory of memory repression is that it's the brain's safety valve to protect our fragile sense of self from recollections that are just too difficult to bear. Just as a surgeon uses anesthesia to prevent postoperative pain, the unconscious brain can use repression to numb the agony of reliving a traumatic experience.

Research shows that memory for negative feelings fades more quickly than for happy ones. In psychology, there's a theory called the mnemic neglect model which contends that people tend to easily recall things that are consistent with their self-perception and more likely to neglect feelings and memories that conflict with the way they perceive themselves. In one study, participants were shown a list of behaviors and asked to evaluate whether they were the sort of person capable of engaging in them. The behaviors ranged from negative, self-threatening actions like "I would not pay back money that I owed to a friend" to positive, self-affirming ones like "I would take care of a sick friend for several days." After some time had passed, the participants tried to list as many of the behaviors as they could remember. They were far better at coming up with the positive behaviors and more likely to conveniently forget the negative ones. For comparison, the researchers conducted a parallel experiment. They showed a second group of volunteers a description of a guy named Chris. They then had the participants evaluate the relevance of the list of behaviors, some positive and some negative, as they may apply to Chris. When the second group tried to recall the list later, they were equally good at recalling the positive and negative actions. It appeared that because the negative actions were referring to someone other than themselves, they were not more likely to neglect them.

The brain often organizes the snapshots of our history in an ego-protective fashion. If the unconscious brain were a news channel, it would be a biased one. Just as many Democrats watch liberal-leaning television and many Republicans prefer conservative talk radio, the unconscious system has a preference for incorporating life experiences that fall in line with our self-perception and worldview. The brain helps maintain that perspective. It makes the story about us, about the things we care about. Sometimes it fudges the time line a little or conveniently omits the subtle details that don't neatly fall in line with the story we'd like to believe. It's not a bad thing. It's a very healthy, adaptive mechanism that protects our conscious thinking and decision-making capacities. Repression is thought to be an extreme example of how the brain protects us with errors of omission. In Eileen's case, however, there were multiple blips in her memory aside from the repression itself. We'll never know just how much of her testimony was true memory and how much came from other sources, but we can safely say that her memory was at least *slightly* affected by the extensive media coverage of the crime.

We know that memories can be altered or even implanted, such as a person made to falsely remember being lost at the mall. It appears that when the brain is arranging the snapshots of time into continuous memories, those snapshots can come from various sources, whether they be personal experiences or memories of a different kind. The unconscious system collects these snapshots, regardless of their origin, and strings them together in a narrative that aligns with our self-perception. We said that memory is not a video recording, but rather a dynamic, evolving process. Now we see that it's also a biased one. But just how far will the brain go to tell a good story?

## "It's Not a Lie If You Believe It"

At Memorial Sloan Kettering Cancer Center in New York City, the psychologist Michael Gazzaniga was preparing to see a patient, a seemingly intelligent woman who was reading *The New York Times* as he entered her room. Gazzaniga introduced himself and asked the patient whether she knew where she was.

"I am in Freeport, Maine," she said. "I know you don't believe it. Dr. Posner told me this morning that I was in Memorial Sloan Kettering Hospital and that when the residents come on rounds to say that to them. Well, that is fine, but I know I am in my house on Main Street in Freeport, Maine!"

The patient was clearly in a state of confusion, but Gazzaniga wanted to test the extent of her delusion. "Well," he began, "if you are in Freeport and in your house, how come there are elevators outside the door here?"

The patient was unmoved. "Doctor, do you know how much it cost me to have those put in?"

When confronted with evidence that conflicted with her belief, the patient fabricated a memory to reconcile her perception of the elevators with her belief that she was lying in her bed at home in Freeport. She called upon a false memory of installing elevators in her New England home and even expressed a hint of frustration about how much it cost. She wasn't lying. She truly believed that this memory was true.

Billy exhibited the same symptom consistently during our many conversations.

DAY 7

ME: I hear your mom came in to help you pay some bills today.

BILLY: Yeah, I paid some big bills today. Took care of my business.

ME: How big?

BILLY: Ten thousand dollars.

ME: Wow, that's a huge bill, Billy. What was that for?

BILLY: Comcast.

ME: Are you sure about that? That seems like a really big bill for Comcast. You can't be ordering that many movies . . .

BILLY: Oh yes I can. I watched thousands of them. I *love* movies.

DAY 11

BILLY: Hey, bro. Wanna go out and pick up some beers with me?

ME: What for?

BILLY: So we can party!

ME: Billy, it's a nice thought, but you aren't allowed to bring beer into the hospital.

BILLY: Of course you can have beer here. This is a Catholic university. All they do is party!

ME: Actually, Billy, we're in a hospital right now, not a Catholic university.

BILLY: Oh. Well, then somebody seriously mixed up my paperwork.

In each of our conversations, Billy filled in the holes in his memory with false claims. When unable to remember what bills he paid, he came up with an absurd $10,000 cable bill and then defended that figure by stressing how many movies he'd seen. When he couldn't remember where he was, he referred to a mix-up with the application he supposedly sent to a Catholic university. These claims were untrue, of course, but Billy wasn't lying. As George Costanza, on *Seinfeld*, once advised Jerry before a lie detector test, "It's not a lie if you believe it." The symptom that Billy continuously exhibited was confabulation, the unconscious fabrication of false memories. People who confabulate are not consciously trying to deceive anyone and are not even aware that what they're saying isn't true. They remember things that never happened.

Brain injury, Alzheimer's disease, drugs, and Korsakoff's syndrome (caused by chronic alcohol use) are among the many causes of confabulation. It is the phenomenon in which the brain creates false memories, apparently to compensate for gaps in a person's recollection, most often for autobiographical information. Confabulation can be spontaneous, meaning the person generates the memory without being probed with specific questions, or it can be provoked by a direct question that forces the person to confront a gap in memory. In a study in London, for example, a group of patients with either Korsakoff's syndrome or Alzheimer's disease read the following story:

Anna Thompson of South Bristol, employed as a cleaner in an office building, reported at the Town Hall police station that she had been held up on the High Street the night before and robbed of 15 pounds. She had four little children, the rent was due, and they had not eaten for two days. The officers, touched by the woman's story, made up a purse for her.

At various time intervals after finishing the story, the patients attempted to recall some of the highlights. Here are some of their answers, immediately after reading the story:

- "She had just come home and two police officers called in to see her about the position as it was."
- "She had had her money and valuables taken. Her confederates—ladies in the office—made up the money to her."
- "Jack Brown took his wife down to Brighton."
- "Anna Thompson of Cane Hill Hospital. She died."

Just seconds after finishing the story, the patients falsely remembered details that were never mentioned, such as Anna's husband, her co-workers, and her death. For comparison, the experimenters showed the story to healthy control subjects, who were able to accurately recall it and tended not to make up any details. When interviewed a week later, however, even the healthy subjects exhibited some false memories:

- "She had a little boy, age two."
- "It happened near a railway station."

Provoked confabulations can happen to anyone, while spontaneous confabulations are almost exclusively the result of brain damage. Either way, why would the brain do this? Why not let the holes in memory stand as they are?

Confabulation can result from damage to any of a number of brain regions, such as the medial prefrontal cortex (associated with self-centered thinking) and the orbitofrontal cortex (emotional gut feelings). The fact that damage to the frontal lobe, the home of higher-level thinking and decision making, is a common culprit has led many neurologists to theorize that confabulation arises when people lose the capacity to decide which snapshots of memory go together, and their stories become distorted mixtures of events from their past.

Some researchers believe it's a form of delusion, as might occur in schizophrenia. There is no consensus at this point, but one of the main neuropsychological theories is that confabulation occurs when fragments of memory are missing or distorted and the existence and stability of the self come under threat. In an attempt to maintain the continuity of our personal history, the unconscious system in the brain takes the various memory fragments and tries to assemble them into a single account, even if that means plugging a few holes with fabricated recollections. The brain creates a unified narrative in any way it can.

In a bit for the television show *Jimmy Kimmel Live*, a woman pretending to be a reporter attended the annual Coachella Valley Music and Arts Festival in Indio, California. The faux reporter, flanked by a cameraman, randomly approached people at the festival to ask them their thoughts on some of the lesser-known indie bands. The trick, however, was that she made up an array of fake band names to see whether the festival attendees would pretend to know their music. She encouraged them to discuss the musical stylings of Dr. Shlomo and the G.I. Clinic, Shorty Jizzle and the Plumbercrunks, and the Obesity Epidemic. The attendees not only pretended to know these bands but freely discussed their "rawness" and "energy" and expressed their excitement at finally getting the chance to see them live.

The attendees were obviously lying, not confabulating. They had never heard of those bands. So why would they pretend they had? Because they thought of themselves as knowledgeable, experienced music lovers, not only when it came to the popular bands, but also in regard to the specialized and up-and-coming groups. The prospect of being caught ignorant of a band was uncomfortable, so the attendees consciously lied.

Perhaps that's what the confabulating brain does on an *unconscious* level. Just as repression protects the ego after emotional trauma, maybe confabulation protects the ego from memory loss or confusion. This would make sense neurologically. Confabulation usually results from damage to the medial temporal lobe—the region responsible for self-centered thinking. It's the same area that fires when hard-core college basketball fans watch and connect with their favorite players. Damage to the medial temporal lobe places our sense of self under threat. Perhaps confabulation is the brain's mechanism to preserve it.

If true, this hypothesis explains the psychological motivation for human beings to confabulate: it's a defense mechanism. It keeps the continuity of our memory, our life story, intact. What the theory doesn't explain, however, is *how* the brain comes up with that story. When it goes about creating false memories, where does the brain get its material?

## Fairy Tales in the Confabulating Brain

DAY 14

ME: Billy, do you remember what really bad thing happened on September 11?

BILLY: Yeah, I remember.

ME: Can you tell me what happened?

BILLY: Yeah. It went like this: there was this plane . . . it was flying, but everything started going wrong, so the pilot had to land *really* carefully. Everyone was relieved.

ME: Are you sure that's what happened?

BILLY: Do you see my face?

ME: Yes.

BILLY: This is the face of someone who knows.

When I asked Billy to recall what occurred on September 11, he correctly remembered that it had something to do with an airplane but not much else. At the time, I thought of his answer as being on the right track but didn't think much of it. In retrospect, however, I wonder if he substituted one memory for another. In January 2009, a US Airways flight collided with a flock of Canada geese and lost power to its engines. In an amazing show of emergency maneuvering, the crew managed to land the plane on the Hudson River with no loss of life. Indeed, thanks to the heroic efforts of the crew, everyone *was* relieved. It's possible that this "miracle on the Hudson," as it would later be called, was the event that Billy was confusing with 9/11. Perhaps his brain filled in the gaps of one memory with a fragment from another.

In virtually all cases of confabulation, studies show that the concocted elements of the story can be traced back to actual events from the person's past or to prior knowledge. The brain is rearranging the snapshots. In one experiment, for instance, Swiss researchers assembled three groups of volunteers: patients with amnesia who did not confabulate, patients with amnesia who *did* confabulate, and healthy control subjects. The experimenters showed the volunteers an array of images, one at a time, and asked them to decide whether they had seen that image before by responding yes or no. Here's an example of a set of correct answers:

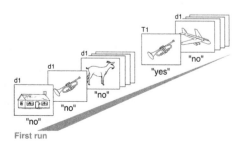

First run

The control subjects had no trouble replying yes at the target (labeled T1): the second presentation of the trumpet. The amnesic patients had some trouble with it, but there was no difference between the confabulators' and the non-confabulators' performances.

One hour later, the researchers repeated the experiment with the same set of pictures but showed them in a different order and used a different image as the repeat. They instructed the subjects to disregard the first round completely and only respond yes if an image was repeated within the new sequence of pictures. A correct set of responses looked like this:

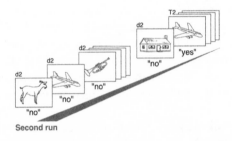

This time, the control subjects and the non-confabulating amnesic patients replicated their performances from the first round. The confabulators, however, behaved very differently: they had a much higher rate of false positives. Rather than responding yes only to the airplane, they also did so to the unrepeated images like the house and the trumpet. Their brains confused the second run with the first, and the patients began to confabulate. They couldn't sort out which pictures in their minds were relevant to their current task. They drew from past experience to create false memories.

In another demonstration of this phenomenon, a research group tested the recall of twelve patients for classic fairy tales or Bible stories. All of the patients in the study had suffered ruptured aneurysms of an artery in the brain that helps supply the frontal lobe. Neuropsychological testing revealed that all of them had memory loss, but only four of the patients exhibited confabulation. The experimenters told the confabulators and the non-confabulators to select any four stories from a list that included such favorites as "Little Red Riding Hood," "Snow White," "Jack and the Beanstalk," "Hansel and Gretel," Moses and the exodus, and Noah's ark. Their challenge was to recite the fairy tales or Bible stories from beginning to end, providing as much detail as they could muster. The experimenters recorded every word of the stories, encouraging the patients to dig through their memories and describe the scenes vividly.

The researchers graded the stories based on their completeness, the number of errors, and the types of errors made, such as distortions of plot details or mixing up plot elements from different stories. For example, one patient said, "The witch built a gingerbread house and took it to Hansel and Gretel." This was a distortion of the actual version, in which Hansel and Gretel come upon a gingerbread house in the woods. A patient in a related study asserted that Little Red Riding Hood was raped. The two groups, confabulating and non-confabulating, made a similar number of these sorts of distortion errors. However, the confabulating patients were much more likely to borrow details from various fairy tales and biblical stories and insert them into others. For example, when attempting to tell the story of Hansel and Gretel, one confabulating patient said, "Hansel and Gretel . . . they walked up the hill to get a pail of water filled up." Evidently, the patient confused Hansel and Gretel with Jack and Jill. Another patient said that Snow White "had two stepsisters and they were mean to her," whereas Snow White actually lived with a group of dwarfs named for their most prominent emotions. It was Cinderella who clashed with her stepsisters.

People with confabulation tend to unconsciously borrow irrelevant thoughts or memories and blend them with ideas they are currently considering. They usually don't invent things out of thin air. A research group tried testing confabulating patients on memories that they were sure they didn't have. They asked them questions about completely invented concepts, such as "Where is Premola?" or "Who is Princess Lolita?" or "What is a waterknube?" Confabulating patients were no more likely to fabricate answers to these questions than non-confabulators were. They would just admit ignorance. Having no experience with such topics, they didn't have any material with which to manufacture a reply. In a similar study, when confabulators were asked to name the capitals of European and African countries, they were far more likely to manufacture names for the European cities than for the African ones. Because they had less experience with the geography of Africa, they were more likely to simply admit ignorance than confabulate.

When Billy spoke about his past, he had no intention of misleading anyone. He was borrowing various snapshots from his life, substituting them, blending them. The way that Billy continuously fabricated memories had a certain pattern to it. He never admitted to not knowing something. It was as if he were protecting his own ego, subconsciously denying that there were any gaps in his recollection. What's more, when answering questions, he plagiarized moments from disparate corners of his life experience and cobbled them together to fill those gaps. Because of some disruption in his brain circuitry, Billy was losing his personal narrative and, in a way, losing himself. It seemed like a classic case of confabulation, but what was the cause?

After weeks of caring for Billy in the hospital, we were stumped. The account of the events leading to his hospitalization remained as cloudy as ever. One afternoon, Billy joined some other patients in a group activity in which all participants were supposed to draw some of their favorite things. "I'm going to draw my favorite chemical reaction!" Billy exclaimed. Because he had worked in a laboratory for years synthesizing chemical compounds, this seemed like a reasonable thing for him to do. Without any hesitation, Billy sketched something on a sheet of notebook paper.

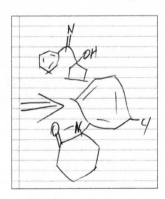

It appeared to be a partial sketch of a chemical reaction. Seeing the drawing, one of the medical students became curious. "What have you drawn there, Billy?"

"It's the reaction to make ketamine. It's nearly there. I just have to make a few adjustments. I used to make it in the lab."

"Why did you decide to draw that?"

"It was fun. Great for parties. I used to eat it all the time."

I didn't know much about ketamine, so I immediately began investigating the substance. Ketamine, for which the street name is Special K, is used medically as short-term anesthesia for brief surgical procedures. Recreationally, it's known as a "date-rape drug" because it's virtually undetectable if you were to put it in someone's drink and it causes confusion and loss of inhibitions, followed by short-term memory loss. If enough time passes after ingestion, routine drug screens can miss it. Apparently, chronic ketamine abuse can wreak havoc on the brain and cause severe memory deficits and confabulation. Indeed, a second MRI of Billy's head revealed diffuse damage in the deep recesses of his brain. Billy was diagnosed with "acute toxic encephalopathy," loosely translated as "drug-induced brain fry." Fortunately, Billy improved day after day. The last time I saw him, his memory was vastly improved, and he was well on his way to recovery. He put his hand on my shoulder, looked me squarely in the eyes, and said, "Hey, man, I'm gonna give you some sound advice: stay away from ketamine." Good advice, but it wasn't the main lesson I learned from him. Behind every seemingly inexplicable act, mannerism, statement, and belief, there is a psychosocial and neurobiological context. Billy said and believed a lot of things that were false, unrealistic, and abnormal and just didn't make any sense. But when these things were interpreted in the context of what was happening in his brain, there was a pattern.

There is an underlying logic to the way the brain interprets our experiences, encodes our memories, and writes our history. The unconscious system creates connections between various snapshots in our lives, it monitors our emotions at each moment to decide what to emphasize, and it organizes those snapshots in such a way as to tell a story that is unified, straightforward, and, most of all, personal and intimate. That story becomes our conscious life.

When parts of the story are missing, however, whether due to brain damage or the confusing nature of an experience, the brain follows the same logical protocol to fill the holes. Just as we might fill in a puzzle with missing pieces, the unconscious brain searches for fragments of memories and ideas, borrowing from our vast bank of knowledge, that fit most neatly and convincingly. Always the egocentric storyteller, the brain relies on our beliefs and personal perspectives, our hopes and fears, to guide its task of inscribing the plot. As we might imagine, however, the more severe the gap in the memory system or the more confusing the experience, the deeper the brain will have to reach to spin its narrative. To outsiders, the story the brain tells in those cases may seem, well, a little weird.

# 5

# Why Do People Believe in Alien Abductions?

*On Paranormal Experience, Narrative, and the Development of Strange Beliefs*

> Most visions of extraterrestrial life are actually steeped in human hubris. The fictional extraterrestrials of *Star Trek* or a hundred other space operas are less alien than many of my neighbors.
>
> —Nathan Myhrvold

"The word of the day is *OVNI*," Madame Dumont said to her ninth-grade French class, "which is the French term for 'UFO.'" She wrote it on the board. "I thought it would be an appropriate word for us to learn today because it's finally come to that time of the year when I tell my story—the story of how I was abducted by aliens."

The students rolled their eyes and exchanged glances. Madame Dumont was infamous for her alien abduction story around the high school and would tell it once a year, each time with the same urgency, promising that it was true and that her students should be wary of the invaders returning to scoop them up next.

"It was eight years ago," she began. "I woke up in the middle of the night because I could sense them coming into my room—the aliens. They came in very quietly, but I could hear their footsteps. They were gray and skinny with big eyes, draped in dark cloaks. They held me down and injected something into my arms and legs to make me weak. I couldn't move. Then they strapped me down and started prodding me with tiny instruments. Electricity shot through my body. I tried to scream, but no sound came out! One of them abused me . . . sexually. The others were doing some sort of experiment. I'm not sure exactly what it was, but they took cell samples from my body. Then they left. I'll never forget the feeling. It changed me forever, and I know it wasn't just a onetime thing. I know they'll be back. That's why I'm telling you all this. So you'll be ready when they come."

## "I Was Abducted by Aliens!"

As someone who took Madame Dumont's ninth-grade French class, and discussed it at length with other students, I can tell you that she told it the same way every time, solemnly and with the body language of someone reliving a terrifying experience, always ending with a warning about the extraterrestrials' inevitable return. She was truly convinced that this event happened.

Why would a tenured high school teacher with an ordinary family and daily routine come to believe that she was abducted by aliens? Waving her off as being crazy is not an answer to the question, especially when one considers the surprising prevalence of this strange belief. When thousands of people were randomly polled about the existence of extraterrestrials, more than 90 percent said they believed that aliens exist in the universe. One in four people thought that aliens had visited the earth. Nine percent said that they themselves had contact with aliens or knew someone who claimed to have such contact. The reason can't be that all of them are crazy. Studies also show that people who believe in alien abductions are no more likely to suffer from psychiatric illnesses than those who don't. Psychological assessments demonstrate that self-proclaimed abductees score high on tests of creativity and that they exhibit a propensity for fantasy, but having these traits certainly doesn't mean they are crazy.

Not only are many abductees ordinary people, but their stories are remarkably consistent. Abductees report that they are lying down and unable to move as the invaders arrive. The aliens are shadowy gray or white figures. They stand over the victim and begin prodding, experimenting with, or otherwise violating the person's body. The abductee may have a variety of sensory experiences, including hearing noises like footsteps or whispers, feeling vibrations or "electrical currents" in the body, and suffering from painful sensations (often in the groin).

Abductees are terrified while the event is occurring, and even when it's over, they may feel scared, depressed, or traumatized. The details differ from person to person, but the overall narrative has the same plot.

Why would an ordinary person, without any trace of psychosis, claim to have had an encounter with space aliens? Where could such convictions come from, and why do people believe them so adamantly?

## Sleep Paralysis

For well over a century, neurologists have known about a mysterious phenomenon called sleep paralysis. During REM sleep, our muscles are paralyzed, and we are immersed in our most vivid dreams. Under normal circumstances, two major changes occur as we wake up in the morning. The first is that we regain our awareness. As if a light switch has been flipped, suddenly we realize we are awake. The second change that occurs is the transition from our paralyzed state to the return of muscle control. Even though different regions of the brain are responsible for awareness and muscle control, those functions reactivate simultaneously as we arise in the morning; at least that's what happens most of the time. In certain cases, it's possible for there to be a delay between the return of awareness and the activation of muscle control. This leaves the person awake and aware but completely paralyzed for a few seconds and up to several minutes, though episodes lasting over an hour have been reported.

In 1876, the American neurologist Weir Mitchell provided the first description of the condition: "The subject awakes to consciousness of his environment but is incapable of moving a muscle; lying to all appearance still asleep. He is really engaged in a struggle for movement, fraught with acute mental distress." The paralysis typically affects the entire body except for the muscles of the eye and throat. In many instances, the respiratory muscles seize up, and the person experiences a feeling of suffocation. Hallucinations, both visual and auditory, often accompany the paralysis. Subjects hear strange sounds that they find difficult to characterize after the fact. They may see ghastly figures and feel the presence of foreign beings in the room. These hallucinations tend to be shockingly vivid and may have a complex narrative arc, making the experience a waking nightmare.

Researchers estimate that sleep paralysis affects about 8 percent of the population. In the United States alone, some twenty million people have experienced the phenomenon at least once in their lifetimes. The severity of the episodes varies widely, so for many people the paralysis lasts for only a matter of seconds and they don't have the extended, hallucinogenic experience. Studies show that people who struggle with anxiety are more likely to feel a foreign presence during sleep paralysis. The stress carries over into sleep, somehow exacerbating the haunting visualizations. People are also more likely to hallucinate during sleep paralysis if they suffer from what's called dysfunctional social imagery, a mild form of social phobia. Those with dysfunctional social imagery feel that they are always being watched and judged by other people. When such people experience sleep paralysis, that sense is magnified as they feel they are being studied and prodded by an alien presence.

The symptoms of sleep paralysis eerily mirror the descriptions of alien abduction: both abductees and sleep paralysis victims get the feeling of being physically pinned down while in the presence of a shadowy invader. Neuroscientists have studied this mysterious phenomenon of "felt presence," and with the help of brain-imaging techniques they've traced it to its source: the temporal lobe.

## Afraid of Your Shadow?

Allison was your average twenty-two-year-old woman. She didn't believe in ghosts or spirits or anything supernatural, for that matter. She did not have schizophrenia or any other psychiatric illness. She did, however, have a neurological condition. Since she was seven, Allison suffered from temporal lobe epilepsy, in which seizures occur in the temporal lobe, located on the sides of the brain. Her seizures were extremely resistant to treatment, so her neurologist referred her to a neurosurgeon to see whether there could be a surgical treatment. Allison told the neurosurgeon everything about her seizure history, including a recent one she had that was different from the rest: she had felt that her mind left her body and then returned.

Allison permitted a neuroscience research group to conduct an experiment as part of her evaluation. To monitor her seizure activity, over a hundred electrodes were planted on her scalp. Then the research group attempted to induce seizurelike activity in Allison's temporal lobe, simulating a seizure. A seizure is hyperactive neuronal activity, like an electrical storm in the brain. With that in mind, the researchers fired precise electrical pulses at regions of Allison's left temporal lobe. Suddenly, after a pulse struck the junction between the temporal and the parietal lobes, Allison had a strange experience: she felt someone in the room, someone who wasn't there before. She described the being as a "shadow." She couldn't tell if it had a gender.

"Where is this shadow person?" one researcher asked.

"He is behind me, almost at my body, but I do not feel him," she replied.

Allison had been lying down during the experiment thus far, so the experimenters asked her to sit up. They fired another pulse at the temporal-parietal junction. Allison shuddered. The shadow person was now sitting next to her, clutching her arm.

Next, the experimenters gave Allison a task: read the words on a set of cards. As she did, they fired a third pulse at the temporal-parietal junction. The shadowy presence returned. Once again, it sat down next to Allison. "He wants to take the card," Allison insisted. "He doesn't want me to read."

Precise stimulation of the temporal lobe can create the perception of a foreign presence in your vicinity. Faced with this strange feeling, the brain seeks out an explanation. Allison consciously knew that the doctors plugged electrodes into her nervous system and were zapping away at her brain, so she didn't attach any mystical or otherworldly significance to the shadow. But what if this stimulation were to happen naturally? Imagine a person who develops a seizure in the temporal lobe, in the same place the neuroscientists targeted in Allison's brain. He would develop the same perception of a shadow in his midst. His brain, too, would seek out an explanation, but it wouldn't be as obvious. He wouldn't be hooked up to any electrodes, and the feeling would not occur in the context of a controlled experiment. He would be left to wonder, who is that shadowy figure lurking?

## Conversations with God

When he was forty-seven, Robert was riding in the back of a pickup truck when suddenly a sedan careened into the side of the vehicle. The collision sent him flying off the back of the truck and headfirst into the pavement. Robert was rushed to the hospital, where emergency physicians identified a skull fracture over his right temporal lobe as well as extensive intracranial bruising. Fortunately, the medical team was able to stabilize him and repair the damage to his skull. Robert was lucky to be alive, but he soon discovered the lasting effects of the injury.

Thirty years later, Robert, now a retired physician, pays a visit to his neurologist to talk about his seizures, from which he has suffered on and off since the car accident. The neurologist asks his family to describe what Robert looks like during an episode. At first, they say, Robert appears to be staring off into space. His face goes blank. Then, abruptly, his body contorts, and his head violently twists toward the left. Finally, he drops to the floor and begins convulsing, his back arched and his limbs flailing violently, until eventually the seizure dissipates and Robert returns to normal.

When the neurologist asks Robert to describe his experience of the seizure, he provides a rather different account.

It begins, he says, with a "beautiful," ever-expanding light on his left side, extending down from heaven. He feels calm. He is "at peace" knowing that "nothing bad is going to happen." The light soon begins to take shape. It forms a tunnel to the sky. His soul enters the tunnel and travels upward, higher and higher, until it meets an angelic figure. "Robert," the angel calls, "it is not your time!" Suddenly a spear of fire strikes him in the chest. To Robert's surprise, he feels no pain—only "unconditional love." "God loves me," he says.

Quite a story. Oddly enough, Robert isn't the first one to tell it. As researchers later discovered, his vision is mysteriously reminiscent of one described by Teresa of Ávila, a Roman Catholic saint and theologian, in 1565. In her autobiography, she described a moment of religious ecstasy:

> I saw an angel close by me, on my left side, in bodily form. This I
> am not accustomed to see, unless very rarely . . . He was not large,

but small of stature, and most beautiful—his face burning, as if he were one of the highest angels, I saw in his hand a long spear of gold, and at the iron's point there seemed to be a little fire. He appeared to me to be thrusting it at times into my heart, and to pierce my very entrails; when he drew it out, he seemed to draw them out also, and to leave me all on fire with a great love of God.

Robert's description of his divine contact is nearly identical to that of Teresa of Ávila. Both descriptions involve a sighting of brightness on the left side and an encounter with an angel. In both visions, the angel strikes them in the chest with a fiery spear yet causes them no pain, rather eliciting a deep love of God.

Robert was raised Roman Catholic and received religious education all the way through high school but knows little about Teresa of Ávila, recalling only that she is a saint. He has no history of psychiatric illness. A recent psychological evaluation returned normal results. However, an MRI showed softening of the right temporal region due to the inflammation he suffered there. EEG monitoring revealed abnormal waves over that same area. The fact that the seizure was on the right side of the brain explains why his vision appeared on the left. Despite what Robert says about his heavenly revelation, the neurologist determines that Robert's experience is nothing more than abnormal activity in his temporal lobe.

Neurologists use the term "hyperreligiosity" to describe a symptom that patients with temporal lobe epilepsy may experience. For every hundred temporal lobe epileptics, between one and four of them will have some type of religious episode or awakening, usually a heavenly vision much like that which Robert described. In some patients, the effects of the seizure can spread to the frontal lobe and exert a lasting effect on behavior: they become devout, practicing believers.

The psychologist Michael Gazzaniga contends that temporal lobe epilepsy could be the reason why certain people claim to have spiritual revelations. He says, for example, that Vincent van Gogh had every symptom of temporal lobe epilepsy and had many religious visions, such as one of Jesus Christ resurrected. He suggests that based on various behaviors they exhibited, spiritual icons like Moses, Muhammad, and Buddha might have had the disorder as well. Could that be the source of their prophecies? Gazzaniga, at least, suspects as much.

In a field of research that has been called neurotheology, neuroimaging studies of people engaged in religious acts show activation of the frontal and temporal lobes. Neuroscientists have successfully induced spiritual experiences by firing electrical pulses in these areas of the brain, just as they elicited the sense of shadowy people by stimulating similar areas of Allison's brain. In one such study, a research group used a helmet that emitted a magnetic field to excite specific areas of the temporal lobe. As a result, the subjects reported having a variety of spiritual experiences. Some claimed to feel the presence of deceased relatives. Others described a feeling of their minds being separated from their bodies, so-called out-of-body experiences. Still others felt the company of "another entity" but could not tell whether it was God or another spiritual visitor. Triggering activity in their brains somehow induced these mystical encounters.

We all know what it's like to sense the presence of someone nearby. Perhaps you turn around to see who's behind you, but nobody's there. You shrug it off and forget about it. We know that targeted stimulation of the temporal lobe can generate this sensation. What if you had a defect in your temporal lobe, and this inescapable feeling washed over you all the time? What sort of explanation might you come up with? If you had attended Catholic school as a child, your brain might go there for answers. Like Robert, your unconscious might latch onto a story you learned long ago about Saint Teresa. Who is that presence you feel? It's an angel who has come to instill in you a love of the Almighty. On the other hand, if you have no religious inclinations, perhaps you'll conclude that it's just your shadow.

When creek water streams along the foot of a hill, it generally flows downhill and around obstacles. It takes the path of least resistance. The same goes for the brain. When you watch a magician perform a trick, your unconscious responds first: he just sliced his assistant in half! That's the simplest, most straightforward account. It's not until more careful, conscious analysis begins that you can start to wonder whether there might be another explanation. Perhaps there are two assistants, one in each side of the box.

The unconscious system in the brain is a straightforward, logical system. When it detects seemingly irreconcilable stimuli, such as the feeling of someone being there when nobody's around, the brain generates the best story it can with the information at hand. It picks out the salient features of what we see and feel, scanning the depths of our memory, our beliefs, our hopes, and our worries to find patterns. It tries to concoct a satisfying explanation. It searches for meaning. By framing our perceptions in a unified narrative, the brain constructs the experience of life. In the same way, given the right person and the right set of stimuli, it might even construct the experience of death.

## The Walking Dead

On an early Monday morning, I was checking on a gentleman who had been admitted to the inpatient psychiatric unit overnight. I had not been on call, so this was my first time meeting with the patient, an elderly man with bipolar disorder who had become withdrawn from friends and family over the previous few months.

"How are you feeling today, Mr. Murphy?" I asked.

"Pretty damn terrible."

"I'm so sorry to hear that," I said. "What's making you feel so bad?"

"Are you kidding me? Can't you tell? I'm *dead*."

Not the answer I was expecting. "What do you mean?" I asked.

"I can't be any clearer. I'm dead. Died three months ago. And, sonny, since you're with me, it looks like you're dead too."

"How can you tell that you're dead?"

"The way I feel. I'm not in the world, not the world of the living anyway. I don't feel anything. I don't know anyone. I'm not here."

This continued for about fifteen minutes. He was completely certain that he was dead. Neither I nor anyone else could convince him otherwise. Defeated, I said, "All right, Mr. Murphy, I'll check on you again soon. Is there anything I can get you?"

"You're mighty generous," he scoffed, "for a dead man."

Mr. Murphy suffered from the Cotard delusion, or "walking corpse syndrome," a condition in which people believe that they are dead. They feel separated from the world, distant from everyone around them, even the people they know most intimately. As Mr. Murphy described it, "I see everyone moving about and doing their business all around me, but I'm in a different world." People with Cotard feel as though everyone in the world were acting in a movie—except them. They are spectators emptily watching from afar.

The Cotard delusion can accompany psychiatric diagnoses like schizophrenia and bipolar disorder, but it can also arise from damage to the temporal-parietal junction, such as a case, years ago, of a man who developed the delusion after a motorcycle accident. As we saw in the case of Allison, the temporal-parietal junction is the area that, when overstimulated, can create the sensation of a foreign presence. Too much stimulation conjures up a feeling of another entity in your midst. A ghost. Not enough stimulation, as from damage in the Cotard delusion, does the opposite. It evokes the feeling that you yourself do not exist. You become the ghost.

Nobody knows exactly how the Cotard delusion arises, but the theory is that it's a failure to connect perceptions with emotions. Neurologically, it's associated with a disconnect between two areas of the brain: the sensory system and the limbic system. The limbic system processes emotion and memory and includes regions like the amygdala and the hypothalamus, which are located at the interior surface of the temporal lobe. When damage to the temporal and parietal lobes interrupts the communication between the sensory and the limbic systems (or if the limbic system itself is damaged), the theory goes, patients will see, hear, and smell the world as they usually do but without having any emotional reaction. When Mr. Murphy saw his wife, he agreed that she looked like his wife, but he did not experience the warm feeling of recognition that one should have when encountering a familiar person, especially a loved one. She looked like his wife but didn't *feel* like her. The broken link between his emotion and his senses extended to every experience in his life.

Consider a person who is suddenly emotionally distant from other people, feels dissociated from reality, and watches the world as if from afar. It sounds a lot like death. At least it sounds like the way death is represented in stories, movies, and many religious factions. Thus, for a lot of people who experience these symptoms, like Mr. Murphy, it's the easiest explanation for the unconscious brain to reach for. Why has his experience of the world been blunted? Why can't he feel anything? Because he's dead.

## Cheating on Your Wife—with Your Wife?

There is a related disorder called Capgras syndrome in which the brain reaches for another, equally bizarre theory. Patients believe that everyone they know has been replaced by a physically identical impostor. As one patient tells her doctor, "Every time you left the room, I thought another person dressed in your clothes was coming back into the room . . . it wasn't scary, just another person dressed in your clothes, doing your job."

In another, especially illustrative case, a seventy-year-old gentleman whom we'll call Mr. Patel developed the belief that his wife had been replaced by a stranger who looked like her, behaved like her, and had the same name. According to his wife, Mrs. Patel, the two of them began having sex frequently, far more than usual. However, after intercourse her husband would beg her not to tell his wife about it. Mr. Patel would whisper to her, saying how much he enjoyed their sex and how much better it was than sex with his wife. He even developed new sexual practices. After forty-five years together, Mr. Patel claimed that sex with his wife was too "ordinary," but it was more exciting with this "new woman."

Mrs. Patel was distraught over her husband's behavior. He treated her as if she were his mistress. Even though her husband wasn't actually cheating on her, he believed that he was, and he assumed he was getting away with it.

A CT scan of Mr. Patel's brain revealed a shrunken amygdala, hippocampus, and temporal lobe—the same regions that are dysfunctional in the Cotard delusion. Like Cotard, Capgras syndrome causes a problem recognizing other people. Mr. Patel agrees that the woman in his bed looks like his wife, dresses like her, and talks like her, yet somehow she doesn't *feel* like her. Therefore, she must be an impostor. Similarly, Mr. Murphy, with Cotard, sees his wife and recognizes who she is supposed to be but doesn't have the feelings he should have when seeing her. Therefore, he must be dead.

Mr. Patel and Mr. Murphy both have trouble connecting their perceptions (especially when it comes to people's faces) to their emotions, yet they come up with different theories as to why. It's as if these syndromes were two sides of a coin, two ways of explaining a thoroughly weird anomaly in the brain. On one side, Mr. Patel points the blame outward and claims that his wife has been replaced by someone else. His brain goes with a paranoid explanation of his symptoms. On the other side, Mr. Murphy points the blame inward, at himself, and decides that he must be dead. His brain takes a depressive, nihilistic approach.

The unconscious system in the brain can generate any number of narratives to explain the same set of symptoms. The narrative that ends up becoming our life experience is the one we are most likely to believe. Mr. Patel was probably more predisposed to developing paranoia, while Mr. Murphy was prone to depression. When concocting a story to reconcile conflicting stimuli, the brain has to dig deep, calling upon our buried convictions, tendencies, and wonders. And the results can seem, well, supernatural.

## Visions from the Brink

Several years ago in Italy, a patient whom we'll call Carlo met with a team of neuroscientists and psychologists, hoping they could explain a mysterious experience he had undergone:

> I was spending my summer holidays in the mountains with my four-year-old child. I had recently separated from my wife; it was a difficult time. One evening, while I was in the room where we were staying, I suddenly saw a great white light . . . Then, some balls of light appeared . . . At the time, I had a profound feeling as if all the beings of the world were within me and, at the same, I felt as if I were within them. The source of light was ellipsoid. It was Love and Joy, and I felt a sort of stream through me . . . I was so enraptured that I had stopped breathing. I was fully lucid, however, and realized that I was not breathing, so I started breathing again, but my breathing disturbed the vision and, after a few breaths, it vanished.

This story appears very much like descriptions that people give of near-death experiences, which often include visions of "bright lights," feelings of contentment, or other notions of a transition from one state of existence to another. In fact, studies of near-death experience have revealed a set of consistent features reported by those on the brink. A Dutch research group, for example, studied 344 patients in ten hospitals who survived a heart attack. Of those, 62 reported having some sort of near-death sensory experience. The table below shows the breakdown of what they saw and felt.

| Type of Experience | Percentage of patients |
|---|---|
| Awareness of being dead | 50% |
| Euphoric emotions | 56% |
| Out-of-body experience | 24% |
| Moving through a tunnel | 31% |
| Seeing bright lights | 23% |
| Seeing colors | 23% |
| Seeing a celestial landscape | 29% |
| Meeting with the dead | 32% |
| Visions reviewing one's life | 13% |

Carlo's account matches several of the visions described by the heart attack survivors, like seeing bright lights, a feeling of euphoria, and possibly the sight of a celestial landscape. The arc of his narrative also seems to parallel what his body was doing. The vision occurred while he was not breathing and dissipated when he began to inhale. However, the major difference between Carlo and the cardiac arrest patients is that Carlo was not on the brink of death at all. He didn't have any serious medical problems and was certainly not critically ill. The only significant source of stress in his life was the divorce process he was undergoing with his wife. He also was not a spiritual person. Though he attended Catholic school as a child, he had since rejected all forms of religion. Carlo was not the kind of person you'd expect to speak of mystical experiences, yet there he was. The incident inspired him to write poetry. He claimed to have overcome his fear of death, realizing it was something to be not dreaded but welcomed as part of the natural order.

The fact that near-death experiences are so consistent from person to person, and that they can happen to someone like Carlo, who is neither dying nor spiritually inclined, suggests that there must be an underlying neurological explanation. As a person is on the edge of death, something must be happening in his brain that creates the vision. More mysteriously, whatever that process is, it must also have the potential to affect someone who is otherwise healthy and in no danger at all.

## Fighter Pilots and Heart Attack Victims

Colonel Dan Fulgham, an air force pilot with over thirty years of experience, recalls an incident that happened to him during a training drill in Arizona early in his career. It was a standard exercise in which Fulgham had to fly in formation with a group of fighters. During the fifth run of the drill, he had an eerie experience. He turned his plane, in a maneuver he had made countless times before, and "the next thing I knew, I seemed to be sitting up on the back of the plane looking down into the cockpit." He felt as if he were suddenly *outside* the plane. "I was watching myself, not knowing it was me. What's going on here? Then just all of a sudden the curtain snaps up . . . it's not a dream. Actually, that's me and I'm flying the aircraft again." Somehow, the maneuver Fulgham made with the plane caused him to feel as though he had separated from his body.

When fighter pilots rapidly accelerate in an aircraft, they expose their bodies to intense gravitational forces, or g-forces. About 10 percent of pilots report that they have lost consciousness while making this kind of maneuver. The high g-forces squeeze blood out of the brain and suck it down toward the feet, temporarily depriving the brain of oxygen. Some pilots, rather than passing out completely, enter into a brief state of altered consciousness.

James Whinnery, a navy physician and aviation researcher, has spent years studying the effects of subjecting fighter pilots to extreme gravitational forces. He gets his data by asking pilots to enter a giant centrifuge machine with a fifty-foot-long arm. It furiously spins the pilot around to re-create the g-forces that the body might undergo during aerial combat maneuvering. In studying the pilots' ability to withstand these forces, Whinnery came upon something interesting. After stepping out of the centrifuge, a number of the pilots reported having strange visions. As Whinnery described them, they were "vivid and frequently include family members and close friends. They commonly have beautiful settings and their content includes prior memories and thoughts of significance to the individual . . . they have a significant impact on individuals who experience them, and remain crystal clear for years after they occur." They saw their families, their loves, and their lives flash before their eyes. Many pilots reported feelings of euphoria, as if they were floating, and some, like Colonel Fulgham, even described having out-of-body experiences.

Pilots exposed to high g-forces also experience another symptom that resembles the near-death experience: they perceive themselves moving through a tunnel of light. The periphery of their vision goes dark for between five and eight seconds, and what seems to be a distant bright light appears in the center.

Fighter pilots at high g-forces and heart attack victims in critical condition both have near-death hallucinatory symptoms. Why is that? What do they have in common? Both have brains that are suddenly deprived of oxygen. For the pilots, the rapid acceleration propels their blood flow away from their brains. In cardiac arrest, the heart loses its ability to adequately circulate blood. No blood, no oxygen. Studies suggest that impaired blood flow to the visual cortex or to the eye itself can cause a loss of peripheral vision and central brightening that creates the perception of a tunnel with a light at the end. The lack of oxygen to the brains of fighter pilots and heart attack victims creates the near-death experience.

The vision that Carlo shared with his doctors in Italy was remarkably similar to descriptions of near-death experiences. Yet he wasn't having a heart attack, nor was he maneuvering a fighter jet. So, what happened to him? It's impossible to say for sure, but what we do know is that he wasn't breathing while it was happening. Could oxygen deficiency in his brain have caused the hallucination? Perhaps. But there may be more to it than that.

Studies of near-death experience have shown that when blood flow to the brain and eyes is compromised, the brain attempts to fill in the gaps of vision. In a process known as REM intrusion, the brain enters a state of activity that resembles REM sleep, the stage in which dreams are the most vivid. REM intrusion is the process by which dreamlike visions enter into consciousness, blurring the partition between reality and fantasy. Have you ever seen or heard things while falling asleep, or right after awakening, that other people did not hear or see? It's actually fairly common. These are examples of REM intrusion: dreamlike states that creep into the waking mind. Research on this phenomenon shows that 60 percent of people who have had a near-death experience have had some form of REM intrusion in the past.

A region of the brain called the locus coeruleus, located in the brainstem, is likely involved in generating these visions. By releasing the neurotransmitter norepinephrine (a cousin of adrenaline), the locus coeruleus helps create the body's physiological response to stress and panic, commonly known as fight or flight. It is triggered by emotions like fear and anxiety and physical stressors such as low blood pressure and oxygen deprivation. Not coincidentally, those are stressors felt by heart attack victims and fighter pilots. Once mobilized, the locus coeruleus initiates a chain reaction of chemical signals, starting with norepinephrine, that constitute what we feel in that stressful moment. Panic sets in. At this point, it appears that in certain people the body tries to relieve the stress. The brain attempts to relax us by sending out competing neurotransmitters that create a sense of calm. Somehow—no one is exactly sure how—this counteraction by the nervous system appears to initiate components of REM sleep, blending our dreams with our waking thoughts.

The hallucination of a near-death experience is a side effect of the brain's attempt to offset fear and panic and foster a sense of tranquillity. Perhaps the tension and misery Carlo underwent while in divorce proceedings fired up his locus coeruleus, and as his body tried to compensate, REM intrusion occurred, and he entered a world of bright lights, beauty, and joy.

Whether or not this is the true explanation, we cannot say. All we know is that near-death experiences are not unique to the dying. They are what our consciousness sees as neurotransmitters battle for control of the nervous system. Near-death experiences are more common in those who are susceptible to REM intrusion, in which people enter dreamlike, hallucinatory states as the brain tries to counter the effects of stress.

There's another group of individuals especially vulnerable to having near-death symptoms: people who have sleep paralysis. Studies show that people who suffer from sleep paralysis are more likely to have near-death experiences as well as REM intrusion. There must be something that links sleep paralysis to heart attacks that creates the proneness for the hallucinatory visions, something that triggers the unconscious to ponder the possibility of death. So, what do they have in common? Fear.

## Hostage Hallucinations

Consider the traumatic experiences of the people in these two cases:

### CASE 1
A twenty-three-year-old male gang member was kidnapped by a rival gang and held hostage for ransom. His captors blindfolded him, tied him to a chair, and beat him. Eventually, his gang paid the ransom and he was released. When interviewed later, he described having eerie hallucinations: "When they were hitting me, I just tripped out, got out of my body. [It was] like a dream, only I kept seeing devils and cops and monsters . . . nightmares, I guess."

### CASE 2
A twenty-five-year-old soldier was held captive for three months by the North Vietnamese. He was trapped in a dark, solitary room, and his arms were bound. Years later, he described seeing "tunnels of lights and tall modern skyscrapers all lit up with colors . . . pictures of the house back home and my buddies like they were right there and I could almost touch them . . . and the room kept on changing, getting funny angles to it." He felt "drained of feelings, like there was a wall between me and what was happening . . . I got pretty religious . . . it was unreal."

In a study of those two people as well as twenty-eight other victims of terrorism, kidnapping, rape, alien abduction, and capture as a prisoner of war, 25 percent of them reported having hallucinations. The hallucinations included visions of shapes and colors, bright lights, movement through a tunnel, floating, out-of-body experiences, vague figures, familiar people, religious icons, and monstrous beings. Though the victims suffered in different ways, many aspects of their trauma were consistent.

The hostages shared three characteristics that render a person vulnerable to hallucinating. First, they were encompassed by darkness. As we saw in chapter 1, hallucinations tend to occur in darkness, as they do in Lhermitte's peduncular hallucinosis. In the dark, because visual stimuli are minimal or absent, the unconscious may fill in the sensory gap with hallucinations. Second, the victims felt trapped and helpless. Being physically restrained by rope or shackles, alone and cut off from human interaction, makes it ever more likely that the mind will wander. Third, and most of all, they were afraid.

This terrifying, restricting setting makes hostages susceptible to developing hallucinations. Not coincidentally, it's exactly the setting created by sleep paralysis, during which people report being abducted by aliens. All three factors are in play. The victim feels trapped and helpless, restrained by her suddenly immobile body. She is in the darkness of her bedroom, and she is terrified.

People who have had sleep paralysis are far more likely to experience REM intrusion than those who haven't. Neuroscientists believe that REM intrusion is a side effect of the brain's trying to calm the nervous system in times of anxiety. Just as the trauma of cardiac arrest is thought to evoke REM intrusion and the resulting near-death visualizations, perhaps the stressful nature of sleep paralysis elicits REM intrusion as well, allowing dreamlike visions of shadowy figures to creep into consciousness.

Regardless of what role REM intrusion plays in creating the hallucinations, sleep paralysis seems like a great explanation for why people believe they were abducted by aliens. Sleep paralysis not only causes a barrage of weird sensations but also, as studies with hostages show, creates an environment perfectly suited for developing hallucinations. As theories go to explain something as baffling as an alien encounter, sleep paralysis is an excellent one.

So, why do people still claim to have had alien abductions? Perhaps some have never been informed about sleep paralysis, but many abductees who do know about it harshly reject the notion that it could be the cause of their paranormal experience. The psychologist Susan Clancy has recorded the responses of many individuals to the sleep paralysis theory. Clancy overheard one abductee outside speaking to a friend on her cell phone about it:

I'm totally pissed. Can you believe the nerve of that girl? . . . [She tells me,] "Oh, what really happened is sleep paralysis." Riiight . . . Did she have it happen to her? I swear to God, if someone brings up sleep paralysis one more time I'm going to puke. There was something in the room that night! I was spinning. I blacked out. Something happened—it was terrifying. It was nothing normal. Do you understand? I wasn't sleeping. I was taken. I was violated, ripped apart—literally, figuratively, metaphorically, whatever you want to call it. Does she know what that's like?

The experience is so convincing that abductees can be steadfast believers even when confronted with a plausible alternative explanation. Why are they so sure of their stories, even though their narratives seem so utterly unlikely? As we saw previously, people recall emotionally intense memories differently from typical ones. They recite those memories with more confidence and are resistant to the notion that there are holes in their story. All of this explains why abductees bristle in response to the suggestion that sleep paralysis is the true cause of their symptoms. All right, so they may not accept sleep paralysis. But why alien abduction? Of all the possible explanations out there, why choose that one?

## Attack of the "Old Hag"

In the 1970s, residents of the fishing settlement of Northeast Harbour, Newfoundland, were haunted by a legend of a phantom spirit who would terrorize her victims during the night. They called her the Old Hag. According to the communal lore, the Old Hag slips quietly into a person's room and sits on his chest, filling him with unspeakable fear. The victim, though completely awake, is pinned down and unable to move, tortured by the immense weight on his torso. As one resident put it, "It's just like you're tied up. Ya know there is some people can put it on you, like a charm." A local fisherman described his own experience this way:

I came up late from the stage [storeroom for fishing gear]. We had beach stones up the path then and I went in and lay down like this [reclining in a chair] and before long I heard steps comin' up the path on those rocks. The outside door opened, then the inner door and I wondered who was comin' in, bein' so late. Then I saw a woman all in white come across the kitchen. She came around the stove and came over to me. Then she put her arms out and pushed my shoulders down. And that's all I know about it. She 'agged me.

Those who have been attacked by the Old Hag, known as being "hagged," report profuse sweating and feeling fatigued or depressed when the apparition dissipates. Some people report that they felt pain after the experience: "Sometimes ya'll see someone comin' in the room and they'll 'ag ya. I've had it when the [Old Hag] gets hold of your privates and you'll wake up all sore and tender. Boy, that's some punishment!"

The Old Hag doesn't appear the same way to every person. Sometimes, the specter takes the form of people or characters that the victim has recently seen. As one resident recalls,

I can feel it comin' on, ya know it's a real uncomfortable feelin' like a fear spreadin' over ya . . . I was 'agged just a few weeks ago . . . ya know those TV chipmunks or TV puppets or whatever you call 'em. I was watchin' those and went to bed and they 'agged me.

Whatever the Old Hag occurrence is, everyone who experiences it describes it in nearly the same way. The story begins with a sudden awakening. The person is paralyzed. There is a ghastly vision of vague, wispy figures. Panic sets in. The apparitions approach and apply pressure to the victim's body. Strange noises emerge all around. The victim experiences pain in the chest, abdomen, or groin. When the lurid vision disappears, the person feels exhausted, confused, or depressed.

The paralysis, the shadowy figures, the feeling of pressure or pain, the fear—we know this story. It appears that the Old Hag phenomenon and the typical story of alien abduction are different ways of describing the same experience.

Most people have not heard of sleep paralysis, so once they experience it, the first thing they do is seek out an explanation. In Newfoundland, they describe it as an attack of the Old Hag, but a variety of other depictions can be found all over the world. In the Caribbean, people refer to the phenomenon as *kokma* and believe it to be caused by the spirits of dead, unbaptized babies that jump on a person's chest and grasp his throat. In Mexico, people call it *subirse el muerto,* or "a dead body climbed on top of me." In the U.K., these spells used to be called stand-stills, and people would describe them as the spirit leaving the body when asleep and not returning on waking. In West Africa, people associate it with witchcraft. Some have even felt it was an episode of rape. As one woman described it, "The tall man with the white hat wants to have sexual contact with me and sometimes lies on top of me. The moment that I fall asleep, he tries to rape me. Then I lie awake, can't move, and I'm scared to death."

When a person experiences sleep paralysis, the unconscious system in the brain creates a story to make sense of it, but what story will it choose? It depends on your culture. It depends on what you believe, what you wonder about, what you fear, what you love, what piques your curiosity, what you remember from your past. In the United States, many people believe in alien abductions, some wholeheartedly, while others just have their suspicions, but everyone has heard of them.

When faced with new or extraordinary circumstances, such as the onset of paralysis and hallucinations simultaneously, the unconscious brain seeks out an explanation. It looks for the path of least resistance. What story best explains the symptoms? For each culture throughout the world, that answer is different, but for many Americans the most fitting explanation is that they had an alien encounter. Not only is it fitting; it's *obvious.* It's a sudden realization, perhaps even a validation of old suspicions, and it puts you in good company: there are lots of believers out there who are just like you and have experienced exactly what you have. For someone open to these sorts of beliefs, alien abduction is a satisfying and logical explanation that brings clarity to a night of confusion and terror.

Every day of our lives, the unconscious system in the brain accumulates countless disparate threads of information and weaves them into an organized, personal narrative. Consciously, we experience that story. However, when there is a miscommunication of signals in the brain, that narrative takes a different arc. In sleep paralysis, because of a lack of coordination between conscious awareness and muscle control, the unconscious is confronted with sets of confusing, conflicting information, so it seeks out an explanation to reconcile them. Similarly baffling scenarios arise when a disconnect forms between perception and emotion in the Cotard delusion, or due to the sudden blood pressure changes at high altitude or after cardiac arrest. When neuronal systems fail to communicate as they should, or when the constellation of our perceptions is new and strange, the story the brain tells edges toward the mystical, the supernatural, and the paranormal.

We typically choose to believe our brain's story unless we can convince ourselves otherwise. If the brain is healthy, we can use education to help to modify and expand our store of knowledge. By adjusting our beliefs, renewing the ground in which the brain's logical system is rooted, we can provide reliable information that may guide the unconscious system toward explanations that are more rational and pragmatic. But what if the brain isn't healthy? What would happen if there were a defect in the brain causing a chronic miscommunication? It would cause the brain to continuously tell the same fabricated story. It would cause a supernatural experience that lasts a lifetime.

# 6

# Why Do Schizophrenics Hear Voices?

*On Language, Hallucinations, and the Self/Nonself Distinction*

If you talk to God, you are praying; if God talks to you, you
have schizophrenia.

—Thomas Szasz

My first encounter with schizophrenia was as a medical student in my
third week of a neurology rotation. The attending neurologist and I
were called to consult on a psychiatric inpatient who had just had a seizure. "Have you taken psychiatry yet?" the doctor asked. I hadn't. The
neurologist insisted that it would be a valuable educational experience
for me to see the patient on my own, listen to his story and medical
history, and report back. So I headed alone to the psych ward, through
the two sets of remote-activated metal doors, and into room 621, where
I met Brandon, a paranoid schizophrenic who suffered from frequent
auditory hallucinations.

At twenty-eight years old, Brandon was a graduate of Cornell University with a degree in history but had been unemployed for years
afterward. He had a fresh-looking, boyish face and floppy brown hair, a
look that conflicted with the disturbing history I had read in his chart.
When first hospitalized three weeks earlier, Brandon repeatedly chased
down staff members and yanked their earlobes. He said he was trying
to "shake out their spy recorders." In the short time he had been on the
ward, he threatened to attack his nurse twice, once with a pen and once
with a pair of tweezers, claiming that she was an FBI agent sent to do
the work of Satan. Before his seizure that morning, he had been rant-
ing that the nursing staff was "making him crazy" and that they were
"putting the angry thoughts in his head" to make him look bad. After

getting the information I needed about his seizure, I asked Brandon about his hallucinations.

ME: Do you ever hear voices in your head?

BRANDON: All the time. Usually I hear him when I'm alone, but sometimes he talks to me at other times. It gets better when I scream at him to shut up. Sometimes he can't speak if I interrupt him.

ME: Who do you mean by "him"?

BRANDON: Gerald. He's such an asshole. He works for the FBI. He spies on me all the time. He knows everything. It happened when I was a kid—you know, when he put the spy chip in my brain—but the doctors here say that they don't see it on their brain scans.

ME: What kinds of things does he tell you?

BRANDON: He says I'm weak and stupid. Calls me a coward. Tells me I should get the hell out of this shithole. He tells me to find my gun—I gotta find my gun and pull the trigger. [To himself:] I told you they confiscated it. I'll never get it back. Stop bothering me.

ME: Can you hear him now?

BRANDON: Yes.

ME: What's he saying?

BRANDON: He's talking about you.

ME: What is he saying about me?

BRANDON [Leaning forward and peering into my eyes]: The devil! He sees the devil in your eyes!

This seemed like a good time to end the interview, but still my mind was flooded with questions. Why does Brandon hear a voice in his head? Where does it come from? Why does it say what it says?

Aside from auditory hallucinations, patients with schizophrenia experience a number of other mysterious symptoms too. Some have delusions, outlandish beliefs that patients will assert with the utmost certainty. The delusions may be paranoid, such as thinking you are being spied on by the FBI, or supernatural, such as believing you are being zapped by aliens. Some schizophrenics believe that their behaviors are controlled by mystical forces outside themselves. One patient

I met in the psych ward, Jenna, told me that her actions were controlled by an electrical force field emanating from her television after she watched *Wheel of Fortune*. Other schizophrenics report instances of "thought insertion," in which they feel as if their thoughts don't belong to them and that someone else—a person, a spirit, or even the FBI—planted those thoughts in their minds. Larry, a patient who had lost his sister to drug overdose, told me that his sister's spirit haunted him. According to Larry, she liked to "lend him her thoughts," which he felt compelled to act upon. That, at least, explained the mystery of his blond pigtails and ladybug hairpin.

Some patients display disorganized thinking, meaning that they tend to make strange connections between ideas. In the movie *A Beautiful Mind*, Russell Crowe plays the mathematician John Nash, a Nobel laureate who suffered from paranoid schizophrenia. In one scene, his wife (played by Jennifer Connelly) discovers his office, finding magazine and newspaper articles strewn throughout, connected by strings and erratically highlighted, with incomprehensible writings scrawled all over the walls. This is a dramatization of disorganized thinking, though to Crowe's character and to other schizophrenics it seems clear-headed and logical.

Brandon not only claims to hear a voice in his head but communicates with it; he and the invisible "Gerald" often have arguments, one of which I briefly witnessed. The voice is so real to him that Brandon gave it a name. Gerald has a personality, perhaps not a very pleasant one (he's an "asshole"), but a personality nonetheless. He has a profession as an FBI agent and an agenda, which includes spying on Brandon and encouraging suicide or homicide. Most disturbing, Brandon is tormented by this apparition, an invader in his mind that mocks him, deceives him, and bullies him to obey its will. The hallucination is pervasive and, when untreated, hopelessly inescapable. How could this illusion be so powerful?

However convincing that experience might be for Brandon, it would seem unlikely that he is actually hearing voices through the processing of sound waves detected by his eardrums. After all, nobody else hears them. The only reasonable assumption seems to be that he is imagining these voices. As we try to answer the question of why schizophrenics hear voices, the initial problem facing us is that the voices are *in their heads*. How, as outside observers, can we attempt to understand the voices they experience internally? Anything we say would seem to be speculation, unless there were some way we could hear the voices for ourselves.

## Whispers from the Microphone

Have you ever had this experience? You are standing in the lobby of an unfamiliar building, various unmarked corridors and elevator banks swimming all around you, and you scratch your head as you attempt to understand the directions in your hand that are supposed to lead you to the main conference room: "Proceed down the second hallway to the left, go through the double doors, and take elevator C to the fifth floor, suite 511." As you ponder which hallway is second to the left, and even begin to question the integrity of your navigational skills, you feel a tap on your shoulder.

"Elevator C is down that way." A friendly passerby points you in the right direction. Apparently, you were thinking so intently about the directions that you began mumbling them out loud. You intended for this mental dialogue to remain only in your mind, and yet you ended up broadcasting your thoughts to a complete stranger. That sort of incident has happened to all of us, but it's really quite odd when you think about it. How does it happen that you accidentally start transmitting your thoughts out loud? The explanation has to do with an idiosyncrasy in the way that the brain processes speech.

When you decide to speak aloud, the frontal lobe sends a command to the temporal lobe (where language is produced) and the motor cortex (which controls the action of muscles). From there, the electrical signaling pathway continues, zipping from neuron to neuron, until it reaches the muscles of the larynx (voice box) that generate your voice. The muscles of your lips and tongue are stimulated in concert as they articulate the words you commanded them to speak. As we've seen before, when we imagine ourselves doing something, such as swinging a golf club, the same areas of the brain light up that would be active if we were actually performing that action. The same is true with speech. When you are reading a text and, in your mind, you think, "Wow, this paragraph makes no sense!" the temporal lobe lights up, because your thought process requires the use of language. But the signal doesn't stop there. Once the temporal lobe neurons are activated, they will inevitably begin to fire, and in doing so, they propel the signal farther along the pathway, shooting it up toward the motor cortex and then back down to activate the muscles of the larynx and perhaps even those of the lips and tongue, occasionally leading you to unintentionally vocalize your thoughts. Luckily, this doesn't happen in every case, or every thought we have would be constantly transmitted to everyone around us like an involuntary Twitter feed. The temporal lobe activation is usually very slight. Generally, when you are thinking *in your head* about something, the brain initiates the speech pathway, sometimes gently flexing the muscles of speech, but softly enough that no audible sound is produced.

This phenomenon is called subvocal speech, and it happens all the time. The brain processes all language, even the private language in our minds, using its distinct linguistic regions and vast neural pathways that transmit instructions to the muscles of speech. Our thoughts turn into subvocal speech when that mechanism goes as far as to rouse those muscles to contract, even though, as I mentioned, that stimulation is usually too weak to generate a voice that anyone could actually hear. In the past, some researchers have suggested that all human thinking is itself a form of subvocal speech and that every time we think of words in our minds, we are actually silently speaking them. That idea has pretty much been disproven after an experiment demonstrated that patients whose vocal muscles are paralyzed are still capable of thinking. Nevertheless, subvocal speech is a real phenomenon that can be studied in the laboratory.

Using a technique called electromyography, or EMG, neuroscientists have seen subvocal speech created firsthand. To obtain an EMG reading, a technician inserts electrodes into the intrinsic muscles of the larynx so she can record the electrical activity of the muscle cells there. Whenever a person speaks, the laryngeal muscles begin contracting, and the EMG recording shows spikes of activity that correspond to the movements of the muscle fibers. The purpose of the EMG is to record when and how hard the speech muscles are working. To test for the existence of subvocal speech, subjects were hooked up to an EMG and asked not to speak but instead to think deeply about something in their minds. As the participants began their inner dialogue, the waveforms in the EMG recording changed: small spikes appeared. The speech muscles were contracting—even though the subjects didn't utter a sound and had no intention of speaking.

In the 1940s, the psychiatrist Louis Gould wanted to know whether auditory hallucinations in schizophrenia have anything to do with the phenomenon of subvocal speech. Are the "voices in their heads" merely the unintentional mutterings of the speech muscles? If so, why would schizophrenics happen to notice their subvocal speech while healthy people do not? Gould designed an EMG experiment. He gathered a group of schizophrenic and healthy patients and, one by one, recorded their vocal muscle activity. When Gould compared the EMG recordings of schizophrenic patients as they experienced auditory hallucinations with those of non-hallucinating patients, he found that while the patients were hearing voices, their EMG recordings showed greater vocal muscle activation. This result meant that while the schizphrenics were hearing voices in their heads, their vocal muscles were contracting; they were engaging in subvocal speech.

Subvocal speech is an activation of the vocal muscles, even though no voice is heard. But why isn't it heard? Is no voice produced at all, or is the voice just very, very quiet? If no voice at all were produced, then subvocal speech couldn't be the source of the hallucinated voice. But what if subvocal speech was just very quiet, and nobody but the patient could hear it? Could it help explain why schizophrenics hear voices?

Gould decided to look for the answer in one of his patients, whom we will call Lisa, a forty-six-year-old woman with paranoid schizophrenia and a set of symptoms closely resembling those of Brandon. She suffered from frequent auditory hallucinations that made her think that the Russian government was spying on her. She was convinced that the Russians were in possession of a ray gun that was gradually sucking the life out of her. Worried that the Russians would attack her in her sleep, Lisa slept with a sword beside her bed. She believed that the voices she heard were transmitted through invisible forces into her mind, claiming, "I am not aware why it is possible with the voltage and rays on my body, but I feel I am connected with the spiritual world and it is apparently done by means of helium current."

If subvocal speech is a slight activation of the vocal muscles, leading to the production of extremely quiet sound, what if we were to make it louder? It should be possible, in theory, to amplify the unheard sound using a microphone. Gould pressed a small microphone to the skin of Lisa's throat, and to his astonishment the subvocal, previously inaudible voice emerged as a soft whisper: "Airplanes . . . Yes, I know who they are . . . Also . . . Yes, she knows it so well." Lisa had just been telling Gould about her recent dream about airplanes. The voice continued:

WHISPER: *She knows I'm here. What are you going to do? She's a voice I know. I don't see where she goes. I know she is a wise woman. She doesn't know what I want. She's wise all right. People will think she is someone else.*

LISA: I'm hearing the voices again.

WHISPER: *She knows. She's the most wicked thing in the whole wide world. The only voice I hear is hers. She knows everything. She knows all about aviation.*

LISA: I heard them say I have a knowledge of aviation.

Gould was taken aback. Whenever Lisa reported hearing the voice in her head, he heard whispers emanating from the microphone. What's more, when asked about what the voice told her, Lisa's description matched the content of the amplified speech word for word. The voice in Lisa's head spoke at the same time, and said the same things, as the subvocal speech she herself generated.

Years later, a research group had a similar interaction with a fifty-one-year-old male patient, whom we will call Roy, who often described his communication with an entity in his mind named Miss Jones. Just like in Gould's experiment, researchers placed a microphone against Roy's throat and recorded the following exchange:

WHISPER: *If you're in his mind, you come out of there but if you're not in his mind you won't come out of there. You want to stay there.*

EXAMINER: Who said that?

ROY: Er she said . . .

WHISPER: *I said that.*

EXAMINER: Are you talking to yourself?

ROY: No I don't. [To himself:] What is it?

WHISPER: *Mind your own business darling, I don't want him to know what I was doing.*

ROY: See that, I spoke to her to ask what she was doing and she said mind your own business.

Yet again, the timing and content of the hallucination matched the patient's subvocal speech, words that were articulated using his own mind, lungs, and muscles. Despite how frighteningly real the "voice in his head" seemed to Roy, Miss Jones did not exist. Apparently, the voice he was hearing all along was his own.

## "He Can't Speak If I Interrupt Him"

On my way out of the psych ward, I heard shrieks emanating from Brandon's room. When I asked a nurse about it, she told me that Brandon did that all the time, claiming that it helped silence the voice in his head. All schizophrenic patients have their own strategies to help cope with their hallucinations. To see whether any of them work, researchers tested five coping strategies to see how they affected the number and length of auditory hallucinations. Twenty schizophrenic patients, each of whom was attached to an EMG, were asked to alert the experimenters whenever they heard a voice in their heads. The research group took note of how often and how long the patients experienced auditory hallucinations. With these data in hand, the experimenters asked the patients to attempt five tasks, one at a time, in order to determine whether any of them improved their symptoms. The tasks were (1) keeping their mouths open, (2) biting their tongues, (3) humming aloud, (4) making a fist, and (5) raising their eyebrows.

The results showed that while most of the tasks either worsened or barely helped their symptoms, humming aloud shortened the length of hallucinations by nearly 60 percent. Later studies found that patients can help rid themselves of the internal voices by counting aloud during episodes. Upon seeing these findings, I was reminded of something that Brandon had said during our conversation regarding his hallucinatory voice, Gerald: "He can't speak if I interrupt him." If hallucinating patients are simply hearing their own subvocal speech, then it should be possible in principle to interrupt it. It's not easy for us to speak with our mouths open or while biting our tongues, but it's far more difficult to speak while humming or screaming or counting aloud.

The fact that Brandon, like others with his condition, can interrupt the voice in his head by interrupting his own subvocal speech is further evidence that *the voice in his head is actually his own voice.* He admits that the voice has surprising access to his knowledge and memories ("he knows everything"). The voice often expresses thoughts that he himself has had. Nobody else hears the voice but him, and he can quiet the voice on occasion by speaking at the same time. Considering the evidence we have seen, it seems clear that Brandon is merely hear-

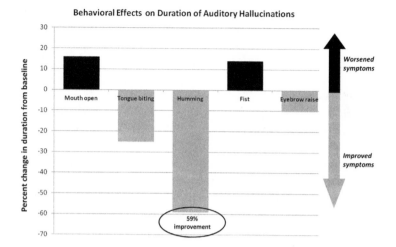

Effect of humming on auditory hallucinations in schizophrenia. Though biting the tongue helped to slightly reduce hallucinations, the effect was negligible. However, having the patients hum aloud reduced auditory hallucinations by 59 percent.

ing his own voice. But why doesn't *he* know that? We mumble under our breath all the time. Usually, we don't notice it, but even if we do, we still recognize that it's our own voice we are hearing, not that of some shady figure trespassing into our minds. Why do schizophrenic patients like Brandon make this mistake often and consistently? Brandon is well educated, he is not an addict, and he has no prior connection to the FBI. Why would he assume that an FBI agent was complicit in planting the voice in his head?

## "Someone Else Is Speaking Whenever I Speak"

In 2006, a research group in Britain designed an experiment to determine whether schizophrenic patients truly have a problem recognizing their own voices. They tested forty-five patients with schizophrenia: fifteen with a current history of auditory hallucinations and thirty who had hallucinations in the past. Both groups were compared with healthy controls. One by one, the experimenters asked the subjects to read words in English into microphones. Connected to the microphone was a machine that distorted each person's voice. The voice was distorted so that it would sound slightly different from the subject's actual voice yet still similar enough that a healthy subject would be able to readily identify it as his own. After reading a word, the participants would immediately hear the distorted version of their respective voices through a set of headphones. They then tried to identify the source of the voice as "self," "other," or "unsure" by pressing a corresponding button.

The control subjects identified their own voices without any trouble. Schizophrenic patients with past, but no current, hallucinations had a little bit of trouble but still did pretty well. Finally, the schizophrenic patients who currently had auditory hallucinations had enormous trouble with this experiment: they were far more likely to identify the source of the voice as someone other than themselves.

It appears that schizophrenic patients not only have trouble recognizing their own voices but also tend to attribute those voices to an external source. The hallucinating patients would say things like "Someone else is speaking whenever I speak" or "I think an evil spirit is speaking when I speak." How does voice recognition happen, and what are schizophrenic patients lacking that renders them helpless to recognize that they themselves are the ones talking? Oddly enough, the answer can be found in a unique species of fish.

## How Are People Similar to Electric Fish?

The mormyrid electric fish is a freshwater species native to the rivers of Africa that has a unique way of communicating: electricity. The mormyrid nervous system has the capacity to release electric signals called electric organ discharges (EODs) into the surrounding water. These signals are like electric fields that project out in all directions simultaneously. For navigational purposes, the fish can fire an EOD at its surroundings (like a flash of lightning), wait for it to rebound off nearby obstacles, and then detect the returned signal using specialized electroreceptors. This allows the mormyrid to create a primitive map of its surroundings much like that created by a bat detecting sound waves as part of echolocation or a submarine using sonar to navigate

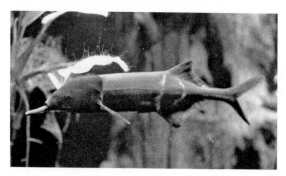

The mormyrid electric fish

the depths of the ocean. The mormyrids can detect EODs sent by other fish using their electroreceptors and then send out their own EODs in reply. This can be used to coordinate the seeking of prey and even for selecting potential mates. It has been shown that mormyrid females are attracted to specific EOD frequencies, and, unfortunately for the males, the lady mormyrids play hard to get: the attractive frequency is different for each one, so you can't use the same moves on each girl. Just like humans, male fish have the challenge of trying to give off the right signals to females in order to generate electricity between them. But that's not the only thing we have in common.

The electrical discharge isn't a targeted linear signal like a laser; it is an electric field that balloons outward in all directions. The signal can be detected by any electroreceptors in range, including those of the fish that sent the EOD to begin with. So the question arises: How do the mormyrids distinguish between signals sent by other fish and ones they send out themselves?

Studies of the mormyrid nervous system reveal that before an EOD is released to communicate with other fish, the fish's brain releases a signal, called the command signal, that instructs the electrical system to fire. In the 1970s, the neuroscientist Curtis Bell and his colleagues tried to study the command signal by deactivating the electric organ with an anesthetic. When he did this, the mormyrid brain was still able to send the command signal, commanding that an EOD be fired, but no EOD would be fired in response. To put it in human terms, if someone paralyzed your vocal muscles but left your brain intact, you could still mentally command yourself to speak, but no sound would come out.

In place of the missing EOD, Bell decided to use his own electric signal, which he could fire at the fish using an external generator. He then connected recording electrodes to the fish's electroreceptors. Whenever he fired an electrical stimulus at the fish, the receptors would spike with activity, meaning the fish detected the pulse. Here's what the electrical recording looked like:

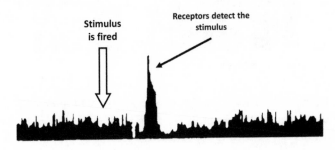

Bell simulated what happens when the mormyrid receives communication from another fish. The receptors detect the incoming electrical signal, and they hum with activity as a result. But what happens when the fish sends out its own electrical discharge? Bell thought of a way to simulate this too. Recall that when the mormyrid intends to fire an EOD, its brain sends a command signal to the electric organ to instruct it to fire. Bell's brilliant idea was to use his generator to stimulate the fish again, but this time do so immediately after the mormyrid's brain sent its command signal. He hoped to trick the fish into mistaking Bell's impostor signal for its own EOD. Here's what happened:

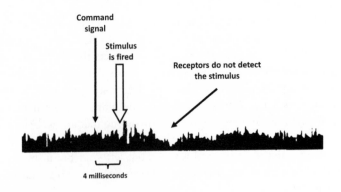

This time, when Bell electrically stimulated the fish, the receptors detected nothing. Why not? Remember that the command signal is the brain's way of telling the receptors, "I am sending out an electric pulse." The receptors are then informed that the pulse is on its way and won't be confused into thinking that the pulse is a message from another fish. In this case, however, Bell was able to fool the fish's neuronal circuitry. Because Bell's impostor electric stimulus arrived at the receptors right after the command signal prepped them to expect that stimulus, the fish assumed that it itself was the one that generated the electricity. The trick worked. Bell discovered that whenever the mormyrid experiences an electric signal within four milliseconds of its intention to fire such a signal, its receptors will not detect it. It assumes that the signal was self-generated and, therefore, not worth paying attention to.

There is more to this story than just the chronological relationship of the signals. We know that if an electrical discharge (whether an EOD or a pulse from the experimenter) is absorbed by the mormyrid within the four-millisecond window, it's canceled out, but how? What dampens its effect? After all, the electroreceptors can't just pick and choose which electric signals to accept and which to reject. They will detect any electrical discharge that reaches them—unless another force intervenes.

On a voltage recording, an EOD looks something like this:

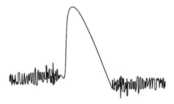

The spike represents a rapid voltage increase in the positive direction that trails off once the electrical discharge dissipates. Bell showed that when the mormyrid fires an EOD, the fish's brain sends a second signal simultaneously to the electroreceptors:

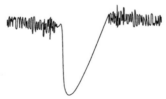

The second signal looks like the first but is upside down. It has approximately the same magnitude and curvature as the first signal but is in the opposite direction. When a negative signal coincides with a positive one of the same shape and size, the signals cancel out. The electroreceptors detect nothing:

This upside-down signal is known as the corollary discharge, and it is part of a crucial neuronal system that allows the mormyrid to distinguish between self-generated and externally generated electrical impulses. Here's how it works. Whenever the fish's brain sends a command to fire an electrical discharge, it sends a copy of that signal to the sensory system, which is responsible for detecting electricity. The copy notifies the sensory system of the command that was just sent out. This process is similar to that of a CEO's sending out an e-mail to her staff. She sends the message about a future product line to her product development department but also CC's the marketing department so it is aware of what's coming. Similarly, the motor command to fire is CC'd to the sensory system so that it knows to anticipate the imminent electrical signal as well as the resulting sensory experience. Once it receives this copy of the command, the sensory system makes a prediction of what sensory input to expect. That's where the corollary discharge comes in: it is the predicted sensory experience that the fish will have when the electricity reaches the receptors.

So, to recap, when the fish decides to fire an electric pulse, it sends out two copies of the command: one goes to the electric organ saying, "Fire away!" while the other goes to the sensory system saying, "FYI, we're firing a signal. Please ignore—it's just us." Right before the signal is fired, the sensory system quickly makes a prediction of what the signal will look like. This prediction is called the corollary discharge. By anticipating what the signal will be like, the fish is ready to recognize it when it arrives.

Now that the relevant sensory systems have been prepped, the motor command is executed: the mormyrid fires an EOD. As the electric field surges outward, the mormyrid compares that signal with the corollary discharge. They are a match. The actual signal and the predicted one have the same shape and intensity, just like the first two recordings shown above. Because the received signal matches the expected one, the fish's brain recognizes it: this is the EOD generated by its own electric organ. Thus there's no need to pay much attention to the signal. It's not an incoming message from a fellow fish. It's simply the effect of having just sent a message *out*. The matching signals cancel out, and the fish's receptors detect nothing. This way, when the mormyrid generates an electric signal, it does not mistakenly identify it as coming from another fish.

If it *were* another fish that sent the EOD, the process would happen differently. In that case, the mormyrid would not be expecting an electric signal, and the received signal wouldn't match the corollary discharge. It wouldn't be expecting a signal, so it would have nothing to compare it with; the sensory system would not be prepped, not CC'd on the e-mail, and no prediction would be made. The signal will not cancel out. Rather, the fish would get the message loud and clear: one of its peers is trying to get in touch. Perhaps a lady friend?

The corollary discharge system allows electric fish to distinguish signals that they generate from those that they receive from other fish. It saves them a lot of confusion. The diagram below summarizes how the system works.

The corollary discharge system is designed for matching experiences to expectations. This system is not unique to electric fish but is found throughout nature. Crickets use it to prevent their own chirping from interfering with the chirps they hear from other crickets. Songbirds like the finch use it to distinguish their songs from those of other birds. And, of course, *we* use the corollary discharge too. And for a surprising number of things. For example, an experiment was done in which subjects lifted a container of water with one hand. As they did so, their grip force on the container was recorded. After repeating this task several times, the subjects drank some of the water from the container using a straw and then attempted to lift the container again. Despite being consciously aware that the container was now less heavy, the subjects applied the same grip force to the container as if it were full. The reason? Based on their numerous attempts with the full container, the corollary discharge system quietly accumulated experience with what it feels like to lift the container (the sensory feedback). Based on that experience, it made a prediction of how much force is needed to reliably lift that container. Because that model was generated before the second

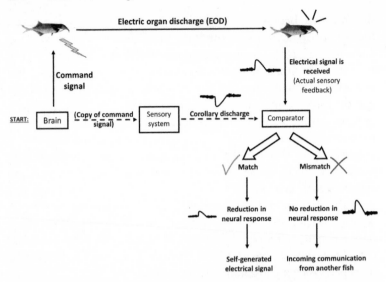

The corollary discharge system in the mormyrid electric fish. Whenever a motor command is sent from the brain, it sends a copy of that command to the sensory system, which in turns generates the corollary discharge (the predicted sensory result of the motor act). This prediction is then compared with the actual sensory feedback brought on by the received electrical signal. If the actual signal matches the prediction, it must have come from the fish in question, and the corollary discharge dampens its effect on the nervous system.

set of trials (with the lighter container), the expected feedback from lifting the container and the brain's prediction of the necessary grip force was out of date. It was based on repeated past experiences with a heavier object. As a result of these unconscious calculations, the subject ended up initially applying too much grip force to the container.

This may be part of how we develop "muscle memory." Try shooting a basketball a hundred times or so from the same spot until you start consistently shooting it well. Then switch to a smaller ball and try again. It will take your muscles a while to adjust to the weight of this new object before you can resume your sharpshooting success.

In humans, the corollary discharge system has also been implicated in helping to maintain the position of our eyes as we move our heads (known as the vestibulo-ocular reflex). We use it to time the movements of our bodies, such as when to extend out our hands so that we will catch a ball at just the right moment. We even use it in our imagination. In chapter 3, we saw that when we imagine having certain motor or sensory experiences, we create those visions based on our internal predictions of what the sensory feedback would be like in real life. Research has shown, for example, that the time it takes to imagine a movement, such as doing a jumping jack, is surprisingly close to the time it takes to physically perform a jumping jack, implying that we are depending on an internal system of prediction.

So, what if that system were broken? Suppose that we encountered an electric fish that had a defect in its corollary discharge pathway. The fish fires its electric signal normally and generates the corollary discharge as usual, but when attempting to match the actual sensory feedback to the prediction, it makes a mistake. Instead of detecting that the two signals match, it determines that they do not. In short, it returns a *false negative* result. How would that affect the way the fish perceives the world? Not only would it fail to recognize its own signals, but it would also falsely believe that other fish were communicating with it.

As is becoming increasingly clear, the corollary discharge has yet another application, and in our discussion it's the most important one of all: the recognition of our own voice.

## System Failure

Let's return for a moment to Brandon, the schizophrenic patient we met at the beginning of this chapter. Consider the following explanation of his symptoms. Often, when Brandon engages in subvocal speech, the corollary discharge predicts what his voice should sound like. When his own voice reaches his ears, the corollary discharge system compares the sound he hears with the expected sound of his voice. Because of a defect in his brain, the unconscious matching system incorrectly identifies a mismatch (false negative) and prevents him from consciously recognizing that it is his own speech that he's experiencing. The corollary discharge does not dampen the voice's effect on the nervous system to prevent distraction and confusion. Instead, the voice exerts its full effect on Brandon's neuronal receptors. His brain now faces two pieces of information to reconcile: first, that a voice has been detected and, second, the false impression that this voice was not self-generated. What does the brain do? It uses its own rationale to make sense of it all—to use limited information to create a complete story. Unconsciously, the brain comes to the most logical conclusion it can: "Well, if I didn't initiate this voice, it must have come from somewhere else."

The defect in the matching system explains why Brandon fails to recognize his own voice and why he believes he hears the voice of a mysterious third party. It explains why this voice seems to know him so intimately; it is, after all, himself. If true, this theory explains why schizophrenics hear voices. But can we prove it?

Recall the experiment we discussed earlier in which healthy subjects and schizophrenic patients were asked to listen to a slightly distorted form of their own voice and identify it as "self," "other," or "unsure." Schizophrenic patients who experience auditory hallucinations were far more likely to incorrectly think their voice belonged to someone else. It has since been shown that a certain brain wave, called the N100, reliably pops up on EEG recordings when a healthy person hears someone

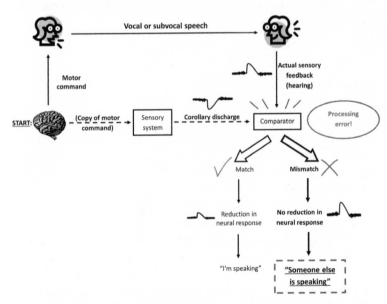

The likely defect in the corollary discharge pathway in schizophrenia. In a schizophrenic patient hearing her own voice, it is thought that the comparator function returns a false negative result. Thus, the patient fails to realize that she is hearing her own voice. Rather, she believes that the voice belongs to someone else. Hence, this circuit provides a basic understanding of the source of auditory hallucinations in schizophrenia.

speaking to her but is consistently reduced when she hears her own voice. Interestingly, this is exactly what the corollary discharge does: it reduces the effect of our own voice on our nervous system. Some neuroscientists believe that the reduction of the N100 signal is a sign of the dampening effect of the corollary discharge. Researchers designed a new experiment in which schizophrenics and control subjects were asked to listen to and identify the source of a number of voices. The first voice belonged to the subjects, the second was their voice with mild distortion, and the third voice was that of a space alien, generated using a computer. The participants listened to the voices while having their brain activity recorded on an EEG.

When healthy subjects heard the alien voice, they correctly identified it as "other," and a strong N100 was noted on the EEG recording, implying that their brains realized it was not their own voice, and therefore did not cancel out the voice's effect on the nervous system. Healthy subjects correctly identified their own voice, even if slightly distorted, and the EEG reading revealed a smaller, dampened N100, meaning that the corollary discharge system detected a match and decided to reduce the signal. When it was just their own voices they were hearing, their unconscious systems knew there was no need to pay much attention. Consciously, they heard themselves speak.

Schizophrenic patients similarly had no problem identifying the alien voice as alien. The N100 in that case was comparable to those seen in healthy patients who heard the alien voice. That makes sense, because schizophrenic patients don't have trouble identifying other people's voices, just their own. But when schizophrenic patients heard their own voice and identified it as "other" as we have seen in the past, the N100 signal was large and intact. *The signal was not dampened.* A defect in the corollary discharge system prevented the match signal from being generated and instead detected a mismatch. This prevented the N100 signal (representing the sensory effect on the nervous system) from being reduced. The schizophrenic patients incorrectly identified the voice as coming from an external source.

A defect in the corollary discharge system prevents schizophrenics from recognizing their own voice, and they instead attribute that voice to a mysterious foreign entity. But does this explanation apply to all schizophrenics? Much of what we have said hinges on the idea that auditory hallucinations in schizophrenia are the patients' own very quiet speech. This is certainly true in many cases, but we don't yet know how far this takes us. Do all auditory hallucinations depend on the patient's ability to hear his or her own speech? Or, put another way, can people who *lack* the ability to hear still have auditory hallucinations?

## Can the Deaf Hear Voices in Their Heads?

Cases of schizophrenia occur in the deaf population at the same rate as they do in the general population, and when they do, the symptoms are quite similar. They display the broad categories of symptoms, including disorganized thinking and speech and social withdrawal. But what about auditory hallucinations? Deaf schizophrenics do claim to have them. Let's consider a few such patients and the way they describe their hallucinations.

PATIENT 1: SIXTY-ONE-YEAR-OLD MALE, BORN DEAF
He hears a ghost speaking to him. It discusses his life at work and his boss. The ghost calls him "snub nose" and advises the patient to be careful about insurance. He says he has actually heard the sound of the ghost's voice.

PATIENT 2: THIRTY-FOUR-YEAR-OLD MALE, DEAF BEFORE
AGE TWO
He claims to have seen Jesus. He often hears a voice communicating to him from London. When asked how he, as a deaf person, could hear someone from London, he replies that he can see the arms and hands of the person signing to him.

PATIENT 3: THIRTY-YEAR-OLD FEMALE, DEAF BEFORE AGE TWO
She hears a man talking "inside of her." She also sees his face. His mouth is closed and he doesn't sign. She occasionally hears the TV actor Patrick Duffy, who insults and threatens her. The voices sometimes come all at once, arguing with each other, but are always saying bad things or laughing at her. She doesn't know how she can hear them, because she knows she "can't hear real people talking."

### PATIENT 4: SEVENTEEN-YEAR-OLD FEMALE, BORN DEAF

She hears a man shouting "Hello, hello!" all day long. She is unsure of whether the man is a ghost. She often signs "shut up" and "go away" to chase away the voice. Sometimes she hears music in one ear and talking in the other, though she agrees that she is "completely deaf" and cannot hear people's voices. She claims that she used to be able to hear a little.

All four patients claim to "hear" voices, despite being deaf since before they were able to understand language. They all attribute the voice to some foreign entity, just like in typical cases of schizophrenia. When pressed on the matter of how they were able to hear, only patient 2 admits that he perceives a person signing rather than actual spoken words. Mysteriously, the others use words like "talk," "shout," and "voices" to describe the experience, insisting that the hallucinations have a vocal quality. They maintain that they can actually hear sound, but we know that such a thing is impossible. Whatever it is the deaf patients are experiencing, it isn't actual sounds. Perhaps they just have difficulty finding the words to describe what they are perceiving and end up using the vocabulary normally reserved for characterizing sound.

The fact that deaf schizophrenic patients aren't actually hearing voices becomes clear when you ask them to describe the acoustic qualities of the voices. What exactly do these voices "sound" like? Deaf patients are unable to describe them meaningfully. They can't recall the pitch, volume, or accent, often replying, "How do I know, I'm deaf?!" Maybe they simply mean something else when they say "voices" and "hear."

Suppose that a friend says to you, "I'm going to go cut down that cherry tree with my ax." What you notice about that statement is not the actual words said, nor is it the sound of his voice. Rather, you picture the cherry tree, consider why your friend would want to cut it down, and perhaps wonder why he owns an ax. You would have that reaction regardless of whether the message were given to you as an e-mail or in sign language (assuming you were fluent) or even through lip-reading across a room. The mode of communication is not as important as the content, insofar as the way it affects your mind. For example, as we saw in chapter 1, sounds from the environment or the echoes of tongue clicking can activate the visual cortex. Similarly, neuroimaging studies of language have shown that the exact same regions of the brain (the prefrontal cortex and the superior temporal gyrus) are activated in a hearing person listening to someone talk and a deaf person watching someone sign. Even though perceiving each language requires a completely separate sensory modality—one is auditory and the other is visual—the same parts of the brain are used to understand what is being communicated.

This is true even for imagined speech. When you look in the mirror after you wake and think to yourself, "Wow, my hair looks surprisingly good this morning," you are engaging in what we'll call "inner speech." As you do so, the left inferior (lower) part of the prefrontal cortex is activated. A study was done in which a group of deaf participants underwent a PET scan while thinking to themselves in sign language, their mode of inner speech. The PET scan revealed activity in the left inferior prefrontal cortex, the same area activated when the hearing abled think in words.

Imagining a visual scene activates the visuospatial parts of the brain. Yet even though sign language is a visual medium of communication, it is *not* the visuospatial regions that activate when someone thinks in signs. Rather, it's the language areas that light up. It doesn't matter whether language is signed or spoken, perceived or imagined, the unconscious system in the brain recognizes the content of the message and treats it in pretty much the same way. This may provide the basis for visual learning. When a student learns a concept through diagrams, pictures, and symbols, the brain treats that information just as it would if the student had read it in a textbook or heard it in class. The student not only remembers the picture but also creates a linguistic representation of the material in his mind.

Patients 1, 2, 3, and 4 are not hearing their own subvocal speech. They are deaf. However, they are having hallucinations of being spoken to. It's likely that what they are experiencing is inner speech, whether that be thinking in sign language or imagining lip-reading (as patient 2 admits). Some deaf schizophrenics eventually agree that the voice they "hear" is actually lip-reading or sign language in their minds but that they can't see the face or hands. Imagine that: seeing sign language performed without hands or reading a pair of invisible lips. No wonder it can be so hard to describe. That is likely what is happening in patients 1, 3, and 4, who insist that they can actually hear the voices.

Their experience is likely analogous to Amelia's corridor of sound that we encountered in chapter 1, except it is vision being substituted for sound rather than the other way around. They imagine sign language or lip-reading, but the picture of the lips or hands is foggy. The words may be unclear, but the content of the message reaches them. Whether it's a greeting, insurance advice, an insult ("snub nose"), or a threat, deaf schizophrenics experience the concept as if it were implanted in their minds by an invader. From the outside, it's difficult to pin down exactly what that experience is like, but this much is clear: it is not like *hearing*. Though the deaf do experience a version of auditory hallucinations, it is from inner speech, not subvocal speech, that the voices arise.

If auditory hallucinations can happen in people who can't hear, that implies that not all schizophrenics are hearing their own subvocal speech. Some are experiencing their own imagined inner speech. That means that the neurological problem posed by schizophrenia, the defect in the corollary discharge system, is bigger than we suspected: Schizophrenics lose more than their ability to recognize their own voice. They lose the ability to recognize their own thoughts.

## A Disorder of Self-Monitoring

The British rock band Pink Floyd, inducted into the Rock and Roll Hall of Fame in 1996, became widely known for its experimental, psychedelic music. As the band emerged to prominence in the late 1960s, its founder, Syd Barrett, began behaving erratically. It started with his having long staring spells and rattling off crazy ideas. Sometimes, Barrett would randomly decide to wear lipstick and parade around in high heels. His fellow musicians really knew something was wrong when they discovered that Barrett had locked his girlfriend in a room for three days, sometimes sliding her a few biscuits beneath the door. In retrospect, though a diagnosis was not confirmed, it's likely that Barrett suffered from schizophrenia, and it shows in his music. On the 1968 album *A Saucerful of Secrets,* Barrett contributed the lyrics to a song called "Jugband Blues." To quote two lines from the song: "I'm much obliged to you for making it clear that I'm not here . . . And I'm wondering who could be writing this song."

These disturbing lyrics led Pink Floyd's manager Peter Jenner to declare the song "possibly the ultimate self-diagnosis on a state of schizophrenia." If there was any shred of truth to the lyrics, Barrett seemingly implied that he was unaware that he was the one who wrote the song. He believed that the artistry he wielded in his mind, his entire painstaking process of composition and lyrical arrangement, was done by someone other than himself. He could not recognize the song as a product of his own thoughts.

One of the more mysterious delusions that schizophrenics may experience is that of thought insertion. Patients believe that their own thoughts do not belong to them and were somehow implanted in their minds by a foreign source. This feeling can be shockingly powerful, as can be seen in this patient's description:

> I look out the window and I think the garden looks nice and the grass looks cool, but the thoughts of Eamonn Andrews come into my mind. There are no other thoughts there, only his. He treats my mind like a screen and flashes his thoughts onto it like you flash a picture.

Just as in auditory hallucinations, patients often attribute the source of the inserted thoughts not only to other people but also to mysterious forces. As a doctor described two of his patients,

> One man said that thoughts were being put into his mind and that they "felt different" from his own; another said that the television and radio were responsible for different thoughts, which were "tampered with electrically" and always felt . . . recognizably different from his own.

The problem with self-recognition goes deeper still. In addition to being unable to recognize their voice and thoughts, schizophrenics may not recognize that they are in control of their own behaviors. For example, patients sometimes describe the feeling that they do not control the movements of their limbs:

> When I reach my hand for the comb it is my hand and arm which move, and my fingers pick up the pen, but I don't control them . . . I sit there watching them move, and they are quite independent,

what they do is nothing to do with me . . . I am just a puppet who is manipulated by cosmic strings. When the strings are pulled my body moves and I cannot prevent it.

It sounds like alien hand syndrome, but it isn't. The patient actually has full control of his body. His brain just doesn't allow him to realize that. Similarly, some patients have trouble recognizing their own feelings. Schizophrenics may even attribute their moods and emotions to external sources:

I cry, tears roll down my cheeks and I look unhappy, but inside I have a cold anger because they are using me in this way, and it is not me who is unhappy, but they are projecting unhappiness onto my brain. They project upon me laughter, for no reason, and you have no idea how terrible it is to laugh and look happy and know it is not you, but *their* emotions.

Schizophrenics have been known to blame external sources for creating the impulses that drive their actions. In the following case, the patient was in a psychiatric hospital as his dinner trolley arrived. Upon seeing the trolley, he dumped a bottle of urine onto it. When the staff member furiously demanded why he had done this, the patient said,

The sudden impulse came over me that I must do it. It was not *my* feeling. It came into me from the X-ray department. That was why I was sent there for implants yesterday. It was nothing to do with me, they wanted it done. So I picked up the bottle and poured it in.

These symptoms seem to follow the same pattern as auditory hallucinations: attributing self-generated thoughts and actions to external sources. A problem in the corollary discharge system elegantly explains all of these strange experiences in a single model. When a defect in the brain prevents a person from recognizing that she is the author of her thoughts, feelings, and behaviors, she is left to conclude that those thoughts and feelings were implanted in her mind and that those behaviors are controlled by someone else. The presence of these symptoms suggests that schizophrenia is not just a problem of hallucinations and delusions. It is a more general disorder of self-monitoring. It is a disease that causes, among other things, the inability to distinguish self from nonself. And the corollary discharge is at the heart of it all.


## Why Can't You Tickle Yourself?

We've known about the mystery of why we can't tickle ourselves since we were kids. Try as you might, you can't induce that tickly feeling in yourself. Yet if a mischievous friend were to wiggle his fingers along your rib cage, you might jump out of your chair. The sensation is much stronger when someone does it to you than when you do it to yourself. Why is that?

Scientists have actually studied the factors that affect whether a sensation is tickly or not. They did this with the help of a tickling machine (yes, really). Each subject in the study used his or her left hand to move a joystick that controlled a robotic arm with a pointed tip, which was to be used as the mechanical tickling finger. Using the joystick, each participant directed the robotic finger to stimulate the palm of his or her right hand. They then evaluated the sensation on a tickliness scale from 0 to 10, with 10 being most tickly. The subjects found that the sensation was not very tickly. Controlling the robotic finger to tickle themselves wasn't any more tickly than using their own finger to tickle themselves. Why would it be? The sensation they experienced matched perfectly with what the brain predicted, so the corollary discharge identified it as self-generated and dampened its effect. That's why it didn't tickle.

Then the experimenters made a modification by gradually introducing a delay between the subject's movement of the joystick and the robotic stimulation of the hand. In addition, the research team caused the movement pattern of the robot finger to differ from the pattern created by the subject, and this discrepancy in pattern got bigger as the experiment went on. As these changes to delay and pattern accrued, the participants reported stronger and stronger sensations of being tickled.

So how does the corollary discharge explain tickling? When you attempt to tickle yourself, a copy of the intended motor action is sent to the sensory system, and the corollary discharge is generated. If the corollary discharge matches the actual sensory experience—the feeling of fingers moving along your ribs at the time and in the pattern that you intended—the brain detects a match and the corollary discharge will dampen the effect of the tickle. In other words, when your brain knows when and how the tickle monster is coming, it's ready to defend itself. The sensation cancels out, and you don't get the feeling of tickliness.

In contrast, when the timing and pattern of stimulation you feel do not reflect the pattern you intend, as in the second part of the tickling experiment, the corollary discharge will not match the sensory feedback from the skin. The brain will therefore treat the sensation as though it were not self-generated but rather produced by someone else. As a result, you feel the tickliness. The defenses are down, and the tickle monster has free rein.

If schizophrenia is a problem of self-recognition, as we have said, then the question arises: Can schizophrenics tickle themselves? Because they attribute their own behaviors to external sources, shouldn't they be unable to distinguish the sensation of trying to tickle themselves from that of being tickled by someone else? When a group of schizophrenic patients compared the sensation of tickling their own hand with that of having their hand tickled by the experimenter, they reported equal levels of tickliness! Because of a global problem in distinguishing self from nonself, schizophrenic patients can do something that the rest of us cannot: they can tickle themselves.

## Déjà Vu

On a recent trip to Mystic Seaport in Connecticut, my wife and I came upon an ice cream shop at the end of a quiet street. There was a picture of a waffle cone topped with a strawberry scoop in the window, and the store had a hanging wooden sign that swayed back and forth in the wind. As I peered at it, I was overcome by a powerful feeling of familiarity. So strong was the feeling that I confidently said I had once been to this exact place as a child while on a trip with my parents. Yet later that week, my father informed me that they had never taken me to Connecticut. My experience is a common one, but why did it happen? How can a never-before-seen place elicit an overwhelming feeling of recognition?

When discussing the defect that leads to auditory hallucinations, I mentioned that the brain generates a false negative match; it incorrectly reports that an expected and an actual sensory experience do not match when in fact they do. So what would a false *positive* match be like? It would be like déjà vu. It would be the feeling of having a personal connection to, or personal ownership of, a certain sensory experience that doesn't reflect a true connection or true ownership in reality. It would be the feeling of recognition when it doesn't belong.

It's amazing how such a simple neuronal misfiring can cause such a profound conscious experience. When we talk about individual circuits in the brain, things can seem simple. If the appearance of an ice cream shop matches one in memory, I feel a sense of recognition. If the sound of a voice matches the sound of your voice, then it's yours. There doesn't seem to be much to it. It is only when false information is passed around that we can really begin to appreciate how much the brain is doing unconsciously.

When my brain misfired in Connecticut, I didn't just have a feeling of familiarity; I made an assertion regarding my personal travel history. The brain is supremely logical: if I recognize the place in which I am standing, if it matches a place in my memory, then the most likely reason is that I've been there in the past. It's hard for me to remember, so it must have happened a long time ago, when I was a kid. Who would have taken me there? Probably my parents. It's a sensible story. Yes, the unconscious system used false information to draw the conclusion, but the reasoning itself is sound. My brain just used the information available to fill in the gaps and created a streamlined narrative to make sense of the situation.

Like other schizophrenics, Brandon has a defect in his brain that causes false information to get passed around. The basic consequence of the defect is that he often fails to recognize his own voice and thoughts. Yet his brain detects a voice. Someone is speaking, but who? Nobody is around, so it can't be someone nearby. It must be someone whom Brandon can't see at that moment. But who? Who could project a voice into his mind who isn't in his vicinity? Perhaps someone with access to impressive technologies—someone with the means and motivation to spy on him. Someone from the FBI? That's possible. If an agent had implanted a chip in his brain, that would explain the voice in his head. If the agent has been spying on Brandon for a while, that would explain why the voice seems to know so much about him.

After receiving misinformation, the unconscious system is left to come up with a story that makes sense out of a remarkably strange situation. Seen in that light, Brandon's explanation for his symptoms is . . . logical. When a person undergoes the confusing and terrifying phenomenon of sleep paralysis, the brain is left to interpret what happened after the fact. An experience that weird deserves an equally weird explanation, so the brain comes up with alien abduction. Oddly enough, it fits the bill. It reflects the unconscious system's tendency to create narratives for emotional experiences and satisfies the person's curiosity about what happened. In the same way, perhaps we can now better understand why many schizophrenic patients report being manipulated by strange technologies (ray guns, helium currents) or religious entities (spirits, the devil), why they report communication from television personalities (Patrick Duffy) or made-up characters (Miss Jones), and why they just generally cite mysterious forces outside themselves for creating the chaos in their minds. The brain creates an explanation that fits with their personality and what they would tend to believe. A religiously leaning person might attribute the voices to divine beings, while a reader of thriller novels might worry about the FBI or the CIA. The brain, through unconscious processes, gathers the disparate fragments of sensory information we accumulate, connects them in the most logical way it can, considering our personal beliefs, fears, and biases, and creates a story to explain it all. Consciously, we experience that story.

When intact, the brain's unconscious architecture provides a scheme with which we distinguish the products of our own minds from those of the outside world. It is the recognition of this separation that allows us to be individuals who interact with the world yet are distinct from it. It endows us with the crucial self/nonself distinction, the foundation upon which our sense of self and personhood is built. Sometimes it takes a disturbance of our normal workings to understand how powerful the brain's logical circuitry is, how much it is really doing behind the scenes, and how easily it can be manipulated. But what if that manipulation were not caused by a simple circuit misfiring, but rather the result of a deliberate scheme?

# 7

# Can Someone Be Hypnotized to Commit Murder?

*On Attention, Influence, and the Power of Subconscious Suggestion*

The conscious mind may be compared to a fountain playing in the sun and falling back into the great subterranean pool of subconscious from which it rises.

—Sigmund Freud

On an eerily cold morning in Copenhagen on March 21, 1951, a twenty-nine-year-old mechanic named Palle Hardrup left work early on his bicycle and headed toward a nearby bank, briefcase in hand. In the briefcase was a pistol and pile of bullets he would use to threaten the bank tellers as he robbed the bank of as much money as he could carry.

As he walked into the bank lobby, the doors clicking to a close behind him, Hardrup pulled out the pistol and fired a shot into the air. He pointed the weapon at the closest teller and bellowed at him to fill the briefcase with cash. Frozen with fear, the teller stood motionless. Hardrup shot him dead. He moved on to the next teller, who instantly bolted away from the counter. Too late. Another gunshot, and Hardrup killed his second victim. Suddenly the alarm system was triggered, and, empty-handed, Hardrup fled the scene. After a brief chase, the police caught up with him. Hardrup did not resist arrest. He allowed himself to be taken and admitted what he had done. It was not until he arrived at the police station that things started to get weird.

At his interrogation, Hardrup explained that he attempted to rob the bank because God had commanded him to do so, in order to raise money for the Danish National Communist Party to prepare for a third world war. Based on the recent pattern of robberies in the area, the police suspected that Hardrup had not acted alone. When pressed on the matter of who gave him the idea to rob the bank, Hardrup replied, "My guardian angel."

It was not long before the police discovered that Bjorn Nielsen, a man with a lengthy criminal record, was the owner of the bicycle used in the robbery. Nielsen and Hardrup had been imprisoned together, as cell mates, for three years. When questioned, inmates at that prison facility recalled that the two had a strange relationship. Specifically, Nielsen had a disturbingly strong influence on his cell mate. Was Nielsen the "guardian angel" that was pulling Hardrup's strings?

Nine months later, as Hardrup prepared to be institutionalized, he wrote a letter to the lead investigator, saying he was finally ready to reveal the whole story behind the bank robbery and resulting murders. When Hardrup first arrived in prison for a prior crime, he wrote, he entered a deep, paralyzing depression. Nielsen, having had more experience serving time, took Hardrup under his wing. Nielsen became his good friend and mentor. He taught him about religion and God and suggested that the two of them have frequent meditation sessions to help become one with the Almighty. Hardrup wrote that eventually Nielsen began experimenting with hypnosis. Each night, in the quiet darkness of their cell, Nielsen would hypnotize Hardrup and command him to act in various ways. He wanted to see how much influence he had over Hardrup's mind and how much that influence could grow over time. Hardrup said that the hypnosis sessions continued regularly until Nielsen took full control of Hardrup's mind. Nielsen, aware of the extent of his new power, decided to use that influence for a new purpose: to commit the perfect crime, with his cell mate as his emissary. The plan was devious—a bank robbery, murder if necessary, accomplished with Nielsen at a safe distance—and Hardrup would be the one to take the fall.

## You Are Getting Very Sleepy

Can external influences such as hypnosis, subliminal messages, and brainwashing undermine our capacity for thinking and decision making? The scenario is reminiscent of the film *The Manchurian Candidate,* in which an army sergeant, Raymond Shaw, is brainwashed and hypnotized by communist agents who attempt to use him as an assassin to help overthrow the U.S. government.

With its status as a tool in clinical psychotherapy, the hype it has been awarded in pop psychology, and its misrepresentation in the media, hypnosis remains poorly understood and seldom exposed to deliberate, scientific analysis. However, as anyone who has ever undergone or witnessed it will attest, the first thing to know is that hypnosis is most definitely *real.*

The most common exposure to hypnosis is probably through watching stage hypnotists, who are able to influence their subjects, usually volunteers from the audience, to behave in strange, embarrassing, and generally humorous ways. A normally straitlaced friend of mine, Ethan, volunteered and was successfully hypnotized at a show I attended. At one point, the hypnotist announced to him that a falcon had just flown into the room and spread its wings in a noble posture. Ethan followed the invisible bird with his eyes and looked visibly awestruck. "The great falcon has taken off again," the hypnotist continued, "and it has just landed on your head." Ethan was frozen with fear. His eyes darted back and forth between the audience and his forehead, and he strained to see the imagined creature's talons clutching his hair. The audience laughed, but Ethan didn't notice. The hypnotist went a step further: "The falcon has risen up again, but now it's flying into your shirt!" Ethan, red-faced and sweating, struggled to fight off his attacker, tearing his shirt half off in the process, until the hypnotist finally told him that the falcon had flown away. When the session ended, Ethan swore to me that he saw the bird as clearly as he saw everyone in the room and that he truly believed that he was fighting with it. Somehow, the hypnotic trance led him to perceive and interact with a creature that wasn't really there.

Hypnosis has become a standard tool in clinical psychotherapy to help foster relaxation, communication, and reflection. Hypnosis helps people manage pain, and its effectiveness appears to go way beyond the placebo effect. In a study of thirty burn victims, patients were given either hypnosis, fake hypnosis (the placebo), or no treatment (the control condition). The patients given fake hypnosis were asked to do things like close their eyes and imagine themselves in a relaxing place but were not actually hypnotized. At the end of the experiment, when asked to evaluate the changes in their pain, the hypnotized patients reported a 46 percent reduction in pain, as determined by thorough questionnaires. The patients given fake hypnosis reported a 16 percent improvement and the control group, 14 percent. Another study showed that hypnosis can alleviate pain in cancer patients undergoing chemotherapy.

During a 2006 episode of her daytime talk show, Ellen DeGeneres was hypnotized to help with her struggle to quit smoking. The hypnotist asked her to name a food she hated. She said she was disgusted by black licorice. After putting Ellen under the trance, the hypnotist convinced her that smoking is just like taking a big bite out of black licorice. Her revulsion was apparent in her expression as she listened to his description. After completing the sessions, Ellen said the experience helped her finally quit after decades of unsuccessful attempts.

In another popularized use of hypnosis, the actress Debra Messing (formerly on *Will & Grace*) worked with a hypnotist to help get over her fear of being underwater while playing an aquatic showgirl in the movie *Lucky You*. The scene involved Messing, dressed as a mermaid, in a giant aquarium tank lip-synching to music and dancing with a variety of underwater critters (that does sound scary). She claimed that hypnosis helped her overcome her fear and get through the scene without panicking.

Hypnosis has also found its way into the military. It was thought, for example, that hypnotizing captured enemy soldiers would make them more likely to disclose confidential information. In one experiment, a steely army corporal with a flawless record was seated in front of a hypnotist and a group of his superiors, who were watching closely to see whether he could be made to reveal military secrets. His captain gave him the secret message: "Company B will leave at 2100 tonight." The corporal was given a strict military order not to disclose that information under any circumstance. Confident and determined, the corporal nodded and turned toward the hypnotist.

Now it was the hypnotist's turn. He put the corporal in a deep, hypnotic trance. Once the hypnotist felt that the corporal's mind was completely under his control, he pretended to be the corporal's superior officer. "I am Captain Sanders," he declared. "I just gave you a piece of information you were not to divulge. I want to see if you remember it,

Corporal. What is it?" The corporal looked at him flatly. "Company B will leave at 2100 tonight," he said, without hesitation. The secret was out. It took less than a minute for the corporal, in this mock exercise, to betray his country.

The hypnotist removed the corporal from the trance. "Did you divulge the message?" he asked. The corporal smiled with the same confidence as before.

"No, and you can't get it out of me."

With just a single question, one of the military's finest had been broken, and apparently he didn't even know it. From here, we can see that in addition to its ability to affect perception and relieve pain, hypnosis can lead people to act in ways in which they wouldn't otherwise act, even if that act is forbidden.

There is a common misconception that hypnotized people are sleepwalking or in some otherwise unconscious state. In actuality, the hypnotized person is completely conscious and might even be described as extremely focused and imaginative. In 1843, James Braid, who coined the term "hypnotism," defined it this way:

> The real origin and essence of the hypnotic condition is the induction of a habit of abstraction or mental concentration, in which, as in reverie or spontaneous abstraction, the powers of the mind are so much engrossed with a single idea or train of thought, as, for the nonce, to render the individual unconscious of, or indifferently conscious to, all other ideas, impressions, or trains of thought.

In other words, hypnosis causes a person to be so focused on a certain train of thought that it leaves him or her vulnerable to external suggestions.

Hypnosis is not a state of unconsciousness but a state of supreme concentration on your imagination. In chapter 3, we saw the power of mental imagery in enhancing performance in things like sports. Mental imagery is a powerful tool. Hypnosis is mental imagery dictated by someone else, experienced without any outside distractions. When you focus hard enough on imagining something, it becomes real to you.

In the movie *Hook,* Robin Williams plays a grown-up Peter Pan who has lost some of his childhood creativity and imagination. In one scene, he is sitting at a table in Neverland with the Lost Boys, who are stuffing their faces with food, but the food is invisible. They hungrily grab handfuls of nothingness from empty bowls and plates as Peter looks on in astonishment. One boy chomps on an imaginary chicken leg, while another grips tightly what appears to be an invisible sandwich as he begins to devour it. When Peter asks, "Where's the real food?" the boys encourage him to use his imagination. He tries. He focuses his thoughts on believing that the food is real, and suddenly it is. Heaping platters of meat and bread and pastries appear before him.

That's what hypnosis is. The hypnotized subject is so deeply focused on the vision elaborated upon by the hypnotist that he begins to believe it. What's more, he becomes so fixated on this vision that he forgets to analyze and filter his own behavior. This gives the hypnotist the ability to provide directives that evade the subject's conscious scrutiny, leading him to behave in ways that, if he were not hypnotized, he would probably find embarrassing. At least that seems to be the best explanation we have so far; there is still controversy in the neuropsychological fields about why and how hypnosis works. But assuming that this explanation is correct, the question arises: How could simply focusing our attention on something have an effect so profound that it prevents other stimuli from reaching consciousness?

## The Cocktail Party Effect

Imagine that you are at a cocktail party in a crowded room. You are standing in a circle of four people, all chatting about the recent trends of the stock market. As the conversation starts to get tedious, your mind wanders. Conversations are going on simultaneously all around you, filling the room with a deafening clamor of voices. You begin to eavesdrop on the cluster of people behind you. They are discussing the eclectic nature of the decor, critiquing the host's taste in curtains and upholstery. Not interesting. Your mind moves on to the group to your left. They are gossiping about people at the party that you know. You listen in. With a smirk on your face, you pay close attention to every detail. Suddenly you hear your name called. The woman standing directly in front of you has been talking to you, but you have no idea what she has been saying because your attention had just been occupied elsewhere.

The selective nature of attention on display in this scenario is known as the cocktail party effect. Within the general hubbub of conversations, you are able to selectively tune in to one discussion at a time while tuning out the rest of the commotion in the room. How does the brain do it? After all, the room is just filled with sound waves. How does the brain figure out which sound waves are important? It seems that you process only one conversation at a time, while the words spoken outside that conversation, even if spoken nearest to your vicinity, fail to enter your mind.

Studies of the phenomenon known as inattentional blindness appear to bolster the point that we only consciously register that which our attention is focused on. In a well-known and very entertaining experiment, the psychologists Christopher Chabris and Daniel Simons asked volunteers to watch a video of two teams of three people passing around a basketball. One team wore white shirts, the other, black shirts. The volunteers were asked to pay close attention only to the team in white and to count the number of passes they make. At the end of the video, they were instructed to report the number of passes by the white team. Then they were asked, "Did you notice a gorilla?" Partway through the video, a gorilla (rather, a woman in a gorilla suit) walked right into the scene, through the basketball players, paused at center stage to face the camera, beat its chest, and walked off. Yet so focused were the volunteers on counting the passes that about half of the people who saw the video did not notice the gorilla. If you find this hard to believe, check out the video on YouTube and try it on your friends.

In a similar study, fifteen pedestrians on the Cornell University campus were individually approached by an experimenter who asked for directions. During the conversation, while the pedestrian and the experimenter were busy looking at a map, two men (who were in on the experiment) rudely walked in between them while carrying a door. As the door was moving by, the first experimenter switched places with the man holding the back of the door and helped carry it out of sight. This left a new experimenter standing with the pedestrian, attempting to get the same directions with an identical map. The original experimenter and the impostor wore different clothes from each other, they differed in height by two inches, and their voices did not sound alike. Nevertheless, again about half of the pedestrians approached did not notice that they were suddenly talking to a different person. They continued to provide the directions as if nothing had happened.

Research on the neurobiology of attention has helped clarify the circuits in the brain that account for the results of these experiments. When we see or hear something, sensory signals are moving from our eyes and ears to the thalamus, the brain's sensory switching station, all the way up to the auditory or visual cortices of the brain. This pathway can be generally called bottom-up signaling. As this is going on, signals from the brain are being sent *down* to the thalamus and even all the way to the original sensory receptors. This is called top-down signaling, which is responsible for filtering the incoming signals, selecting the important components, and synthesizing them into a meaningful visual scene or a coherent conversation. You might think of top-down processing as a courtroom judge trying to settle a dispute about a car accident. The involved parties present her with myriad different reports as to what happened. Witnesses who were standing at unique vantage points present their accounts of the collision, and once all the evidence is presented, the judge has been given many different pieces of information, but she still wants to get the real story. That is her challenge: to take the disconnected fragments of information with which she is presented, filling in the gaps when necessary, and use the wisdom of her experience with such cases to create a sensible narrative.

That's what the brain is doing with the overload of sensory information it receives from moment to moment. It takes in the information, evaluates it, identifies the most salient features based on past experience, and finally synthesizes it into a single, unified experience.

In the video of the basketball players, there's a lot going on: people moving in many directions, black shirts, white shirts, balls flying around, walls of the room, the floor, the features on the players' faces. What's significant? What should the brain prioritize in creating its visual narrative? Considering that the challenge is to count the number of passes by the white team, it makes sense that the brain would use top-down processing to focus only on these aspects. However, the brain, like a judge, has limited resources. If the white team's activity has been tagged as most significant, then the brain assigns a secondary importance to the black team, and the unconscious system softens the impact of those stimuli on the conscious mind. The black parts of the visual field fade into the background. Not coincidentally, the gorilla suit is black. Because the brain is not expecting to find importance in black parts of the visual field, the gorilla is unconsciously attributed to background noise, and as a result 50 percent of people fail to notice it. Had the gorilla suit been bright yellow rather than black, it would not have blended as well into what the brain had deemed to be visual background noise. Nobody watching the video would have missed it because the brain would have picked out the bright stimulus and separated it from the rest of the scene.

The same system is at work during the experiment with the pedestrians. Half of them did not notice that the person in front of them was suddenly switched, because the limited resources of their brains had been allocated to the task of providing directions. However, had the replacement experimenter been wearing a pink birthday hat or a Santa Claus suit, every pedestrian would have noticed the change. The sudden addition of those features to the experimenter's appearance would have caused the brain to assign an increased importance to those aspects of the visual scene. The experimenter's appearance would have acquired a greater degree of salience, and the pedestrian would have been far more likely to notice.

This is also the reason why, at the cocktail party, your attention may be immediately diverted when you hear phrases uttered nearby like ". . . and then she ran into the elevator completely naked!" It's a phrase we tend not to hear too often, as much as we might like to. It also has content that may be significant and interesting to some people, and the brain recognizes that. The same goes for the abrupt shift in attention that occurs when you hear your name called. From its long history of processing the stimulus that is the sound of your name, the brain considers that an important signal, and your attention is briskly redirected to locate the source.

A 2007 neurological study of the cocktail party effect examined the neuronal activity in the brain of certain bird species called the zebra finch while it listened to a mishmash of sounds. The goal was for the finch to selectively pay attention to a familiar birdsong recorded from another finch. However, at the same time, the research group played recordings of background noise that at times included a chorus of other birdsongs. This would be the bird's version of the cocktail party: sounds coming simultaneously from birds in all directions, though, unfortunately, no cocktails are being served. Nevertheless, recordings of the finch's brain activity revealed something fascinating. On the one hand, it was clear that the finch detected the overload of sound—a confusing barrage of interfering signals was detected in the auditory cortex. However, each time a syllable of the familiar birdsong was played, one series of waveforms remained markedly tall, while the rest of the brain waves shrank. It was as if the finch recognized the relevance of one bird's voice amid the hullabaloo of sounds and selectively listened to the voice while suppressing the rest of the sounds and relegating them to background noise. The human brain works in a similar way: it identifies the importance of certain stimuli and directs attention toward them while recognizing the irrelevance of other stimuli and downgrading their impact on the nervous system, a process that is, not surprisingly, reminiscent of the corollary discharge system.

The lesson from the neuroscientific study of attention is not that the brain detects only certain parts of a visual landscape or acoustic harmony and leaves out the rest. The brain receives pretty much everything that our eyes and ears (and other sensory receptors) detect. But the amount of information is overwhelming. Attention research demonstrates that our unconscious has the ability to select which facets of the sensory bombardment are *relevant* and to synthesize a singular, consistent narrative that becomes our conscious experience. The fact that you respond to your name at a cocktail party, while your attention is occupied with other conversations, implies that *something* is getting through, even if you are usually oblivious to it. In fact, the brain gets nearly all the information, but we are consciously aware of only a fraction of it. It makes you wonder about all that information we are *unaware* of and how it might affect us subconsciously.

## Overcoming the Stroop Effect

Let's try an experiment. Take a look at the words below and, as fast as you can, identify the color of the font in which each one is typed:

**BLACK** WHITE **GRAY** **BLACK** WHITE **GRAY** **BLACK** WHITE

How long did that take you? I imagine not very long. Now try the same thing with the set of words below. Remember, just identify the colors of the *font:*

BLACK **WHITE** **GRAY** BLACK **WHITE** GRAY BLACK **WHITE**

That probably took considerably longer, as it does for most people. The reason, of course, is that the colors of the words conflict with the words themselves. Even though you are charged with the task of identifying the font colors, the meanings of the words themselves distract you and interfere with your ability to complete the task quickly. As a result, you take significantly longer to identify the second set of colors than the first.

This is known as the Stroop effect, named after John Ridley Stroop, the psychologist who came up with the test. Present in more than 99 percent of people, the Stroop effect has been extensively studied and well established over many years. It's not something we can control. Practice may help with our reaction time a little, but we will still be far slower when the colors don't match the names than when they do. This is because the effect is derived from the creation of a conflict in the brain between competing perceptual signals. The words say one thing; the colors of the font say another. Before we can correctly identify the font color, the brain has to sort out these competing representations, and that takes time—hence the increase in reaction time that we call the Stroop effect. There isn't much that can be done to modulate this effect, though there is one thing: hypnosis.

When hypnotized subjects attempt the Stroop task, their reaction time is much improved. In fact, they are so proficient that there is little discernible difference in reaction time between the task in which the colors match the words and the task in which they don't. Hypnotized subjects are able to identify the color of the font without being burdened by the interference of what the words mean. So focused are they on the task at hand that the conflicting stimulus is ignored. In short, *hypnosis can eliminate the Stroop effect*. Somehow, the hypnotic state blocks the conflict in the brain that causes a slowing of reaction time, but how? Where does this conflict resolution take place in the brain, and how does hypnosis intervene?

Neuroimaging studies of the brain, using techniques such as fMRI and PET scans, have demonstrated that the anterior cingulate cortex, a region located below the prefrontal cortex, is active while subjects engage in the Stroop task. The anterior cingulate has many functions, including emotional processing and helping with focusing attention.

We encountered it in chapter 1, where we discussed its role in discovering the distortion in the question "How many animals of each kind did Moses take on the ark?" That question tries to trick you by structuring the sentence so as to refer to Noah but instead substitutes the name Moses. Similarly, the Stroop task pits your color perception and your word recognition against each other. In both cases, the anterior cingulate appears to help you sort out the contradiction.

A multitude of studies of the anterior cingulate have demonstrated that it is the site of conflict monitoring in the brain. Whenever we are struggling with conflicting perceptions as in the Stroop task, or weighing options on a multiple-choice exam, or dealing with errors that we make, or trying to think of the right word to say when several come to mind, the anterior cingulate is hard at work. The anterior cingulate is responsible for sorting out those kinds of situations, all of which involve some kind of conflict monitoring.

If hypnosis can eliminate the Stroop effect, which is processed by the anterior cingulate, then presumably hypnosis has some effect on the anterior cingulate. So, how does hypnosis fit into this neurological picture? John Gruzelier, a neuroscientist and psychologist, ran an experiment to answer that very question.

Using a screening tool known as the Stanford Hypnotic Susceptibility Scale, Gruzelier identified and assembled a group of highly hypnotizable participants. He then had them attempt the Stroop task twice, once in their normal state and once while hypnotized. In both cases, Gruzelier monitored their brain activity using fMRI.

The imaging data revealed that hypnotized subjects showed significantly stronger activity in the anterior cingulate cortex after being hypnotized than before. This seems counterintuitive. We might assume that the anterior cingulate would be *less* active in hypnosis because the brain fails to detect the conflict and focuses only on the font color. However, the anterior cingulate, the hub of conflict resolution in the brain, actually appears to be working overtime. So how do hypnotized subjects overcome the Stroop effect?

That's where Gruzelier's second finding comes in. In control subjects (who were not hypnotized), the anterior cingulate cortex illuminated together with the frontal lobe, implying that the two brain regions were in communication. Presumably, in control subjects, the anterior cingulate detects the conflicting signals unconsciously, but then has to report them to the frontal lobe so conscious analysis can sort out the contradiction. This makes the control subjects consciously aware of the challenge of the Stroop task, but it slows them down. Hence, their reaction time is worse when the colors of the font and the meanings of the words don't match.

In hypnotized subjects, however, the brain activity is different. The anterior cingulate illuminates alone. The frontal lobe stays quiet. The two regions fail to work in concert as they normally would. Gruzelier's discovery is that hypnosis uncouples the unconscious conflict monitoring of the anterior cingulate from the conscious analysis of the frontal lobe. Consequently, the frontal lobe never gets the message that the anterior cingulate detects the conflict between the written words and the font colors. In the meantime, the anterior cingulate realizes that its message is not getting across, so it begins to work harder. That's why the fMRI reveals enhanced activity there. Unaware that there is a block in communication, the anterior cingulate ramps up its efforts to report the conflict that the frontal lobe is ignoring.

Hypnosis eliminates the Stroop effect not by preventing conflict monitoring but by interrupting conflict *reporting,* a feat it accomplishes by disconnecting two regions that would otherwise communicate. Consider what this means. By decoupling the activity in the anterior cingulate cortex from that of the frontal lobe, hypnosis modifies the way the brain sorts through our perceptions, recognizes conflicts, and deals with errors. Gruzelier says that this is why hypnotized people may do outrageous things that they wouldn't do otherwise.

Hypnosis changes the way our brains process information. That is how hypnotists can exert such a powerful influence on the people they hypnotize. Suggestions that are received while in a hypnotic trance are not subjected to the same rigor of conscious scrutiny by the frontal lobe. It is for this reason, Gruzelier says, that a hypnotized person may do ridiculous things like believing he is fighting with a falcon and nearly tearing off his shirt. Though the hypnotist's reference to a falcon conflicts with my friend's visual perception of a falcon-free environment, his conscious mind is not made aware of the conflict, and his imagination fills in the gaps. His conscious defenses are down, and the hypnotic suggestion can sneak in under the radar. A hypnotic suggestion has greater influence—greater *access*—than a typical suggestion, but how much greater? What could a hypnotist make a person do?

We've seen that once a person is properly hypnotized, hypnotic suggestions can enter a person's head without being monitored by consciousness. At this point, they take on a power that would seem similar to subliminal messages, which also work by avoiding conscious analysis. The topic of subliminal influence has a long and fascinating history that can help shed light on the question of how subconscious influence can affect our behavior.

## Eat Popcorn, Drink Coca-Cola

In the 1950s, soon after the Korean War and just before the release of the film *The Manchurian Candidate,* an advertising expert named James Vicary undertook a secret experiment. In a movie theater in Fort Lee, New Jersey, he placed a device by the movie projector that, every five seconds or so during the film, caused the words "EAT POP-CORN" and "DRINK COCA-COLA" to flash across the screen. The words appeared for only three-thousandth of a second each time, too briefly for people in the audience to consciously notice them, but perhaps long enough that the words would still have an impact on their nervous systems unconsciously. By the end of six weeks, after nearly forty-six thousand people had seen the movie, Vicary claimed that Coke sales rose by 18 percent and popcorn sales shot up by almost 58 percent.

When this finding was reported in the newspaper, readers were left with a sense of foreboding. People felt violated. *Newsday* called it "the most alarming invention since the atomic bomb." How could someone infiltrate their minds and manipulate their decision-making process without being detected? To make matters worse, it was thought that the use of these subliminal messages could be expanded to create devices of full-scale mind control. As one respondent to the newspaper article wrote, "If the device is successful for putting over popcorn, why not politicians or anything else?" Even Aldous Huxley, author of *Brave New World,* joined the conversation, stating that it would be possible within a few years to "abolish the free will almost completely."

And so began an era of fear about the possibility of subliminal mind control—a fear that exploded in the summer of 1990, when the rock band Judas Priest and CBS Records were put on trial for allegedly inserting a subliminal message into one of their songs. Five years earlier, the teenage boys Ray Belknap and James Vance had listened to the song, titled "Better by You, Better Than Me," and immediately afterward headed to a nearby playground with a sawed-off shotgun and shot themselves in the head. At the trial, it was revealed that, hidden in the heavy metal track and repeated numerous times, was a message: "Do it." To make matters worse, hidden in the album cover was the image of a projectile passing through a person's exploding head.

In the end, CBS Records won the case. Between the two of them, Ray and James had a history of drug use, shoplifting, and even violence. The judge concluded that the evidence regarding the power of subliminal messaging to influence human behavior, especially choices of that magnitude, was insufficient to rule in favor of the boys' families. What's more, it didn't help their case that one of their expert witnesses was a man named Wilson Key, who published a number of books on how subliminal sexual messages pervaded all products and forms of communication. He cited examples of advertisements for gin with the word "sex" in the ice cubes, Ritz crackers with the word "sex" baked into them, and a restaurant ad showing a plate of food that Key claimed was a subliminal image demonstrating a group of men engaged in a sexual act with a donkey. When Key was cross-examined in the Judas Priest trial, it was clear that his views on subliminal messaging crossed the boundary into paranoia and were not based in reality:

ATTORNEY: You have seen "SEX" embedded in Lincoln's beard on a $5 bill?
KEY: Yes.
ATTORNEY: And you believe that to be done purposely by the U.S. government, the Mint, the Department of the Mint?
KEY: Yes.
ATTORNEY: The same is done in Canada with Canadian money?
KEY: Oh, yes.
ATTORNEY: You believe that the cover of *Time* magazine, the publishers, use subliminal messages?
KEY: Yes, yes.
ATTORNEY: Hilton hotel menus?
KEY: Yes.

ATTORNEY: Elementary school textbooks?
KEY: Yes, yes.

As it turns out, Vicary's Eat Popcorn/Drink Coca-Cola experiment wasn't real either. It was never published in a scientific journal, nor could it be reproduced by other researchers. In one attempted replication, the Canadian Broadcasting Corporation subliminally flashed the message "Phone Now" more than 350 times during a popular Sunday night television show. However, not a single call came in. Later, the station asked its viewers to guess the message that was hidden in the broadcast. Nearly five hundred letters were received, but none of them contained the correct answer. Nearly 50 percent of the respondents claimed that they became hungry or thirsty while watching the program. Evidently, it was thought that the hidden message was another food-related one like the popcorn/Coca-Cola experiment that audience members had already heard so much about.

It was even discovered that the theater supposedly used for Vicary's experiment was too small to accommodate the audience that Vicary claimed it did, and the theater manager had never heard of the study. The experiment was a hoax.

Nevertheless, the concept of subliminal messaging is still out there, and it presents a question that has consequences for our discussion. How real is subliminal messaging? How does it influence us, and how far does that influence extend?

## Invisible Faces

Though its influence has been greatly exaggerated by Vicary and others, subliminal messaging is real, and neuroscientists have used it in various forms as part of research. One such technique, known as backward masking, involves the presentation of two images one after another. The first picture, called the prime, is shown for less than fifty milliseconds before it is replaced by the second picture, called the mask, a neutral image like a rectangle or other basic shape that is presented for several seconds. Fifty milliseconds is too brief of an exposure time to reach conscious awareness, so, as long as the mask replaces the prime within the fifty-millisecond window, subjects will not see the first image at all. They will only see the second, masking image. Yet what scientists have discovered is that even though the priming image is practically invisible to the subject, information about that image is somehow registered deeply within the unconscious parts of the brain.

A team of psychologists tried out this technique in two experiments, one with practicing Catholics and the other with psychology graduate students. The Catholic participants were asked to read a sexually suggestive passage about a woman dreaming of an intimate encounter. After having some time to process what they had just read, the participants were exposed to one of two priming images. Half of them were flashed a picture of the pope staring at them disappointedly, and the other half were shown an unknown person's face. The priming images, by definition, were shown for only a few milliseconds before they were replaced by an image of neutral shapes.

Once they had been shown the subliminal images, the participants filled out a questionnaire to evaluate their level of religious commitment. The researchers then compared the questionnaire answers with an earlier set of self-assessments that the participants filled out before seeing the images. Among the Catholic subjects who were flashed the unfamiliar face, their self-evaluation was unchanged. The answers from before and after exposure to the face were about the same. However, the subjects who were flashed the pope's disappointed face gave themselves lower ratings of religious commitment on the second evaluation, even though none of them consciously registered the faces. As far as they knew, they had just seen some pictures of shapes.

The graduate students underwent a similar treatment. They were asked to evaluate their own research ideas after being subliminally primed with either the disapproving face of their department chair or the face of a random person. As before, the subjects who were flashed the department chair's face gave their work lower ratings. The students who were shown a random person's face did not show this effect. In both experiments, the participants' ability to assess their own feelings or ideas was affected by stimuli that they themselves did not see or even know existed.

Imagine that as you are leaving the supermarket, the cashier flashes you a dirty look because you paid for your chips and soda with only coins. You don't notice the look and continue to go about your day. An hour later, you find yourself becoming quickly frustrated with your friend on the phone. You aren't sure why. For some reason, you're just in a bad mood. It's possible that the dirty look that you never consciously saw acted like a subliminal message, provoking an emotion that you can't seem to trace back to a specific cause.

Now consider the way body language affects us. Someone stands an inch closer to you than usual. You don't really notice it, but later you wonder, was she flirting with you? On another day, a new client's handshake is a bit too firm . . . just ever so slightly. When he leaves your office, he leaves you with a bad vibe. He seemed a little arrogant, but you can't seem to put your finger on it.

Research on backward masking shows that unseen moments in our lives can influence the way we judge other people. In one experiment, twenty-six people were primed with images of fearful, disgusted, or neutral faces. As before, these images were shown for only a few milliseconds, and the participants were not consciously aware of them. After being shown the primes, the volunteers were asked to look at a number of pictures of people with neutral faces and judge how genuine they thought those people appeared. The results showed that the subjects exposed to subliminal fearful or disgusted faces were significantly more likely to judge the neutral faces as being ungenuine than those exposed to the subliminal neutral faces were. In another study, volunteers were primed with angry or sad faces and then asked to analyze descriptions of tragic events. Those primed with sad faces were more likely to appraise those events as being caused by unfortunate circumstances, whereas those primed with angry faces were more likely to blame the actions of people involved in the story for causing the trouble.

From a behavioral standpoint, it's clear that techniques of subliminal priming such as backward masking can influence the way we perceive ourselves, the way we perceive others, and the way we judge a situation. Subliminal messages do work, but how? What is going on in the brain that allows these images to affect us even though we are consciously unaware of them?

Studies using fMRI show that when a person consciously sees an image such as a scary face, regions throughout the brain begin firing. The signal is initially sent from the receptors in the eyes, winding along the optic tract, to the occipital lobe (responsible for vision) in the back of the brain. From there, it travels to the frontal and parietal lobes, where a flurry of intensifying neuronal activity allows for interpretation and analysis of what is being seen. The amygdala (responsible for emotional processing) is also activated because the image has a fearful quality. When the dust has cleared, the person in question consciously perceives the face, notices that it has a threatening gesture, feels the feeling of fear, and perhaps even wonders why the guy in the picture is making that face and whether he might be in need of psychotherapy.

In contrast, if the same image is shown using backward masking, the brain activity has a very different pattern. The beginning of the pathway is the same: the signal travels from the receptors in the eyes, zipping along the optic tract, through the relevant visual nuclei, until it arrives at the occipital lobe. What happens next, however, differs from the previous scenario. The signal does not become amplified in the frontal lobe, and the fMRI does not show that same explosion of activity. The frontal lobe is relatively quiet. But another area suddenly goes to work. Deep within the brain, the amygdala lights up as it begins processing the fearful content of the unseen image.

The person in question does not consciously see the picture. His frontal lobe does not initiate any analysis or interpretation. As far as he knows, no image of a scary face was ever presented to him. Yet the subliminal image left an imprint in his brain, and his nervous system, specifically the amygdala, was busy unconsciously processing the emotional content of an image that he didn't even know he had seen.

This implies that any moment in our lives can affect us without our even being aware of it. A passing glance from someone in your subway car. A single lyric in a song on the radio. A poster in the corner of your eye. Anything that reaches our sensory receptors can potentially and ever so subtly manipulate our emotions, and our resulting decisions, without our taking notice.

How powerful are these effects? This is controversial. Some say subliminal influence is weak. In one experiment, two groups of undergraduates were assembled, half of whom claimed to be terrified of spiders and half of whom claimed to be unafraid. Both groups were subliminally primed with either happy faces or scowling faces and then asked to evaluate the unpleasantness of pictures of spiders. In the non-fearful group, there was some effect. Priming with happy faces made the spider pictures seem more tolerable, while scowling faces made them seem more abhorrent. However, this effect was not shown in the group afraid of spiders. The subliminal images did not do anything, presumably because they were too weak to significantly affect an emotion as visceral as arachnophobia.

On the other hand, a number of department stores have tried using subliminal messages to reduce shoplifting. Embedded in the stores' background music were words of moral encouragement like "I am honest, I will not steal" repeated over and over again. Some stores claimed that the incidence of shoplifting fell dramatically as a result. Is this connection real or coincidental? Would a potential shoplifter be subliminally deterred from his crime because of hidden words in department store music? Probably not. It's hard to say anything definitive, but the consensus seems to be that there is *some* effect of subliminal stimuli but not to the extent that it will radically change behavior.

Despite all the hype it has been awarded, the influence of subliminal messaging is subtle. Yet the influence of hypnosis is remarkably clear and profound. It could be that the difference lies in the ways that the two techniques interact with consciousness. Subliminal messages avoid conscious awareness completely. But this immediately restricts their ability to modify our thinking. If we don't consciously see the image, we can't make the decision to obey it or incorporate it into our behavior. The neurological repercussions of a subliminal message are limited to isolated activation of the amygdala, which translates to a slight alteration in one's emotional state. Maybe this will have some slight impact on a person's behavior, such as by affecting his or her responses on a self-assessment, but maybe it won't have much of an effect at all. Without the ability to access consciousness, the power of subliminal messaging has a low ceiling. It's like trying to change the path of a bowling ball by hitting it with marbles.

Hypnosis, on the other hand, changes the way the bowling ball is thrown. It doesn't avoid consciousness. Subjects are well aware of the suggestions being given to them. Hypnosis changes the way we *use* consciousness. Subjects are so focused on the imagery being narrated that they become more vulnerable to blindly accepting what they are told. Rather than circumventing conscious awareness, hypnosis lulls subjects into being less scrutinizing, less analytic. It encourages them to use their minds for the purpose of imagination, to allow them to absorb the experience passively, rather than for the purpose of monitoring their behavior.

My friend was well aware that the hypnotist was talking to him about a falcon. It wasn't subliminal; he was conscious of the suggestions the whole time. He had no problem remembering the event, unlike those who are flashed masked faces. The power of hypnosis was that it suppressed his ability to reflect on the weirdness of the suggestion and the conflict with his better judgment.

Hypnosis is more powerful than subliminal messaging because it *does* access consciousness, as well as the decisions, thoughts, and associations contained therein. What's more, it maintains this access while our instruments of self-monitoring and conflict resolution are engrossed with the pictures and sounds that the hypnotist presents.

It appears that James Vicary was wrong not only because his research was fake but also because he thought that advertising would be more effective if it could elude conscious awareness completely by using subliminal techniques. As it turns out, successful advertisements might actually have a lot more in common with hypnosis.

## Brand Names in the Brain

There are many different styles of advertising. Some commercials appeal to a product's practicality, such as infomercials for the cleaning agent OxiClean, which demonstrate its ability to eliminate hard-to-clean stains from fabric. Other advertisements focus more on creating positive associations around a product in the minds of their viewers. That can be done in an obvious fashion, as in an ad showing a man spraying himself with Axe body spray and immediately noticing hordes of bikini-clad women flocking to him. It can also be done in a more subtle manner, such as a successful 1984 commercial for British Airways in which, though the narration was about the wideness of its airplanes' seats, the power of the ad was derived from the very relaxing background music it featured. Describing all the various categories of advertisements and the theories of why they work is beyond the scope of our discussion. What we will focus on, however, is how certain kinds of ads affect brain activity and what that reveals about the mechanisms and extent of hypnotic influence, as there are a number of similarities.

Michael Yapko, a clinical psychologist and expert on the therapeutic uses of hypnosis, argues that advertising is a lot like hypnosis in the way that it often encourages us to use our imagination. He says that like a hypnotist ads often present a vision that we are asked to embrace.

Through this vision, the ad presents suggestions of products that will supposedly make our lives better. He writes,

> Advertisers begin by creating a need for a product . . . using techniques such as promoting identification with a person in the ad so that you'll solve your problem by using the product in the same way he or she modeled it for you. Then they strengthen your buying habit by telling you how [much more] bright, masculine, [or] feminine . . . you are for having made such a fine choice . . . The entire field of advertising uses words and images in a way that is intended to influence your buying behaviors.

Similarly, hypnotists attempt to create a vision for their subjects using as much sensory terminology as possible. They tend to use phrases like "you feel that you are becoming hot and sweaty" or "you can see the green fields of grass and the lush trees and hear the sound of the burbling brook." Yapko writes that suggestibility is "an openness to accepting and responding to new ideas, new information." The more you identify with the scenario depicted in the commercial, the more open you will be to accepting its suggestions. One approach to advertising is to try to make the viewer imagine herself as if she were the person in the commercial, who, for example, has yellowish teeth, and feel the things that this imagined character is feeling, such as the pain of being ignored by potential romantic partners. If this vision can be attained, perhaps the viewer will be more open to considering the product being advertised, in this case teeth-whitening strips.

Whenever we find ourselves watching TV at 1:00 in the morning, we get to experience a deluge of commercials for workout equipment that claim it takes only one simple rowing motion to get you from that unfortunate before picture to the super-toned (and tanned) after picture. Tired and slumped on the couch, with potato chip crumbs littering our clothes, this might be the only moment in the day at which we might think, "I should order one of those!" Even though the ad makes outrageous claims for the contraption's effectiveness, we are tired, so more suggestible, and are feeling lazy and out of shape. We identify with the character in the commercial who wants to get fit, and suddenly an otherwise unconvincing ad has a greater influence on us.

Yapko has done a lot of research on the elements that make for a good hypnotic suggestion, but how would one design a hypnotic television commercial? Yapko defined thirty-five qualities that empower an advertisement with hypnotic influence. Here are some examples:

- The carrot principle: The ad creates an expectation of reward from using its product. *Use our mint gum and you'll get kissed by a tall blonde.*
- Rapport: The ad sets a warm ambience, creating positive associations with the product. *Peacefully lying on the beach, drinking a beer.*
- Positive suggestion: The ad uses positive rather than negative words. *Eat our low-calorie sandwich and you'll get thinner* rather than *you won't get fat.*
- Dominant effect: The ad appeals to a prominent emotion in the viewer to convey its message. *Are you depressed? Bored? This car will set you free.*
- Chaining suggestions: The audience is told that it should do something in response to something else it should do. *The more kids you have, the more you need to save for college, and the more you need to save for college, the more you'll need to invest in a college savings program.*
- Confusion: The audience doesn't understand what's happening until the product is ultimately revealed and the built-up tension is relieved. *A man appears to be robbing a bank, but he's actually showing off his comfy ski mask.*
- Visualization and/or analogy: The ad describes a sensory experience associated with the product. *The juicy burger with tangy mustard is like a party in your mouth.*

So, let's think of a familiar TV commercial. Take the standard Olive Garden commercial, for example. If you watch it carefully, you'll notice a lot of these hypnotic elements. The commercial opens with a crowded table of good friends laughing and chatting as they study the menu, jazzy music subtly playing in the background. The camera zooms in so you are at eye level, as if part of the group. As the friends exchange smiles and witty banter, the warm, inviting voice of the narrator begins describing the delicious sauces and fresh bread sticks. A heaping bowl of tomato-herb fettuccine appears. A ladle drizzles steaming Alfredo sauce over the pasta. Olive Garden. *We're all family here.*

In the span of fifteen seemingly innocuous seconds, the ad employs at least five of Yapko's manipulative tactics. The music, the laughter, and the warm voices establish *rapport,* creating a positive association with the restaurant. By connecting the happy group of friends to the bowl of pasta, the ad fulfills the *carrot principle:* if you come here and eat our food, you too will enjoy friendships like these. The ad also uses the principle of *dominant effect* by providing an antidote to our innate sense of loneliness. When the food is finally presented on-screen, the *visualization* stage works its magic as we salivate over the sensory buffet. Finally, the commercial ends with a moving analogy: going to Olive Garden is like being welcomed into a family. These elements come together to generate a vision so engrossing, so hypnotizing, that the viewer becomes vulnerable to suggestions about where to get dinner.

In a 2007 study, Yapko took a selection of twelve television advertisements (for things like food, drinks, clothing, communication, and toiletries) and, using his thirty-five guidelines, ranked them in order of how much hypnotically suggestive content they contained. Next, he showed the commercials to 173 volunteers and asked them to rate the effectiveness of each one. What he found was that the more the commercials fit his guidelines for hypnotic suggestions, the higher the effectiveness ratings they received from the viewers.

It does seem that there are some parallels between advertising and hypnosis, but are they visible neurologically? The effect of advertising on the brain is a complicated area of research because commercials make an enormous variety of appeals, whether practical, emotional, or otherwise. Many regions of the brain, including the frontal lobe, the anterior cingulate cortex, and the amygdala, can be activated. Because no two commercials are alike, it's hard for scientists to study how all commercials affect the brain. However, neuroscientists have been able to learn a lot by simplifying the experiments to look at the effects of just the brand names alone.

Suppose that you want to buy a car and are debating between a Toyota and a Porsche. Before you head out to the dealerships, you watch television during breakfast. Suddenly a commercial for Porsche comes on. It shows a sleek-looking car cruising through Las Vegas on a summer evening and ends with a display of the recognizable Porsche shield in the center of the screen. What is going on in the brain at this moment?

A 2007 neuroimaging study monitored the brain activity of fourteen volunteers as they were shown different brand names of cars. One finding that stood out was the pattern of brain activation that occurred in response to luxury brands. When subjects were shown the logos of Porsche, Mercedes-Benz, and other luxury brands, fMRI data revealed enhanced activity in the medial prefrontal cortex, located near the front of the brain. We encountered the medial prefrontal in chapter 4, when discussing sports fans who strongly identify with their favorite players. This region is known to be associated with self-centered, selfish forms of thought. At least on the surface, this provides some insight into why you, once you visit the dealership, might have the urge to indulge yourself by purchasing the Porsche rather than the Toyota. Just the image of the brand is enough to spark selfish urges and edge you toward choosing luxury over practicality.

Activity in the medial prefrontal cortex (specifically the ventromedial prefrontal cortex) has also been implicated as a cause of the phenomenon known as the Pepsi paradox. Research shows that in blind taste tests people reliably prefer the taste of Pepsi over Coke. Yet Coca-Cola sells nearly twice as well as Pepsi and has outsold it consistently for a long time. In a neurological study of this phenomenon, two groups were asked to take a blind taste test of Coke and Pepsi. One group comprised people with damage to their ventromedial prefrontal cortex (due to injury or surgery), while the other group contained healthy control subjects. When given the blind taste test, both groups showed a tendency to prefer Pepsi over Coke, the same finding seen in the general population. Next the experimenters brought out two new cups of Coke and Pepsi, but this time with the cups labeled. Both groups did the test again, this time knowing which one was Pepsi and which was Coke. The responses of the control group revealed that their preferences had been dramatically shifted from Pepsi to Coke. Apparently, seeing the brand name had a significant impact on their declared preference, thereby illustrating the Pepsi paradox. However, the patients with damage to the ventromedial prefrontal cortex still preferred Pepsi and did so at approximately the same rate as they did in the blind taste test. The presence of the brand name did not affect their preference. The experimenters concluded that the medial prefrontal cortex is responsible for processing the effects of brand names on our decision making. It's the neurological source of the Pepsi paradox. To the average consumer, no matter how good the taste of Pepsi might be, it just can't compete with Coca-Cola's brand name, unless the medial prefrontal cortex is compromised.

Hypnosis changes the pattern of activity in the anterior cingulate cortex, while brand names in advertising affect the medial prefrontal cortex. These areas are near each other but are not the same. Yet what both techniques have in common is that they change the way the brain processes information, whether or not we are aware of their influence. Like hypnosis, certain forms of advertising use imagery and narrative to increase the suggestibility of their target audience and offer propositions for future behavior. Of course, hypnosis is by far the more powerful technique because the level of imagination and distraction is much deeper, so much so that the subject falls into a trancelike state, but the similarity with some types of ads is notable nonetheless. There is also a third characteristic they have in common, one that they share even with subliminal messaging: they are targeted outside influences that can affect our behavior in ways we are not aware of. As long as these techniques avoid the security system that is our deliberate, conscious reflection, their influence is free to blend into the background buzz of unconscious information processing that contributes to our decision making. So, if some unconscious foreign influence were to change our behavior in any way, it would be up to the brain to come up with a convincing explanation for why we decided to act the way we did.

## When the Brain Makes Excuses

As we saw in the previous chapter, schizophrenic patients who experience auditory hallucinations have gaps in the information processed by their brains. When a patient hears a voice, fails to recognize it as his own, and sees that there is nobody around who could have uttered those words, his brain has to get creative to try to conjure up a sensible explanation. What it comes up with are possibilities like spying agencies, technological mechanisms, or spiritual deities—all of which could in theory gain access to his mind through invisible forces. So, in a sense, these seemingly bizarre explanations are rational attempts by the schizophrenic patient's unconscious mind to fill in the gaps of a very incomplete story.

Similarly, research shows that when external, subconscious influences affect a person's behavior, the brain creates a story that attributes that new behavior to his or her own reasons and motivations. This applies to hypnosis, too. For example, in one experiment, a hypnotized subject was instructed to open a window upon hearing the word "Germany." Several minutes later, the hypnotist said the word. The subject paused for a moment and said, "It is awfully stuffy in here, we need some fresh air. Do you mind if I open the window?" The subject did not have the urge to open the window on his own. The feeling of stuffiness didn't naturally come over him, and he didn't think of the idea to open the window. That thought was given to him through hypnotic suggestion, and it thereby evaded his conscious analysis. So, suddenly, his brain is confronted with an urge to open the window, yet the source of that urge is unknown. How does the brain explain it? It must be stuffy in here. Logical.

Now consider the other examples we have seen of external stimuli subconsciously affecting our behavior. Recall the backward-masking experiments involving practicing Catholics and psychology graduate students who were shown subliminal images of disapproving faces. Suppose you asked the Catholics why they gave themselves such low ratings on the religiosity scale and asked the students why they didn't think their dissertations were in perfect order, as they expressed in their self-assessments. What do you think they would say? They probably would *not* tell you that those feelings suddenly appeared within them, as if inserted into their minds by some unknown source. The Catholics might cite their recent transgressions or how they believe they need to give more to charity. On the other hand, the graduate students would point out the flaws in their research model or the revisions needed to fix their writing.

When we buy products or services that we have seen advertised, we often don't cite the advertisements themselves as the reason for our purchases. If I head to a car dealership and buy a Porsche, it's because I want a car that handles well with comfortable seats and a powerful engine. If I buy a Toyota, it's because I want something safe and affordable to get me from point A to point B. These reasons are all valid, I'm sure, but they aren't the whole story. How did I come to associate Porsche with luxury and Toyota with practicality? Certainly, the countless ads I've seen since early childhood have something to do with it. Yet my immediate tendency is to provide my own reasoning as the sole motivation for why I choose the car that I do.

In the same way, if an unseen dirty look from a cashier puts you in a bad mood, you might try to come up with an explanation for why you are feeling down. Maybe it's the situation at work. Maybe it's the cold weather. Unaware of the true cause, you come up with an explanation that fits.

Targeted external suggestions, whether from hypnosis, advertising, or subliminal messaging, certainly have the ability to affect our brain activity and behavior. We have seen that backward masking can trigger isolated activity in the amygdala to process emotions we don't know we're having, hypnosis can dampen the process of conflict monitoring in the brain, and advertising icons can activate the medial prefrontal cortex and feelings of selfish preference. And once these effects have taken hold, our brains incorporate them into what we believe are our own self-generated motivations.

Yet of all these techniques of influence, hypnosis seems by far the most potent. After all, it can cause a person to perceive things that aren't there or do things they wouldn't otherwise do in ways more overt than these other methods. If it can make a straitlaced volunteer humiliate himself in front of an audience or an army corporal reveal military secrets, can it make an ordinary person into a murderer?

## "The Knife Went In"

Anthony Daniels worked for many years as a psychiatrist and prison doctor in Winson Green Prison, located in inner-city Birmingham, England. One of his major roles at the penitentiary was to run a methadone clinic to help treat the addictions of certain inmates. In doing so, he came across many of the most dangerous criminals incarcerated there. One day, a murderer came into his clinic office for a methadone dose and, during the meeting, said, "It's just my luck to be here on this charge." Confused by this comment, Daniels thought to himself,

Luck? He had already served a dozen prison sentences, many of them for violence, and on the night in question had carried a knife with him, which he must have known from experience that he was inclined to use. But it was the victim of the stabbing who was the real author of the killer's action: if he hadn't been there, he wouldn't have been stabbed. My murderer was by no means alone in explaining his deed as due to circumstances beyond his control. As it happens, there are three stabbers (two of them unto death) at present in the prison who used precisely the same expression when describing to me what happened. "The knife went in," they said when pressed to recover their allegedly lost memories of the deed.

"The knife went in." There is a stark contrast between this statement and another way the murderer could have put it: "I stabbed him." The latter declaration implies willful control over the act, while the former has a tone of passivity, as if the act just happened, irrespective of his conscious intentions. Underlying the killer's words was an excuse for his crime. He was implicitly claiming that the murder was not an act that he himself initiated but a product of the situation. Forces external to him caused the murder; the knife just happened to be in his hand when it occurred.

In discussing the murders that took place in Copenhagen in 1951 and the possibility that Nielsen used hypnosis to make Hardrup a murderer, we saw an extreme example of external forces being used to make a person do unspeakable things. But we never finished the story. Danish authorities eventually brought Nielsen in for questioning. Interrogators went back and forth between Nielsen and Hardrup, trying to make sense of this disturbing series of events and their terrifying implications. The police interviewed them together as well as in isolation. The interrogators analyzed not only the details of their stories but also their behavior, their body language, and the subtle features of their interactions. As the investigation progressed, it became increasingly clear that Nielsen did not have the character profile of a criminal mastermind. In fact, he was surprisingly dull-witted. What's more, the examiners realized that Hardrup was far more clever and manipulative than he pretended to be.

Investigators eventually determined that Nielsen did not hypnotize Hardrup to commit robbery and murder. It's true that the two of them had experimented with hypnosis, but that did not cause Hardrup to walk into that bank with a gun. Hardrup very much intended to do that himself. The hypnosis story? Well, it made for a good story. It kept the Danish authorities busy for a while and temporarily helped divert the blame away from Hardrup. Just like the prisoner who said "the knife went in," Hardrup wanted to cite situational or subconscious phenomena as the cause of his actions (though Hardrup was certainly more devious about it). But in truth, he was the author of his own actions, and he was responsible.

Hypnosis is a state of intense concentration on one train of thought. Subjects are so focused on the fantasy created by the hypnotist that they don't scrutinize the suggestions being covertly passed to them. So why couldn't one of those covert suggestions be to commit murder? The answer takes us back to the cocktail party effect. When you are at a cocktail party, focusing on one conversation prevents you from being consciously aware of other discussions in your vicinity. However, hearing your name, even from a distant conversation, jolts you out of your state of concentration. As we discussed, the same thing occurs when you hear the phrase ". . . and then she ran into the elevator completely naked!" Even when we are focused on one conversation, the brain still processes the other information coming in and alerts us when something is pertinent or significantly out of the ordinary. If jarring enough, a stimulus, even at the periphery of consciousness, can knock us out of our current state of narrow attention and return to us our better judgment.

The same goes for hypnosis. A hypnotized person may be distracted enough by his imagination that he accepts the suggestion that there is a falcon in the room, but that's not likely to be the case if the suggestion were to obtain a gun, put it in a briefcase, march into a bank, threaten the tellers, fill the briefcase with cash, and kill everyone in his path. Even in a highly suggestible person, ideas like those raise a red flag. They jolt a person out of that state of focused attention. In this way, the unconscious processes in the brain alert us whenever we need to shift our attention to something important, just as a near-collision might startle a preoccupied driver to snap out of his daydreaming and slam on the brakes. It's the brain's way of looking out for us by giving us a heads-up.

Even if we are not conscious of all of our perceptions, the brain is still diligently sorting through them. Hypnosis may modulate the activity in the anterior cingulate cortex, but it does not shut down the frontal lobe. A hypnotized person is still conscious and still able to apply some degree of scrutiny to his or her behavior. The unconscious system in the brain just has to detect that an issue is critical enough to merit immediate attention, and then it will rouse the conscious mind to action.

So, just to be clear: Can someone who is mentally healthy, with no traces of psychosis or other neuropsychological disorder, be hypnotized to commit murder? Probably not, unless he was planning to do it anyway. It would take a person for whom the command "find a gun, kill the tellers, and rob that bank" is not an idea that would raise a red flag. That would be the kind of person who has much experience with crime, someone who doesn't think much of it and could probably be persuaded to commit the act without hypnosis. In contrast, anyone who would consider such a proposition jarring could not be hypnotized to commit murder, or robbery for that matter.

## One Brain, Two Systems

At any given moment in our lives, innumerable unconscious processes are occurring in our brains. There are subconscious stimuli streaming through the nervous system of every person, leaving unique and often unforeseen neurological footprints. Whether they consist of the jingles or slogans of advertisements, the words we don't pay attention to at a cocktail party, or the subtle emotions we have whenever we meet someone, visit a new place, or have a distinctive experience, those stimuli have real effects on the way we think and make decisions, but they don't control us. The totality of these effects, combined with our conscious sensations, knowledge, and memories, is what constitutes our life experience. It helps create the fabric of our vast background knowledge from which we draw our wisdom and insight. Whenever our perceptions are incomplete or whenever we face a scenario in which we don't have all the facts, the brain unconsciously draws on this background knowledge to help supply the rest of the story. The way we make associations between ideas is guided by the unconscious mind, and we need that perspective to help narrow down the field of choice and, ultimately, to make the best decisions we can.

In this book, we have followed two brain systems, the conscious and the unconscious, to see how their interaction engenders our thoughts and behavior. The conscious system gives rise to our life experience. It's what allows us to feel our senses and emotions, reflect on our thinking, and deliberate our decisions. The conscious system creates our sense of self.

The unconscious system, on the other hand, has an extraordinary ability that we have seen demonstrated again and again. It recognizes patterns, using context to anticipate events before they happen. It fills in the gaps, reconciling disconnected elements of our experience in order to maintain a complete personal narrative. The unconscious system does this when stitching together the plotlines of our dreams or generating gut feelings. In memory disorders, it may confabulate, bridging holes in recall by substituting related anecdotes from the brain's store of knowledge. In schizophrenia, it ventures as far as to fabricate elaborate stories, featuring government conspiracies or supernatural intrusions, to cover up an internal defect in self-recognition. It helps us rationalize our thoughts and behavior, even if we act because of external influences such as hypnosis, subliminal messages, or advertising.

The unconscious system in the brain goes to great lengths to fill in the gaps, to rationalize irrational behavior, and to concoct logical explanations for thoroughly illogical situations. Throughout this journey of ours, we've seen case after case and study after study that demonstrate that, but the question is, why? Why maintain a complete narrative? Why is it necessary to invent an explanation that reconciles confusing or conflicting experiences? The reason, as we will see, is to preserve our sense of self.

As human beings, we have a need to understand the order and organization of the world around us, as well as our place in it. In order to contemplate our needs and desires, as well as to set goals and devise plans to fulfill them, we each must appreciate our personal history, be able to reflect on it, and gain insight into ourselves. Losses of memory, gaps in our perceptions or thinking, conflicts in our experience, external subversions—these are all threats to our personal narrative, and the brain endeavors to protect it. The unconscious system maintains the unity and continuity of the self and will go to extremes to secure that end. There is one circumstance, however, in which the brain goes so far in pursuit of this goal that it actually breaks apart the self in order to preserve it. This brings us to Evelyn.

# Why Can't Split Personalities Share Prescription Glasses?

*On Personality, Trauma, and the Defense of the Self*

> I learned to recognize the thorough and primitive duality of man; I saw that, of the two natures that contended in the field of my consciousness, even if I could rightly be said to be either, it was only because I was radically both.
>
> —Robert Louis Stevenson

Evelyn was in bad shape when she was admitted to the inpatient psychiatric unit. A thirty-five-year-old single mother, she was legally blind and traveled the city with the help of a guide dog. The cause of her blindness was unknown. An old file in her chart listed the diagnosis as "congenital blindness due to bilateral optic nerve injury," yet there was no proof for that. No medical work-up was documented and Evelyn couldn't confirm that she had ever undergone testing to determine why she lost her vision. But it wasn't Evelyn's eyes that brought her to the psych ward. It was her skin.

Carved deeply into her forearms were the words "FAT PIG" and "I HATE YOU." She had no idea how they had gotten there. Neither could she explain why her skin had evidence of old burn injuries. A review of hospital records revealed that Evelyn had come to the hospital one year earlier with the words "DUMB SHIT" and "MAD" cut into her skin. She claimed she didn't do these things to herself and she couldn't think of anyone else who could have done so. After all, she lived only with her young son.

Why couldn't Evelyn identify her abuser? Perhaps it had to do with an anomaly she described with her memory. When she first noticed the cuts, Evelyn couldn't remember what had happened to her in the prior hours. Throughout her life, she had experienced "blackouts" or "lost time," hours missing from her memory. As Evelyn described it, "I have noticed, since I can remember, that I have lost periods of time, and they were very frightening when I was young, and mysterious as I grew older, and I was afraid to tell anyone about it because I thought they would lock me up and throw away the key."

She could never know for sure what happened during those missing hours, but occasionally she would discover clues: "When I come to I might find toys, like my son's preschool toys. I have found grocery or shopping bags full of several items that I would not buy."

Evelyn traced these problems to her childhood. She had a horrific upbringing. As an infant, she had to be taken from her biological mother because of physical and sexual abuse. Child protective services discovered her locked in a closet and immediately put her in foster care. She was adopted at age two by parents who had finalized their divorce by Evelyn's tenth birthday. Her adoptive father physically and sexually abused her just as her biological mother had. Evelyn's adoptive brother, nine years older than she was, used to tie her up and try to strangle her. The entire family blamed Evelyn for the divorce, citing the difficulty of managing her visual problems.

When Evelyn turned eight years old, her doctor arranged for her to transfer to a school for the blind. Before her doctor explained that there was probably something structurally wrong with her eyes, Evelyn had assumed that her visual impairment and struggles in school were her own fault. Soon after beginning classes at her new school, just following her adoptive parents' divorce, Evelyn had her first episode of "lost time." Later that day, she discovered bruises and small abrasions on her arms and legs, but she had no idea how they got there. She couldn't say what had just happened to her or how much time had passed since her last accessible memory.

What was happening to Evelyn? Who cut the messages into her arms? Was someone assaulting her and she was just forgetting it? Or, alternatively, was she harming herself? Back at the hospital, doctors would soon discover that in a certain sense the answer was a little bit of both.

Evelyn was diagnosed with dissociative identity disorder, the mental illness formally known as multiple personality disorder. Her condition left her with several alternate personalities. There was the adult female character "Franny F." Franny F. held a baby named Cynthia. There was the "scary-looking" ten-year-old girl Sarah, who had "red, stringy hair," brown eyes, and freckles. Finally, there was Kimmy, the "angelic-looking" four-year-old girl, with blue eyes and short blond hair. Her mannerisms changed depending on which personality was in play. As Evelyn, she came across as intelligent, mature, and remarkably articulate. As Kimmy, her voice suddenly became childish, and she mispronounced common words, such as calling a purple shirt "poiple." She said the president was "her daddy" and excitedly expressed the discovery that the word "orange" refers to both a color and a fruit. She said her older brother was teaching her how to print her name. Here's an excerpt of a conversation Kimmy had with her psychiatrist:

> PSYCHIATRIST: How old are you?
> KIMMY: I be four.
> PSYCHIATRIST: You be four? My goodness, what a big girl! What are you doing right now, Kimmy?
> KIMMY: Um, just trying to sit here and be a good girl.
> PSYCHIATRIST: Oh, is it important to be a good girl?
> KIMMY: Yes.
> PSYCHIATRIST: Why is it so important?
> KIMMY: 'Cause when I be bad I get hurt.
> PSYCHIATRIST: Oh, I am sorry. Who hurt you?
> KIMMY: My mommy and daddy.

As she spoke about this abuse, Kimmy shut her eyes tightly and clutched her teddy bear. Later, in a more sunny part of the conversation:

> PSYCHIATRIST: What games do you like to play?
> KIMMY: Ring around the roseys and we all fall down, and the bridge, and take the keys and lock 'em up, and suck the goose, and I like play with bears.
> PSYCHIATRIST: Real bears?
> KIMMY: No, but they are my friends.

As Evelyn switched between alter egos, it wasn't just her personality that changed. For example, Kimmy used a pencil with her right hand, yet Evelyn was left-handed. The greatest shock came when the psychiatrists tried a vision test. When evaluated with a standard vision chart, Evelyn's vision was 20/200, which qualifies as legally blind. Franny F. and Cynthia were also 20/200. Sarah's vision, however, was 20/80. As for Kimmy, she had a visual acuity of 20/60. That difference between 20/60 and 20/200 is the difference between needing a pair of mild prescription glasses and being legally blind. Evelyn had a Seeing Eye dog, but her alter ago just needed glasses. How is that possible? After all, both personalities have the same set of eyes.

That's just a fraction of the problem. How can a person have more than one personality in the first place? Are these just extreme fluctuations in mood, or are they truly separate, independently functioning identities? If the latter is true, if the alter egos are indeed discrete conscious entities, then the most glaring question seems to be, which one is truly Evelyn?

We all have a rich sense of *self.* It's not simply that we understand ourselves or know our tendencies. We feel as if we are somewhere in our heads, looking out onto the world. We seem to have an inner essence that numbs with pain or trembles with excitement. That internal identity is not just a passive experiencer but an active agent. We reflect on our thoughts, deliberate on decisions, and wield actions—all from what seems to be a central controller within us. There is something in our heads that the word "I" refers to, and it appears to be singular, unified, and consistent through time. Yet Evelyn's case seems to imply that the self can be fragmented. It can be broken down, split apart, separated into component personalities that grow and develop individually.

Throughout this book, we have witnessed the interaction of the conscious and the unconscious systems in the brain that together bring about our thoughts and behavior. Somewhere amid these two processors there emerges the human self, leading so many of us to ask the elusive question, where exactly am I in my brain? Before we address the issue of multiple selves, let's start with just one. What do we really mean by the concepts of self and identity? From where in the brain might such a phenomenon arise? It's perhaps the greatest mystery of neuroscience, and answers are not easy to come by, but we can approach it as best we can. In fact, we have been implicitly doing so since the very first page of this book. So, where do we begin? As is the practice in neurology, the first step in investigating any brain system is to see what happens when it's broken.

## Finding One Self

On a cold November evening in Poland, a gynecologist named Peter got into his car after a heated argument with his wife. Fuming, Peter was preoccupied as he drove through the darkness, replaying the fight over and over in his mind. He was having trouble staying on the road. Suddenly he realized he had edged into the wrong lane. A delivery truck was rocketing directly toward him. He spun his wheel to the right, his car swerving and spinning off the road, and ran head-on into a tree. Then everything went black. Peter was in a coma for sixty-three days.

When Peter finally awoke, he wasn't the same. Before the accident, he was a fun, witty, and personable guy. At the age of forty-three, he had a wife and three children and loved to play with his dog. Now, tragically, he didn't know who he was. He could easily name famous public figures yet didn't know his own name, and that was only the beginning. Over the next decade, a group of psychologists tracked Peter's mental state, as his neurological deficits took a number of different forms, all seemingly related to damage to his identity and sense of self.

For starters, Peter was unable to recognize his own appearance. When a therapist named Jacek had Peter stand in front of a full-length mirror with him, they had the following exchange:

JACEK: Who is that, Peter? Who do you see there?
PETER: I don't know. Oh my God! That monster is staring at me!
JACEK: And who else do you see in the mirror?
PETER: I don't know, but maybe Jacek. I think you said so, isn't that right?

Peter was able to identify a man he barely knew yet could not recognize his own reflection. Tragically, he also couldn't recognize those closest to him.

When Peter's family came to visit, he began shouting, "I don't have a family. My family was all killed in an accident. I don't know these people . . . They are body doubles . . . doubles of my entire family or I don't know!" You may remember that this is Capgras syndrome, the condition in which people believe that those around them have been replaced by physically identical impostors. As we discussed in chapter 5, Capgras syndrome (like its counterpart, the Cotard delusion, in which people believe themselves to be dead) is a symptom of feeling oneself to be dissociated from the world. When people with Capgras syndrome see their loved ones, they don't feel that emotional connection they are supposed to, and their brains concoct a story to explain the disconnect. In that sense, Capgras syndrome is a manifestation of a faded sense of self.

Peter's next symptom was another one we've encountered before: gaps in his memory. He couldn't remember basic facts about his life. For example, he denied ever having had a dog. When his therapist brought the dog over to convince him otherwise, Peter exclaimed, "A lump of fur like that! I don't own a dog. I wouldn't want such a rubbishy thing! I'm afraid of this dog. It wants to bite me!" He similarly didn't remember that he was a gynecologist, but he had an excuse for that too. "I'm too young to be a doctor," he claimed. "Everyone thinks that I'm 40 when I'm really 20." To explain this discrepancy, Peter cited an alleged government conspiracy:

> The government has not only changed the money and I can't recognize it, but also the calendar to avoid paying the life annuity . . . they added 30 years to the established calendar and as a result I am supposed to be 45 years old, but really, I'm 25. They want to get rid of me. I'm scared.

Peter had developed confabulation. His brain was unconsciously bridging the gaps in his memory, concocting stories to explain his various deficits as logically as possible. He didn't remember owning a dog, so he touted the excuse that the animal was "rubbishy" and had the intent to bite him. He wouldn't own a rubbishy or violent pet, so that couldn't possibly be his dog. When he couldn't remember his profession, he confabulated the idea that the government manipulated the calendar and that his true age rendered it impossible that he could be a doctor.

For each element of his identity that Peter lost, his unconscious brain was quick to generate an explanation to cover up the void. His personal identity was broken, yet his brain was trying to put the pieces together.

It seemed, however, that Peter's injury was too severe, his loss of personhood too profound, to be mended by these patches. The gap was too large to fill. Peter's brain had to look elsewhere to fix his loss of self. Unable to extract enough information from its own store of knowledge and memory, with Peter's fragile identity hanging in the balance, his brain began to borrow from other people.

While in the hospital, Peter shared a room with a patient named Jurek, who had just undergone knee surgery. One morning, when the staff came by his room, Peter demanded that he be brought a wheelchair. He said he couldn't walk because of his knee operation. He also mentioned that his name was actually Jurek. Later, Peter was approached by a twenty-nine-year-old art therapist who explained that his job was to use art to help teach self-expression. Peter grabbed the brushes from him and refused to return them, claiming that he needed them for his profession. He also stole the art therapist's name and claimed to be twenty-nine years old.

The changes that Peter underwent all appear to be related to his sense of self. So the question is, what parts of his brain did he lose in the car accident that caused these deficits?

An MRI of the brain showed that Peter had suffered damage to his frontal and temporal lobes, together known as the frontotemporal region. The worst of it was in the right hemisphere.

Not recognizing oneself in the mirror, Capgras syndrome, and confabulation are all associated with right frontotemporal lobe damage. That pattern of brain damage is consistent with a slew of cases from the annals of neurology of patients who lose their sense of identity. For example, consider the condition of asomatognosia, in which people lack the feeling of ownership over a limb that has been paralyzed. They claim that the immobile arm or leg doesn't belong to them. Todd Feinberg, a neurologist at the Albert Einstein College of Medicine and an expert on asomatognosia, recorded the following exchange with such a patient, named Shirley, who denied ownership of her left arm after it had become paralyzed:

SHIRLEY: It took a vacation without telling me it was going. It didn't ask, it just went.
FEINBERG: What did?
SHIRLEY: My Pet Rock. [She lifted her lifeless left arm with her right arm to indicate what she was talking about.]

FEINBERG: You call that your Pet Rock?

SHIRLEY: Yeah.

FEINBERG: Why do you call it your Pet Rock?

SHIRLEY: Because it doesn't do anything. It just sits there.

Patients with asomatognosia will usually declare that the limb is an inanimate object such as "a piece of rusty machinery," "a bag of bones," or "my dead husband's hand." Most often, they'll claim the limb belongs to someone else, such as their doctor or someone in their family.

Asomatognosia is a lot like Capgras syndrome, except instead of feeling dissociated from other people, you feel dissociated from your own body. It's yet another case of neuro-logic at work. The damaged brain is unable to recognize that the paralyzed limb is part of the body. The unconscious system therefore has to reconcile two conflicting pieces of information. First, there is a nearby object that looks like a hand and always seems to be nearby. Second, that object doesn't respond to motor commands. What logical explanation can the brain generate? It must be someone else's hand or at least an inanimate object that is always by one's side, like a Pet Rock.

Asomatognosia results from damage to the right frontal, temporal, and parietal cortices. Again, the right frontotemporal network appears to be involved.

Studies of self-identity seem to agree with the clinical cases. Experiments using fMRI have shown that the right prefrontal cortex (part of the frontotemporal region) is active as we engage in self-reflection but not while we think about other people. The literature on locating the neural correlates of the self is vast and could easily fill an entire book, but the consensus seems to be that we don't know exactly where the self lives in the brain. Broadly speaking, it's probably in the right frontal lobe because the activity of that region is highly correlated with self-referential activity, as we have just seen. However, that contention has to be considered with skepticism, because it is by no means the only region that contributes to the emergence of identity.

Nevertheless, Peter's case reveals the many aspects of human identity that can be expunged by brain injury: the ability to recognize ourselves and those we care about; the memory of our personal history; a consistent sense of our personality and how we differ from others; a feeling of control over our thoughts and actions. When Peter was asked to draw a picture to help express himself, he drew a ladybug, explaining, "My insides remind me of a ladybug. She's looking for something, because it's empty inside her, like it's empty inside me."

We know that our sense of self can be destroyed by brain damage, but how can it be split apart? Evelyn didn't have any apparent source of brain damage, yet her body was at various times under the control of different personalities. How is this possible? If we suppose, as many neurologists do, that human identity is localizable to a rough area of the brain, then it would seem that we could surgically separate the self into parts by cutting up the brain. If, under anesthesia, we were to slice a person's brain in half, who would wake up after the operation? Would it be one person or two?

## A Brain Divided

There is a surgery available for severe, uncontrolled epilepsy called a corpus callosotomy in which the corpus callosum, the thick nerve bundle that connects the right and left sides of the brain, is cut. Because seizures are electrical storms that propagate along nerve bundles in the brain, detaching the two halves of the brain prevents the electricity from crossing over and overtaking both hemispheres. This last-resort procedure can do wonders for someone with otherwise uncontrollable seizures, but it can have some strange side effects.

The well-studied split-brain syndrome is the most infamous. Just ask Vicki, who had the procedure done in June 1979. During the months after surgery, the two sides of her brain would act independently. For example, while shopping at the supermarket, she noticed that as she would reach toward a shelf with one hand, her other hand seemed to have a mind of its own. "I'd reach with my right [hand] for the thing I wanted," she says, "but the left would come in and they'd kind of fight. Almost like repelling magnets."

The same thing would happen each morning as she tried to get dressed. She would intend to select one outfit, but one of her hands might decide to pick a different one. "I'd have to dump all the clothes on the bed, catch my breath and start again," she says. Once in a while, Vicki became so frustrated that she just gave in and left the house wearing three outfits at once.

Split-brain syndrome is a condition in which the disconnected hemispheres of the brain begin acting independently of each other. Vicki was experiencing alien hand syndrome, which we discussed briefly in chapter 2 as one of the possible consequences of frontal lobe dysfunction. It's also a prevalent symptom of split-brain syndrome, because the right brain controls the left hand and the left brain controls the right. This cross control also applies to vision: the right side of the brain processes vision from the left visual field and vice versa. What's more, the left brain (in a right-handed person) controls language production. Because of this lateralization, each hemisphere of a split brain has its own set of abilities and perceptions that it cannot share with the other. For example, if Vicki's left hemisphere sees a written word in the right visual field, she is able to say the word aloud, because the left brain controls spoken language. However, when that same word appears in her left visual field, where only her right hemisphere will see it, Vicki is unable to vocalize it but can take a pen and write it down.

The neuroscientist Michael Gazzaniga, the leader of split-brain research, has been running these studies for five decades. Throughout his research, aside from discovering how our various cognitive abilities are assigned to each hemisphere, Gazzaniga wondered whether each individual hemisphere has its own sense of self. Certainly, each half brain has access to sensations, perceptions, and skills that the other does not, but does each side have its own self-reflective, decision-making consciousness?

Gazzaniga thought so when he began his research in the 1960s. After all, when two halves of the body are wrestling in a supermarket aisle, that conclusion seems completely reasonable. Since then, however, it has become apparent to him that the two sides actually do share one sense of self. Despite having no access to what the other side knows or does, the hemispheres seem to cooperate in trying to sustain that singular identity.

In one experiment, Gazzaniga showed the word "walk" to a split-brain patient's right hemisphere by placing it in the left visual field. The patient stood up and began walking. When the patient was later asked why he began to walk, he provided a reason: "I wanted to go get a Coke." The left brain, responsible for language production, generated that explanation, yet it did so without knowing that the instruction "walk" was ever displayed. Only the right brain saw that. The left brain simply made up a reason.

In another illustration, Gazzaniga flashed a picture of apples to a woman's right brain. Upon seeing the image, the woman laughed. When asked why she laughed, the woman replied that "the machine was funny, or something," referring to the machine displaying the picture. When Gazzaniga showed the same image to her left brain, she laughed again and quickly pointed to the depiction of a nude woman that was hidden among the apples.

Finally, in one of his favorite experiments, Gazzaniga displayed the word "smile" to a split-brain patient's right hemisphere and the word "face" to his left. He then verbally asked the patient to draw whatever words he had just seen. The patient drew a smiley face. When Gazzaniga asked him why, the patient replied, "What do you want, a sad face? Who wants a sad face around?" The left brain never saw the word "smile," so it fabricated an explanation for why the face had to be smiley.

In all of these cases, the left brain (which was doing all the talking) was ignorant of what the right brain was seeing yet tried admirably to concoct logical explanations for the behaviors of walking, laughing, and drawing a smile. Faced with utterly confounding circumstances, it was filling in the gaps. If the two halves of the brain were separate conscious selves, why would they try to cooperate in this way? Why not just plead ignorance?

Even when surgically separated, the two halves of the brain don't behave as separate entities. They somehow find a way to preserve a unified sense of self by trying to reconcile each other's behavior. Gazzaniga attributes this phenomenon to the efforts of the left hemisphere, because that's the side of the brain that came up with all the excuses in his experiments. He hypothesizes that there is a "left-hemisphere interpreter," a region of the left brain that tries to pull together all of our daily experiences and construct a single, unified narrative to make sense of them. He acknowledges the extensive research we saw that seems to imply that the sense of self emerges from the *right* hemisphere (specifically the right frontotemporal region, as we saw earlier) but argues that self-processing is actually spread throughout the brain—and the left hemisphere plays a crucial role. It binds our experiences to create our personal stories, our internal, unconscious rationalizations that we've been calling neuro-logic. At least in the split-brain experiments, the left brain is filling in the gaps.

Whether there is a left hemisphere interpreter, and how it might work, is a question that remains under investigation. Nevertheless, what we can say is that there is an unconscious system in the brain that, when faced with conflicting pieces of information, generates a narrative to reconcile them. It's the same scenario we've seen over and over again throughout this book. It happens in asomatognosia and Capgras syndrome. It causes the Cotard delusion and alien abduction stories. It's the reason why people with schizophrenia believe they are being watched by the FBI or controlled by supernatural forces. It's the source of confabulation and false memories. It composes the narrative of our dreams.

The brain has a tendency to fill voids in our thinking and perceptions whenever they may be incomplete. Each time the brain fills in the gaps, it does so with a purpose: to preserve our sense of self. The unconscious system is thoroughly focused on protecting our personal narrative, the stability of human identity, and its efforts are never more evident than in cases of emotional trauma.

## See No Evil

It was a day the Ackermans would have prayed to forget. It was the worst car accident they could imagine, and they were right in the thick of it. The collision involved more than one hundred vehicles. The injured lay everywhere. Several people died. After smashing into the vehicle in front of them, the Ackermans were briefly trapped in their car. As the husband and wife watched someone burn to death outside their window, the realization set in that they might die within moments.

But they survived. Mr. Ackerman, adrenaline pulsing through his body, broke open the windshield and, after climbing through the shattered glass, pulled his wife out of the car and led her to safety. After escaping the wreckage, the Ackermans were rushed to the hospital for evaluation. Luckily, neither of them had been injured, at least not physically. Mentally, they were traumatized. The psychological toll of the accident was severe, but it affected Mr. and Mrs. Ackerman in different ways.

During the collision, Mr. Ackerman felt his mind switch to overdrive. A surge of fear and anxiety. The desperate search for an escape route. The chaos in his mind paralleled the chaos beyond his windshield. In the days that followed, he began having terrifying flashbacks. Nightmares awoke him regularly in a cold sweat. He felt wired at work and couldn't concentrate. He was easily startled, recoiling at the sound of loud noises, and became a nervous, hyperaware driver.

Mrs. Ackerman, on the other hand, had the opposite reaction. During the crash, she sat as if entranced, numb to the outside world. She felt somehow distant from the events occurring around her. She was "in shock." She perceived the pandemonium and recognized that she was in imminent danger, yet the emotional force of the trauma did not seem to impact her mind.

The Ackermans' reactions represent two extremes of a spectrum used to classify a person's response to trauma. Mr. Ackerman had the stress reaction known as hyperarousal, which is characteristic of posttraumatic stress disorder (PTSD). Mrs. Ackerman, on the other hand, exhibited dissociation, the feeling of distance between oneself and one's emotions and experiences. Two people, one traumatic event, two very different psychological reactions. What could have happened in their brains to account for these divergent responses?

The couple agreed to participate in a short fMRI study in which their brains were scanned as they reimagined the day of the accident. The results revealed drastic differences in brain activity between husband and wife. Mr. Ackerman showed activation in his frontal, temporal, and parietal lobes, among other regions. What's more, his heart rate increased significantly, and he reported feeling anxious and "jumpy" during the session.

In contrast, Mrs. Ackerman didn't feel anxious during the study. Her heart rate remained steady, and she reported feeling extremely "numb" and "frozen" while recollecting the accident. On the fMRI, the BOLD signal did not highlight the swath of brain tissue that was active during her husband's session. Only a tiny part of her occipital lobe was illuminated on the fMRI as she mentally visualized the accident. It was as if her brain blocked the hyperarousal response from occurring, instead anesthetizing her emotional reaction.

Psychological trauma is perhaps the greatest threat to the human sense of self. It can destroy the will to act, relegating the physically healthy to sit idly in their beds because of psychological paralysis in depression or grief. It haunts veterans with PTSD. It can even nullify the will to live, as it can tragically lead to suicide.

Alternatively, psychological trauma can result in the feeling of dissociation from oneself. In psychiatry, there is a spectrum of dissociative disorders in which people, to varying degrees, feel separated from the world around them or experience what feels like a loss of their own identity. For example, in depersonalization disorder, people feel detached from themselves and their surroundings, as if they are just watching the world rather than experiencing it. In dissociative fugue, a more dramatic form of dissociation, people completely forget who they are and where they live (it usually happens after traveling far away), and they tend to take on a new identity. Dissociative identity disorder, which is what Evelyn had, is the most severe of these conditions, in which a person's personality and sense of self become fragmented into what seems like several discrete identities.

Dissociative conditions usually result from emotional trauma, and like the trauma that causes them, they are extremely difficult to bear. To feel separated from the world, to constantly feel as if you were watching from afar, seems like a cruel curse. Yet it has a purpose: it protects victims from having to relive the pain of their trauma. The feeling of dissociation is an unconscious defense mechanism. Most commonly exhibited by victims of long-standing abuse, it insulates the fragile psyche from having to endure the emotional toll of the past.

Our brains are equipped to defend against the destructive potential of psychological trauma. As we saw with memory repression (chapter 4), the mind can distance itself from memories or feelings that are too agonizing to bear. The feeling of dissociation is a side effect of the brain's self-defense mechanism. Consider, by analogy, the way the body may react to a bacterial infection. To prevent the foreign invader from spreading, the immune system walls off the infection, forming an abscess. Once encapsulated, the bacteria are quarantined off from nearby tissue. This defense mechanism is not without side effects, however, because abscesses are excruciatingly tender.

Dissociation similarly quarantines the traumatized portion of the psyche. It redirects attention away from all that is painful, attempting to isolate the poisonous thoughts from the conscious self. But the emotional damage never quite disappears; it's just locked away in some deep cavern of the mind. Researchers have termed such regions the "emotional parts" of the brain, the abscess of haunted thoughts and memories. The emotional parts represent the traumatized aspects of the self that have been buried. In contrast, the areas spared by the trauma are known in the literature as the "apparently normal parts." Ideally, just as an abscess shouldn't rupture, the emotional parts and the apparently normal parts should remain isolated from one another, never making contact. But that isn't always the case. When a damaged part of the mind is segregated from the rest, there is always the risk that it will not remain dormant. The haunted aspect of the self might reemerge from its exile, resurfacing as an alternate personality, the Mr. Hyde to your Dr. Jekyll.

Enter dissociative identity disorder. It is the tendency to switch back and forth between formerly disconnected aspects of personality. On the one hand, there is the everyday, neutral self (the "apparently normal parts"), who functions well in society but feels dissociated from himself and the world. On the other hand, there is the haunted self (the "emotional parts"), which has been distorted by emotional trauma. It is as if a person switches between Mr. and Mrs. Ackerman's reactions to trauma. We might think of Mr. Ackerman, who had the hyperarousal reaction, as the emotional parts. Haunted by the car accident, he developed nightmares, severe anxiety, and a loss of emotional control that made it difficult to function. His wife had a reaction reminiscent of the apparently normal parts: emotionally blunted and dissociated. Though calm during the accident, she felt an emotional barrier develop in her mind.

When reimagining the car accident, the Ackermans exhibited drastically different stress levels that paralleled their reactions during the incident itself. As we know from chapter 3, mental simulations tend to be very true to life. Studies show that, just as the Ackermans did during the experiment, patients' alternate personalities will develop different stress levels while picturing their traumas. While mentally reliving the traumatic incident, one personality may respond with a pounding heart rate and rapid breathing, like Mr. Ackerman, while another personality will show no change in vitals, like Mrs. Ackerman. Thought of this way, dissociative identity disorder is a combination of dissociation and hyperarousal, where the dissociated self is the default and the hyperaroused, unstable alter ago emerges sporadically.

When Evelyn arrived at the hospital with insults carved into her arms, the immediate task was to determine who her abuser was. It seems clear that the abuser was herself, or rather an aspect of herself. Her disorder developed as an adaptive mechanism. The goal? To protect her sense of self from the psychological destruction wreaked upon her mind by years of abuse. Each alter ego represented a fragment of her personality and history that had been quarantined long ago but would suddenly reawaken.

Perhaps this explanation seems plausible on the surface, but is there any neurological evidence? After all, we've seen how difficult it is to break apart the self. Even when a surgeon cuts a brain in half, forcing the cerebral hemispheres to operate on their own, a person's sense of self does not split. The unconscious system digs deep to think up ways to maintain the continuity of identity, even in the midst of a divided brain. It has no idea that the corpus callosum has been severed, only that there is a schism between thought and behavior that must be bridged.

In someone with dissociative identity disorder, however, there is no obvious brain damage. Evelyn never fell on her head or suffered a car accident. She certainly never had her brain cut in half. Yet her identity was fragmented into various alter egos, each of which had no knowledge of the other. These apparently discrete personalities shared no memories and obtained radically different results on tests of vision. How could this be? How can you divide a mind without physically slicing up the brain?

## The Fragmentation of the Mind

What happens in the brain as a person cycles between multiple personalities? To investigate that question, a group of researchers in the Netherlands recruited eleven patients with dissociative identity disorder to participate in a neuroimaging study. Their plan was to provoke the patients to switch personalities while a PET scanner monitored for any changes in brain activity. After thorough interviews with the participants, the researchers developed eleven personalized scripts that would encourage each of them to imagine traumatizing events in their lives. It has been well established that stress is a trigger for personality switches in dissociative identity disorder, and what could be more stressful than reimagining the very suffering that brought on the condition?

While the volunteers were hooked up to the PET scanner, the researchers used the scripts to incite the personality changes. For most of the volunteers, it worked. Their heart rates suddenly quickened, their blood pressure rose, and they felt as if they inhabited their alter egos. So what did the PET results show?

When the subjects were their neutral personalities, their brain activity looked like that of someone experiencing a dissociative state. The activity was blunted, reminiscent of Mrs. Ackerman's dissociative reaction after her car accident. If the switch occurred, however, several brain regions suddenly ignited on the scan, especially the amygdala, the brain's emotional center. This reaction was more like Mr. Ackerman's hyperarousal state after the accident. The emotional system in the brain illuminated while the haunted self was active but quieted down while the neutral self was in play. That implies that while in their neutral state people with dissociative identity disorder are protected from their harmful emotions and may be able to confront their past without incident. However, should their defenses fail and the haunted self reemerge, their emotional system becomes vulnerable, and painful feelings may overtake them.

But that's not all that the researchers noticed. There was another part of the brain that behaved differently with each personality switch: the hippocampus, the hub of episodic memory (memory for life events). The PET signal illuminated different parts of the hippocampus depending on which identity was in play. It was as if each alter ego had access to some memories but not to others.

Unfortunately, Evelyn never had brain imaging to confirm whether such findings applied to her, so we can only hypothesize that her personality divisions were reflected in her neurologic activity. Evelyn, Franny F., Sarah, and Kimmy certainly did seem independently compartmentalized in one person. They not only had unique patterns of behavior but were unable to access one another's memories. Kimmy was a child still learning to print her name, yet Evelyn was a mature adult. One of the personalities was carving obscene insults into her own skin, but Evelyn reported amnesia for those periods of time. Because we know that Evelyn's hippocampus was not physically cut into quarters, creating four separate memory stores, the only other explanation is that each personality was using different parts of one memory bank. Evelyn's neutral self had access to the regular, untainted memories but not to any traumatic ones. That access was blocked. The ugly heads of the alter egos emerged when those inactive parts of the hippocampus (and other quarantined brain regions) were suddenly activated, perhaps by stress or some other trigger.

In fact, alternate personalities even have different reactions to threatening *unconscious* stimuli. In a 2013 experiment, neuroscientists showed patients with dissociative identity disorder images of angry faces using backward masking. If you remember from our previous chapter, backward masking is the technique by which images are flashed so briefly that we do not consciously see them, yet the images exert effects on the unconscious. Using fMRI, the researchers discovered that when they showed the angry faces to the haunted personalities, there was a burst of activity in the parahippocampal gyrus, a region that works with the hippocampus in recalling autobiographical memories. That didn't happen when the neutral personalities were shown the images. No memories were activated. The neuroscientists explained this difference by hypothesizing that while the haunted self is in play, the threatening faces unconsciously trigger the emergence of traumatic memories. In contrast, while the neutral identities were active, those memories were not accessed. The brain shielded them from any association with the masked faces.

If it's true that each alternate personality has different and unique access to our emotions and memories, that would suggest a neurological basis for the development of multiple personalities. It is not simply that the mind, in an abstract sense, quarantines parts of the psyche. Rather, the brain segregates its actual neuronal processing to prevent volatile memories and emotions from overlapping with self-reflective cognition.

What's more, the unique way in which dissociative identity patients process memory and emotion appears to shape the anatomy of their brains. The laws of brain plasticity dictate that frequently used areas of the brain experience neuronal growth and get bigger. Neglected regions of the brain experience neural atrophy and shrink. In theory, if you were to quarantine a fraction of your memories and emotions, cutting off access to the involved neurons in the hippocampus and amygdala, then those brain regions should gradually shrink over time due to underuse. Using MRI, researchers have shown that this is indeed the case. In people with dissociative identity disorder, when compared with controls, the hippocampus is 19.2 percent smaller, and the amygdala is 31.6 percent smaller on average. So, not only do the alternate personalities exhibit reduced brain activity in the memory and emotion regions, but that activation pattern is also reflected in the brain's physical structure. Because the emotionally traumatic memories are accessed only by the haunted personalities, which seldom emerge, the brain regions that store those memories become neglected and shrink in size.

We've seen that memories may be repressed, forgotten, and falsely remembered. Now we wonder whether they can split apart, become accessible to one personality but not another. Is that really possible? In addition to the studies we've seen, in several isolated cases neuroimaging has demonstrated unique patterns of activity in the hippocampus, temporal lobe, and prefrontal cortex that change simultaneously as patients cycle between personalities. Studies also suggest that people with the disorder have reduced activity in the orbitofrontal cortex. If you recall from chapter 3, that's the site of somatic markers, which dictate emotional memories and gut feelings. In short, the memory system behaves differently in people with multiple personalities, lending support to the idea that each personality has only partial access.

The idea that multiple systems within one brain can have different access to memory isn't entirely new. In fact, we need to look no further than the habit and non-habit systems in chapter 2. The habit and non-habit systems in the brain use different forms of memory (procedural versus episodic) that are stored and accessed in different places (the striatum versus the hippocampus). When the preoccupied driver is using his habit system to steer, he remembers how to drive just fine, because the habit system uses procedural memory. However, because the habit system has no access to episodic memory, the preoccupied driver forgets that he has to pick up a gallon of milk on his way home from work. If, even in someone without a trauma history, two brain systems are unable to share certain memories, then conceivably the same might happen for Evelyn's alter egos.

The research on these issues is still in its infancy. Concrete data are limited, the findings are vague, and seemingly every aspect of the diagnosis is a point of controversy among psychiatrists. Yet with the help of neurological studies, we can cautiously say that dissociative identity disorder arises when formerly latent regions of the memory and emotional circuitry are reanimated, the previously dormant neurons reawakened. The brain decommissioned those regions to protect the self from the pain and anguish of the past, but new emotional stressors can reactivate them. Stress changes the brain from within, leading to the reemergence of haunted aspects of the self that were meant to be locked in some dark vault of neuronal isolation.

However, there may be another way to draw out the alter egos. What if we could, from the outside, bring forth the haunted personalities without inducing stress? While she was hospitalized, something happened to Evelyn that, at first glance, appears to challenge the very concept of multiple personalities. There's another chapter to her story.

## The Hypnotist Within

Back at the hospital psychiatric ward, Evelyn and her alter egos were having their eyes checked. Each identity had a different visual profile, with unique and reproducible scores on tests of eyesight. In running the testing, however, the examiners didn't simply wait around for each personality to arise. They brought them out, one at a time, using hypnosis.

After speaking with Kimmy for a while and testing her vision, one of the examiners said, "Switch and let us talk to Sarah for a few minutes."

Kimmy hesitated. "She is scared." After some encouragement, Sarah's more mature voice emerged, replacing Kimmy's.

"I'll talk to you," Sarah began. "I'm feeling better since Kimmy's my friend now. It was hard for me to give her a hug, it was scary."

Did you notice what happened there? Kimmy and Sarah acknowledged each other's existence. How did they know about each other? If they are separate conscious identities, who don't share thoughts or memories, Kimmy could not have known that Sarah was scared. How could she have known who Sarah was in the first place?

One of the defining characteristics of Evelyn's condition is that the alternate personalities are unaware of each other and do not share memories. Yet, somehow, hypnosis breaks this barrier, granting the characters access to each other's thoughts and inclinations and even allowing them to interact. For this reason, hypnosis is one of the main treatment options for dissociative identity disorder. It allows for the traumatized alter egos to emerge in a controlled environment. Hypnosis helps soothe patients, helps get to the root of the trauma, and can even help merge the alter egos to rebuild one single personality. It certainly helped Evelyn. After hypnosis, she said, "I feel better. It's like trying to put a jigsaw puzzle together, putting the pieces together, and I feel like the first piece is there."

Hypnosis can also worsen the symptoms of dissociative identity disorder, reinforcing the construct of multiple personalities. For that reason, some psychiatrists subscribe to the belief that the condition does not arise internally, but rather is induced by therapists who encourage patients to acknowledge these alter egos and talk about their respective feelings, giving credence to the bizarre idea that they exist. Another interpretation, however, is that dissociative identity disorder is a true illness that arises internally but does so through a mechanism neurologically similar to hypnosis.

If you remember from the previous chapter, it is believed that hypnosis works by focusing a person's attention on a certain idea or vision. The subject, guided by the hypnotist, focuses so intently on this single train of thought that he ignores the rest of his perceptions. Like someone concentrating on one conversation at a cocktail party, he tunes out the rest of the room. What also gets tuned out is the person's capacity to carefully reflect on his behavior, which is why, supposing he's a subject at a hypnosis show, he fails to notice the peculiarity of his dancing a jig onstage or wrestling with an imaginary falcon in front of an audience.

The essence of hypnosis is focusing on one set of thoughts or perceptions to the exclusion of others. Can we not say the same thing about dissociation? In dissociation, the brain moves the spotlight of attention away from traumatic memories and emotions, focusing instead on more pleasant meditations. It appears to be a similar process. If true, that would explain why hypnosis has such a powerful effect on dissociative identity disorder, but can we find any evidence in the brain?

Studies using fMRI reveal that while in a dissociative state the brain exhibits heightened activity in the anterior cingulate cortex—the same region that we found to be hyperactive in hypnosis. The anterior cingulate is involved in sorting out conflicting information, such as in the Stroop task or in detecting the distortion in the question "How many animals of each kind did Moses take on the ark?" The anterior cingulate prevents us from thinking on autopilot and accepting things at face value. It helps us detect errors and expose conflicting concepts in our environment.

As we know, hypnotized subjects relinquish this shrewdness when they enter a trance. The theory is that in hypnotized subjects the anterior cingulate fails to communicate with the frontal lobe, so it tries to work harder to send its message. It fruitlessly doubles its efforts to report the conflict in the environment. This futile hyperactivity may be why people are willing to do more embarrassing things while hypnotized without realizing that those acts conflict with their typical behavior. It's also what allows them to, without protest, accept the hypnotist's commands at the expense of their other thoughts and feelings.

The same neurological pattern appears in dissociation, which is also a state in which we accept a vision of the world by focusing on one set of ideas to the exclusion of others. This makes the comparison to hypnosis all the more viable. In a sense, people experiencing dissociation are in a hypnotic trance that protects them from traumatic memories. When the trance breaks and the mental walls come down, those traumatic memories return. In the brain, the anterior cingulate activity dissipates as the harsh reality of the past kicks in.

Hypnosis can induce dissociative identity disorder by accentuating the divide between alter egos. Alternatively, it can cure the disorder by reuniting the disparate identities and reconstructing the self. What's more, we now find that hypnosis and dissociation exhibit similar neurologic activity. The evidence seems to suggest that dissociative identity disorder is itself a form of hypnosis.

The difference is that in hypnosis it is the external suggestions of the hypnotist that guide the subject's attention and focus his imagination. In dissociative identity disorder, however, the suggestions come from within, generated by the unconscious system. Given all the reasons we discussed, many psychologists have concluded that dissociative identity disorder is an "auto-suggestive" condition, a syndrome of self-hypnosis. It is as if Evelyn's subconscious were her own hypnotist.

After years of trauma, her brain tried to protect the integrity of her identity by focusing attention away from its troubling aspects. Perhaps hypnosis was the mechanism of this process. Her mind created a mental state that was at once hyper-focused and ignorant, excluding swaths of mental experiences from meeting with consciousness.

As Evelyn's case makes clear, compartmentalizing the mind after trauma is not the most precise process. It has side effects. When the brain attempts to quarantine harmful emotions or memories, part of the self goes with them. That's why the feeling of dissociation is so unpleasant. The unconscious system has effectively broken off a fragment of the self in order to protect the larger whole of human identity. Luckily, that fragment tends to be small. Perhaps that's why alternate personalities are often immature, younger characters. Evelyn's alter egos Kimmy and Sarah were ages four and ten, respectively. They don't have access to the brain's higher cognitive powers and years of accumulated wisdom.

Through hypnosis, Evelyn's doctors were able to draw out each of her alter egos. As each identity emerged, it came with not only a different personality and behavior but also a unique visual acuity. Evelyn was legally blind. She couldn't travel without her Seeing Eye dog. Doctors had come to the conclusion that there was something anatomically wrong with her optic nerves. Yet how is it that when her alter ego inhabited her mind, all she needed was a pair of mild prescription glasses?

As we said, the process of dissociation excludes more than just traumatic memories from consciousness. It takes part of the self with it. But suppose the unconscious were to go even further, cutting off access to a greater portion of the brain. Could it suspend perception itself?

## An Eye for an I

There is a mysterious condition that doctors occasionally see in the hospital that always seems to stump them. Patients come in after suddenly experiencing neurological symptoms such as numbness, weakness, and blindness. Mysteriously, despite the dramatic symptoms, the patients don't seem all that worried. Their demeanor is surprisingly, disturbingly relaxed. When doctors run tests to narrow down the field of possible diagnoses, they find that the tests repeatedly come up empty. There doesn't seem to be an underlying medical cause, no physical evidence of the problem. Yet the symptoms are all too clear. It's almost as if the patients were faking it.

But they aren't. The diagnosis is conversion disorder, a condition in which psychological stress manifests as physical symptoms, masquerading as a neurological illness.

All her life, Evelyn thought she was blind, yet in an instant her blindness was cured by switching to her alter ego Kimmy. That couldn't have possibly happened if the cause had been damage to the visual pathway. Structural defects in the eyes or brain do not spontaneously repair themselves without surgery. Rather, especially given her history of emotional trauma, conversion disorder is the most likely explanation. That's why no doctor ever found a medical reason for her sightlessness. Her blindness was psychological. That's not to say that she was pretending to be blind. Conversion disorder is different from Munchausen syndrome, in which people intentionally feign symptoms. People with conversion disorder aren't faking anything. The conversion from psychological stress to physical symptoms occurs unconsciously.

How does the conversion happen? No one knows exactly how, but researchers in London tried to answer that question by imaging the brain. They recruited patients with blindness due to conversion disorder as well as volunteers with intact vision. The goal was to compare the brain activity of the two groups to see if there were any major differences. And there were.

Compared with the healthy controls, the patients with conversion blindness exhibited heightened activity of the prefrontal cortex and blunted activity in the visual cortex. It was as if the higher processing centers in the brain were suppressing the visual system. The eyes were working. The visual circuitry was intact. But the mind's eye was denied access. The brain was blocking conscious vision, leaving the subjects with only unconscious visual detection reminiscent of blindsight, which we encountered in chapter 2.

But neuroscientists have also noticed something else: patients with conversion disorder have an overactive anterior cingulate cortex—the same region that is overworked in hypnosis and dissociation. In hypnosis, as we discussed, it is thought that the anterior cingulate is working extra hard because its message is not reaching the frontal lobe. As a result, the brain loses its capacity for conflict monitoring, and hypnotized subjects may act silly without paying any mind to the fact that their behavior is out of character.

In conversion disorder, patients display a similar apathy about their condition. The brain blocks their perceptions or motor control, yet despite the terrifying symptoms patients appear unperturbed. This common finding in conversion disorder is called *la belle indifférence*, which is French for "the beautiful indifference." So, why do people with conversion disorder seem indifferent to their symptoms? Perhaps it's for the same reason that hypnotized subjects seem unmoved by their embarrassing antics onstage: ineffective anterior cingulate activity. People with conversion disorder cannot discern the peculiarity of their condition any more than a hypnotized subject can identify the peculiarity of his behavior. Their blindness is just as "in their heads" as was the imaginary falcon that flew at my hypnotized friend. In both cases, their conscious systems are convinced. It's as if conversion disorder were itself a kind of hypnotic state, but rather than being implanted by a third party, it is generated from within as a result of psychological stress.

The great French neurologist Jean-Martin Charcot, who is considered the founder of modern neurology, was the first one to propose that hypothesis in the late nineteenth century. Noticing how deeply intertwined conversion disorder (historically called hysteria) was with hypnosis, he wondered whether conversion disorder may be, like dissociation, a condition of autosuggestion. To prove it, he used to do public demonstrations in which he would use hypnosis to cause conversion paralysis.

Neuroscientists today have similarly shown that hypnosis can *induce* the symptoms of conversion disorder. In one case, researchers used hypnosis to induce left leg paralysis in a twenty-five-year-old volunteer. They then asked him to try moving each leg, one at a time, while a PET scanner monitored what his brain was doing. The results showed that as the man moved his right leg (the one unaffected by the hypnosis), the motor cortex illuminated on the PET scan. That's what we would expect for any healthy person. On the other hand—or other leg, I should say—when the man tried and failed to move his left leg, his motor cortex was quiet. Just as the visual cortex is suppressed in Evelyn's conversion blindness, the motor cortex can be silenced in hypnotic paralysis. The man's anterior cingulate, however, was overactive, just as it is in conversion disorder. So, not only can hypnosis cause the symptoms of conversion disorder, it also creates the same pattern of brain activity, just as we saw with dissociation.

But the question is this: Can hypnosis *cure* conversion disorder, as it appeared to do for Evelyn when hypnosis brought out her alter egos? Consider the case of Brett, a young man in his twenties, living in Texas, who believed that he went gradually blind after taking a blow to the head two years earlier in a boxing match. After running a gamut of tests, however, doctors could not find any medical reason for Brett's condition. They began asking some questions about his emotional state and psychological history. It turned out that Brett had unresolved feelings of guilt about two incidents from his past. The first happened when he was fourteen. His parents had asked him to babysit his younger sister, but Brett decided to go out with his friends instead, leaving his sister by herself. While he was gone, hoodlums dropped a package containing bullets through the family's mail slot and set it on fire. When Brett's sister tried to put out the fire, a bullet flew out and struck her in the left eye. That eye became permanently blind. Brett felt responsible for his sister's injury, and he never let go of his remorse.

The second incident was Brett's decision to quit boxing, to the grave disappointment of his father. In retrospect, his having gone blind provided a useful excuse, helping relieve the onus of quitting. Together with the guilt about his sister, as well as the lack of medical evidence, doctors decided that conversion disorder was the most likely cause of Brett's blindness. He was referred to a psychologist for treatment. After only a few sessions, Brett's vision was restored. Hypnosis cured his blindness, just as it did for Evelyn.

Hypnosis has worked for others as well, regardless of their type of conversion disorder. The blind can regain their sight, the paralyzed recover their strength, and the numb recoup their sensations. In guided hypnotic sessions, patients focus on addressing their traumatic past and on regaining whatever ability was disrupted. And it works.

From the clinical standpoint, hypnosis can cause or cure conversion disorder the same way that it can cause or cure dissociative identity disorder. From the neurological standpoint, both conditions exhibit brain activity reminiscent of a hypnotic trance, involving an overactive anterior cingulate cortex. The evidence points to the theory that just like hypnosis conversion disorder and dissociative identity disorder focus the brain's attention in such a way so as to exclude certain information from reaching consciousness. The anterior cingulate not only is responsible for conflict detection but also helps with emotional processing and attention. So, it's plausible that the emotional effects of abuse would interfere with this region, thereby modifying the way our attention and conflict-monitoring systems work. Just as it can cause dissociation, emotional trauma can divert our attention away from certain sensory information, causing blindness or numbness, or it can ignore motor information, causing conversion paralysis. By unconsciously modulating our brain activity, both conditions manipulate our conscious experience by guiding the mind in one direction at the expense of others.

Evelyn's blindness was a result of conversion disorder, caused by years of emotional trauma. Her multiple personalities emerged from that same history of abuse. As her alter egos shifted, so did her vision. She had a unique visual acuity for each identity, an "eye" for every "I." And hypnosis granted her examiners access to everything. It allowed them to elicit each of her identities, break down the barriers between them, and cure her conversion blindness.

Evelyn isn't the only one to have these two diagnoses simultaneously. People with dissociative identity disorder often have a component of conversion disorder because the two conditions arise from the same cause. What's more, the alter egos in dissociative identity disorder and the visual or motor changes in conversion disorder emerge in the same way: autosuggestion, or self-hypnosis. To protect human identity from traumatic memories and emotions, the brain focuses our attention away from them, interrupting their access to consciousness.

When it quarantines these dangerous ideas, however, the unconscious system in the brain can go too far. Most often, it leaves a person with a sense of dissociation, a feeling of disconnectedness between her and the world. Evelyn and others feel as if they lose a part of themselves along with the trauma. Worse, the unconscious system can sever the connection between consciousness and our sensory or motor circuitry, causing conversion disorder. Evelyn lost her sight, but still others have been left paralyzed, numb, or otherwise disabled by the brain's attempt at self-preservation. When an alter ego arises, however, reactivating the harrowing recollections of the past, these essential faculties can return as their access to the conscious mind is reestablished.

That's why alter egos in dissociative identity disorder can have different capacities for vision. The unconscious system in the brain was forced to break the self in order to preserve it, even though doing so left Evelyn vulnerable to the tragic consequences that followed.

Perhaps we can now see why cutting the corpus callosum in split-brain patients does not lead to two distinct selves, yet Evelyn, with no brain injury at all, had her personality fragmented. The answer may lie in the different role of the unconscious system in each case. In a split-brain patient, the unconscious system tries to fill in the gaps, as it would in anyone else. It attempts to reconcile all aspects of experience into a single narrative, even those generated by the opposite hemisphere, in order to preserve the integrity of the self. For those with dissociative disorders, however, the unconscious system in the brain has a different goal. For once, it doesn't want a single narrative. The single narrative is dangerous, as it would expose the self to toxic information. So, the brain intentionally splits the story. It segregates harmful emotions and memories from the person's sense of self in order to protect it. For once, the brain *doesn't* fill in the gaps.

The self. It's been such a nebulous, elusive concept in science. In part, this is because nobody has agreed on a definition for it. Are we talking about memory? The experience of feelings and emotions? Self-control? Self-reflection? When discussing human identity, we tend to bundle these all into one, even though they are not necessarily part of some singular process. Perhaps that's why, when we employ the rigor of neurological analysis to locate the self, we end up having to break it into parts. Human identity cannot be pinpointed in the brain. It emerges from the cooperation of many brain regions and processes. These processes can be broadly divided into two systems. There is the conscious system, with which we are intimately familiar, and then there's the unconscious system, which operates discretely through mysterious programming that we have affectionately referred to as neuro-logic.

## NeuroLogic

This book ends just as it began: with a discussion of a woman suffering from blindness. Neurologically, each woman's story is completely different. Amelia was blind because of a defect in her visual circuitry. Her unconscious system was unable to process photons of light and convert them into a picture of the world. In contrast, Evelyn's visual pathway was intact. She was blind because her conscious system was unable to gain access to her picture of the world. Two parallel systems, two causes of sightlessness.

The brain's process of creating vision is much like that of constructing identity. For one thing, the experience of vision is made up of component parts: distance, shape, color, size, and speed. They are all calculated by different parts of the brain and therefore have to be fused with ultimate precision. Similarly, the experience of selfhood has component parts: autobiographical memory, feelings, sensations, control over our thoughts and behaviors. These are also managed by different brain regions, and yet they ultimately coalesce to create one unified experience of the world.

Vision and identity also depend on the cooperation of our two fundamental systems in the brain. Without the unconscious visual system, we are blind because the brain cannot process light into images. On the other hand, without the conscious visual system, we cannot experience our surroundings, only detect them unwittingly through blindsight.

So too, identity is dependent on both systems. The conscious system is what allows us to experience selfhood. Pain and pleasure happen to *us*. We have intentions to act, willful control over our minds and bodies. The conscious system allows us to live out the narrative that the brain creates.

And the unconscious system? The unconscious system creates that narrative. It takes disconnected fragments of our experience, filling in the gaps when necessary, and chronicles our life story. It builds our sense of self. What's more, it maintains and protects that sense, even using dissociation to oust harmful thoughts and memories.

Why do this? What's so sacred about human identity? From an evolutionary perspective, self-reflective organisms are more likely to survive. We care about our own survival and are invested in protecting ourselves and our lineage. By maintaining the integrity of our personal narratives, the brain helps us gain insight into our own thinking. It helps us understand our intentions, reflect on our reasoning, deliberate our decisions, and act in a way that is consistent with our goals and desires. Having a sense of identity allows us to better understand our own nature and advance our place in the world.

It's no wonder, then, that the brain places a premium on maintaining the health of our personal narrative. Each waking moment we spend, the brain's underlying logical circuitry absorbs the experiences we accumulate, scrutinizing them to mature and refine human identity. Even outside wakefulness, during our dreams each night, our unconscious may be fixated on this same objective. Some neuroscientists theorize that the function of dreaming is to help develop our sense of self. Perhaps that's why dreams always take place in the first person. Dreams rehearse the feeling of being in the action, observing it firsthand, and being the protagonist in a story. Dreams may be a crucial part of developing our sense of self, even in those who were born blind.

The idea of representing the brain as two parallel systems, one conscious and one unconscious, is actually a controversial one in the neurosciences. It's not that scientists deny that consciousness exists or that there are processes in the brain that operate below the conscious threshold. Rather, research studies are seldom designed in a way that acknowledges this parallel processing infrastructure. Rarely do scientists use their research to elucidate the interactions of the brain's two systems of behavioral control. It may be that they believe that consciousness is not a concept fit for translation into rigorous, quantitative analyses. True, it may be difficult to investigate, but neuroscience is as in need of big-picture, system-oriented studies of the brain as it is of insights into the minute structure of one enzyme in a single neuron. Perhaps the reason for avoiding the question of consciousness is that for some the mountain seems too tall to climb.

Often in the history of the sciences, mysteries have been declared impenetrable—touted as a black box—because researchers did not have the right framework. Breakthroughs require that we pose the right questions. The route to discovery begins by knowing what to look for. Representing the brain as consisting of conscious and unconscious systems is not the answer to the mysteries of consciousness. It is just the beginning of the journey. It is a platform with which to approach many of the baffling questions in neuroscience that perhaps today seem unanswerable. While some might elect to keep the focus of research on straightforward extensions of what we already know, others may try to open the black box by thinking outside it and asking something that might initially seem outlandish.

That was the approach we took together in this book: to take a step back and look at the breadth of neurological research conducted by some of the greatest historical and contemporary thinkers. It was to try to see how we might amass scores of disparate, seemingly unrelated studies and examples from all corners of neuroscience and discover the underlying logic that connects them, organizing them into a single narrative.

As the study of the brain moves forward, let's continue to journey into the black box, using our collective ideas, finding the points at which patterns of thought and behavior meet the mechanisms of neuroscience. The evidence is out there. It's now up to us to fill in the gaps.

# Appendix

*Maps of the Brain*

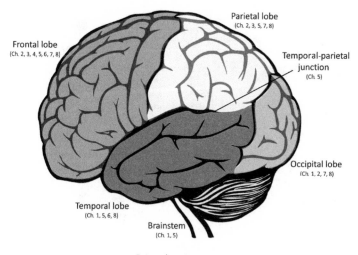

External anatomy

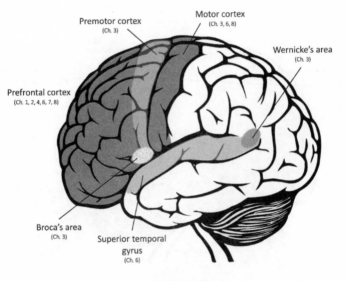

Premotor cortex
(Ch. 3)

Motor cortex
(Ch. 3, 6, 8)

Wernicke's area
(Ch. 3)

Prefrontal cortex
(Ch. 1, 2, 4, 6, 7, 8)

Broca's area
(Ch. 3)

Superior temporal
gyrus
(Ch. 6)

Detailed external anatomy

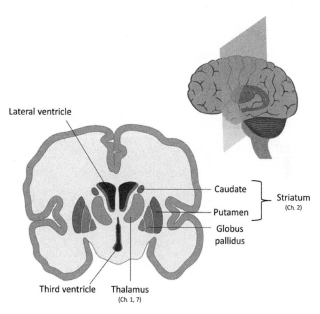

The basal ganglia (coronal section)

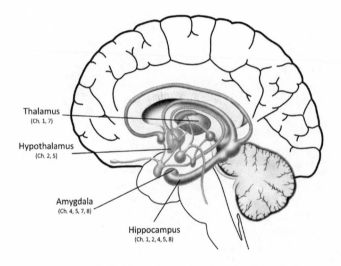

The limbic system—select anatomy (sagittal section)

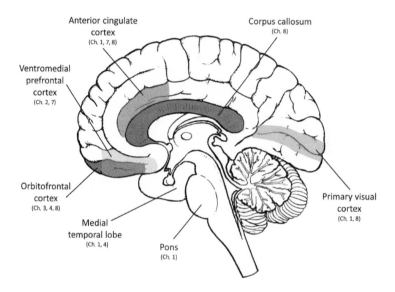

Anterior cingulate
cortex
(Ch. 1, 7, 8)

Corpus callosum
(Ch. 8)

Ventromedial
prefrontal
cortex
(Ch. 2, 7)

Orbitofrontal
cortex
(Ch. 3, 4, 8)

Medial
temporal lobe
(Ch. 1, 4)

Pons
(Ch. 1)

Primary visual
cortex
(Ch. 1, 8)

Other internal anatomy (sagittal section)

# Acknowledgments

This book would not have been possible without the help and contributions of many people. I would like to thank my agent, Kirby Kim, who brought his insight and experience to bear on this manuscript at its earliest stages and continued to be there for me throughout the process. Thanks to my editor, Dan Frank, who helped elevate the text to its current form. Thanks to Betsy Sallee for her attention to detail at every stage. I am grateful to the neurologists, psychiatrists, and neuroscientists who read over the manuscript and gave helpful comments: Chaya Bhuvaneswar, Hal Blumenfeld, Joseph Burns, John Lisman, and Morris Moscovitch. I want to express special thanks to John Lisman, with whom I co-authored a paper in the *Journal of Cognitive Neuroscience* that became the inspiration for this book, especially chapters 2 and 6. Thanks also to Jeff Alexander, Rachel Gul, Lindsay Hakimi, Bita Nouriani, and David Spiegel for their valuable contributions. I'd like to thank my father for his sage advice as well as the rest of my family for their support. My utmost gratitude also goes to all the patients I interviewed, for sharing their stories and for educating me.

Most of all, I want to thank my incredible wife, Sharona. Aside from everything else she does for our family, she read through the manuscript for this book countless times, becoming something of an expert in the process and guiding me with her amazing clarity of thought. She was my partner in bringing this book to fruition, as she is in everything in my life.

# Notes

12    Most dreams incorporate aspects: Domhoff 2015.

12    same areas of the hippocampus: Peigneux et al. 2004.

12    thalamus begins behaving differently: McCarley, Benoit, and Barrionuevo 1983.

13    neurologists have picked up on unique waves: Hobson, Pace-Schott, and Stickgold 2000; Hong et al. 2008.

13    these regions are working together: This model of dreaming is certainly not comprehensive. It is the theoretical basis of the dream pathway, which likely involves many other brain regions.

13    form their own visual pathway: Hobson and Friston 2012.

13    attempts to connect disparate signal fragments: Hobson and McCarley 1977; Franklin and Zyphur 2005.

14    the prefrontal cortex . . . is utterly quiet: Hobson 2009.

15    Lucid dreamers have access: Dresler et al. 2012.

15    a treatment for nightmares: Spoormaker and van den Bout 2006.

15    Most dreams are not simple replays: Fosse et al. 2003.

15    more likely to discover creative shortcuts: Wagner et al. 2004.

15    neurons that have worked together: Murphy et al. 2011. In fact, in another experiment Tononi tried restraining a participant's arm in a sling for a while and then recording her brain activity that night. Just as he hypothesized, the overnight EEG *didn't* show slowing in the areas of the brain controlling that arm movement. See Huber et al. 2006. See also Miller 2007.

16    "I sort of feel as though": Kew, Wright, and Halligan 1998.

17    "So Alice ventured to taste it": Carroll 2013, 11.

17    First described in 1952: Lippman 1952.

18    "Then there was a horrible state": Drysdale 2009.

18    Some scholars have speculated: Podoll and Robinson 1999.

18    represents incomplete processing of visual signals: Brumm et al. 2010.

18    suddenly perceive objects around them as shrunken: Cohen et al. 1994.

19    first reported in 1922: J. Lhermitte 1922.

19    neurologists in Italy described a disturbing case: Vita et al. 2008.

19    Bernardo had endured inflammation: Ibid.

20    complain of particularly vivid dreams: Manford and Andermann 1998.

21    a diagnosis of Charles Bonnet syndrome: Jacob et al. 2004.

21    vision of blue and green eyes: Ricard 2009.

21    "elongated face": Kumar 2013.

21    seen in about 10 percent of people: Teunisse et al. 1995.

22    "release hallucinations": Burke 2002.

22    On September 3, 2004: Kleiter et al. 2007.

23    generate its own visions: Neuroscientists have tested this hypothesis in animals by temporarily deactivating an area of a cat's retina, rendering it partially blind. When they did so, the area of the visual cortex corresponding to that part of the retina began firing spontaneously. Eysel et al. 1999.

24    it may cause visual hallucinations: Ibid.

24    mistake their own imagination: Heilman 1991.

25    Consider the case of Mr. Pasche: Colon-Rivera and Oldham 2013.

25    "auditory Charles Bonnet syndrome": Ibid.

27  category-specific responses to the images: Kreiman, Koch, and Fried 2000.
27  the researchers found . . . Tower of Pisa: Adapted from Quian et al. 2005.
27  but also spoken words: Quian et al. 2009; Quian 2012.
27  Jennifer Aniston neuron often fired: Ibid.
28  Anatomical studies of primate brains: Suzuki 1996; Saleem and Tanaka 1996.
28  causes them to see colors: Head 2006.
28  vanilla brings to mind rounded shapes: Hanson-Vaux, Crisinel, and Spence 2013.
28  That's the McGurk effect: McGurk and MacDonald 1976.
28  reverse McGurk effect: Spence and Deroy 2012.
30  "It is the same process bats use": Kremer 2012.
30  Using fMRI . . . human echolocation: Thaler, Arnott, and Goodale 2011.
31  neuroscientists in Denmark published a study: Kupers et al. 2010.
32  sleep study: Bértolo et al. 2003.
34  phenomenon known as alpha blocking: Also called alpha attenuation.
34  brains of people who are meditating: Stinson and Arthur 2013.
35  harnessing visual imagery in his mind: Barrett and Ehrlichman 1982.
35  alpha blocking peaking during REM sleep: Cantero et al. 1999.
35  processing more visual imagery: Bértolo et al. 2003.
35  direct critique of Bértolo's study: Kerr and Domhoff 2004.
36  those who go blind before the age: Hurovitz et al. 1999.

## 2.
## CAN ZOMBIES DRIVE TO WORK?

38  "For if habit is a second nature": Proust 1982, 781.
39  "When you drive by habit": "Driving You Crazy," 2012.
40  "physically identical . . . dark inside": Chalmers 1995, 96.
42  cell phone group didn't even notice them: Strayer et al. 2003.
43  Here's what happens: Parton, Malhotra, and Husain 2004.
43  As the photographs in the figure: Prasad and Berkowitz 2014.
44  Neurologists theorize . . . see there anymore: Mark, Kooestra, and Heilman 1988.
44  known as blindsight: Weiskrantz et al. 1974.
45  whether it is moving or stationary: Cowey 2010.
45  Accuracies of up to 100 percent: Weiskrantz, Barbur, and Sahraie 1995.
45  focus on the locations of the targets: Poppel et al. 1973.
45  A 2008 study: de Gelder et al. 2008.
48  left turn without hesitation: Packard and McGaugh 1996.
49  westward toward the food pellet: Yin and Knowlton 2006.
49  Neuroscientists have traced the habit system: Ibid.; Packard and McGaugh 1996.
49  travel west to score itself a snack: Yin et al. 2004.
50  "If you're aiming": Twersky 2011.
51  In a study of skilled golfers: Beilock et al. 2004.
52  mark of a fake smile: Duchenne 1990.
53  giving me an inappropriate response: Lisman and Sternberg 2013.

54   these forms of memory: Both types of memory have been studied in the mouse as it navigates through the plus-maze. Before it is trained to run through the maze and make a left out of habit, the mouse has to find its way using episodic memory. It has to remember what its goal is (to find the food pellet), which directions it has already seen (and which are dead ends), and which directions it still needs to investigate. Monitoring the untrained mouse's brain activity as it looks around the maze confirms that the neurons in the hippocampus are firing away during this process. In fact, the hippocampus exhibits unique signal activity depending on the mouse's position in the maze, a finding that has led to research on "place cells." Place cells are poorly named because they are not actually biological cells. Rather, they are specific neuronal firing patterns in the brain that represent positions in the environment, allowing us to visualize where we are in the world with respect to a gradually expanding mental map (O'Keefe 1979). Neuroscientists can actually see these place cells activated sequentially as the mouse moves through the maze. This means that the mouse is visualizing its path as it travels. What's more, as the mouse stands at the intersection trying to decide which way to turn, the place cells are activated yet again, implying that the mouse is recalling its previous trip through the maze to inform its decision of where to go. Johnson and Redish 2007.

54   make a left as usual: Packard and McGaugh 1996.

56   generated in the hypothalamus: Tataranni, Gautier, and Chen 1999.

57   transformed it into something automated: Tricomi et al. 2009. In another experiment, a group of rats was trained to pull on a metal chain that caused a food pellet to be released. The rats then ate the food pellet. Early in the rats' training, before any habits could develop, the experimenters tried feeding the rats before placing them in front of the chain. They did so to see what would happen when the rats were already satiated. Would they still pull on the chain? They didn't. The rats felt full, so there was no need to. However, once the rats were trained further, after many more repetitive sessions doing the same task, their behavior changed. When the now well-trained rats were fed before being placed in front of the chain, they yanked on it without a moment's delay, and did it over and over again. It was clear that the rats weren't actually hungry; they had just been fed until they refused additional food. Yet they continued to pull on the chain and consume the pellet that was released. Rather, their extensive training caused them to develop the habit of pulling on the chain whenever it was near. Their habit caused them to eat despite not being hungry (Balleine and Dickinson 1998).

58   young Russian engineering student: Goldberg 2001, 119–20.

59   tried to strangle her: Spence and Frith 1997.

59   alien hands grab objects: Y. W. Park et al. 2012.

59   hung the picture on it: F. Lhermitte 1983.

59   In another experiment: F. Lhermitte et al. 1986.

60   same automated response: F. Lhermitte 1983.

62   not guilty on both counts: The account of this case was taken from Broughton et al. 1994.

62   "Although the word 'automatism'": *Rabey v. R.*, [1980].

63   Stage 3 is known as: The old categorization included stages 3 and 4, which are now together called stage 3.

63 share the following characteristics: *International Classification of Sleep Disorders,* 2005.

63 "sexsomnia": Béjot et al. 2010.

64 60 percent of the time: Chellappa et al. 2011.

64 thoughts than actual dreams: Cicogna et al. 2000.

64 episodes of sleepwalking: Five of the subjects had night terrors rather than sleepwalking. Night terrors also occur during slow-wave sleep.

64 The table below: Oudiette et al. 2009.

66 "I know what good piano playing is": Joel 2012. The quotes that follow are also from this interview.

67 allows for multitasking: Lisman and Sternberg 2013.

67 exactly this kind of experiment: Maclin, Mathewson, and Low 2011.

70 "I'm trying to pare down decisions": Lewis 2012.

3.
## CAN YOUR IMAGINATION MAKE YOU A BETTER ATHLETE?

71 "Golf is a game": Ross 2008, 222.

71 His daily routine: "Tiger's Daily Routine," 2014.

71 "We'd drive to the site": Diaz 1998.

72 "Before every shot": Nicklaus 1976, 45.

72 Backley won silver: Price and Price 2011.

72 claimed to employ the technique: Downing 2011, 166.

72 same pair of socks: "The 10 Most Interesting Rituals in Sports," 2011.

73 one second of each other: Decety, Jeannerod, and Prablanc 1989.

73 imagine yourself drawing a triangle: Decety and Michel 1989.

74 nearly indistinguishable: Lacourse et al. 2005.

74 similarly accurate mental simulations: Barr and Hall 1992; Decety, Jeannerod, and Prablanc 1989; MacIntyre and Moran 1996; Oishi, Kasai, and Maeshima 2000.

74 neuroscientists in France: Gentili, Papaxanthis, and Pozzo 2006.

75 increased by 13.5 percent: Ranganathan et al. 2004.

76 as much as physical repetition: Ibid.

76 the acronym PETTLEP: Holmes and Collins 2001.

77 study of thirty-four golfers: Smith, Wright, and Cantwell 2008.

78 led to higher scores: Guillot et al. 2013.

78 It helps soccer players: Seif-Barghi et al. 2012.

78 improves shooting percentage: Hemayattalab and Movahedi 2010.

78 archery: Chang et al. 2011.

78 gymnastics, weight lifting: Schuster et al. 2011.

78 improve her actual piano performance: Pascual-Leone et al. 1995.

78 played their pieces faster: Bernardi et al. 2013; Brown and Palmer 2013.

79 "infant in a woman's body": J. B. Taylor 2006, 35.

79 "Imagery has been an effective tool": Ibid., 128.

79 help injured athletes: Hamson-Utley, Martin, and Walters 2008.

80  increase athletes' recovery rates: Driediger, Hall, and Callow 2006.

80  motor recovery after stroke: Butler and Page 2006; Zimmermann-Schlatter et al. 2008.

80  study of 121 stroke patients: Ietswaart et al. 2011.

80  imagery exercises can be disrupted: Mast, Merfeld, and Kosslyn 2006.

81  study of mental imagery: Van Elk et al. 2010.

82  even feel it moving: Henderson and Smyth 1948.

82  patients experience phantom pain: Sherman, Sherman, and Parker 1984.

82  case of an elderly gentleman: Jacome 1978.

83  "mirror box" therapy: Ramachandran and Rogers-Ramachandran 1996.

83  experiment with four amputees: Ramachandran and Brang 2009.

84  replicated in larger studies: Goller et al. 2013.

84  active neuronal groups were identical: Gallese et al. 1996; Di Pellegrino et al. 1992.

85  mirror neurons in human brains: Shmuelof and Zohary 2008.

85  activates the same region: Gangitano, Mottaghy, and Pascual-Leone 2001.

85  movements in a different direction: Kilner, Paulignan, and Blakemore 2003.

85  located in a network in the brain: Buccino et al. 2001; Sakreida et al. 2005; Filimon et al. 2007; Lui et al. 2008.

85  In a 2011 study: Kim et al. 2011.

86  most publicized findings: Jarrett 2013.

86  The sound of yawning: Arnott, Singhal, and Goodale 2009.

86  videos of other primates yawning: Anderson, Myowa-Yamakoshi, and Matsuzawa 2004; Massen, Vermunt, and Sterck 2012.

86  response to human yawns: Joly-Mascheroni, Senju, and Shepherd 2008.

86  more than half the time: Provine 2005.

87  the mirror system was quiet: Haker et al. 2013.

87  "Yawn, Yawn, Yawn": Platek 2010.

87  the act of mutual grooming: Palagi et al. 2009.

87  affectionate social relationships: Silk, Cheney, and Seyfarth 2013; Sakamaki 2013.

87  If the results of this study: Recent studies have shed doubt on the finding that there is any connection between yawning and emotional closeness or empathy. See Bartholomew and Cirulli 2014.

88  we ourselves were in pain: Hutchison et al. 1999.

88  excludes the regions: Singer et al. 2004; Jackson, Meltzoff, and Decety 2005; Morrison et al. 2004.

88  cringe-inducing experiment: Avenanti et al. 2005.

89  own system for withdrawal: Ibid.

89  EMG matched the expression: Dimberg, Thunberg, and Elmehed 2000.

89  less likely to recognize: Niedenthal et al. 2005.

90  people with Moebius syndrome: Cole 2001.

90  more likely to imitate: Chartrand and Bargh 1999.

90  exhibit greater activation: Schulte-Rüther et al. 2007.

90  more active his mirror neuron system: Pfeiffer et al. 2008.

90  porn industry earns more: Ackman 2001.

90  Neuroscientists in France: Mouras et al. 2008.

91  broken mirror theory: Ramachandran and Oberman 2006.

91   other people's existence: Sigman, Spence, and Wang 2006.
91   "tried to remove the foot": Kanner 1943.
91   psychological tests of empathy: Baron-Cohen and Wheelwright 2004; Baron-Cohen 2010.
92   did not shrink away: Minio-Paluello et al. 2009.
92   Erotica has a minimal impact: Mathersul, McDonald, and Rushby 2013.
92   fifty-six children: Helt et al. 2010.
92   Some researchers suspect: Senju et al. 2009; Usui et al. 2013.
93   A 2010 fMRI study: Martineau et al. 2010.
93   study in the journal *Neuron:* Dinstein et al. 2010.
94   neurologist Antonio Damasio: Damasio 1994, 173–75.
94   Every time we have an experience: There are bodily experiences associated with sadness, joy, anger, and the other emotions.
95   "no longer Gage": The account of Phineas Gage's accident and recovery was taken from Damasio 1994, chap. 1, and Gazzaniga, Ivry, and Mangun 2002, 537–38.
95   Damasio recalls: Damasio 1994, 35–44.
96   "gambling task": Bechara et al. 1994; Bechara, Damasio, and Damasio 2000.
96   Elliot had described: Damasio 1994, 214–16.


4.
CAN WE REMEMBER THINGS THAT NEVER HAPPENED?

99    "He was still too young": García Márquez 1985.
102   As we accumulate new experiences: Bliss and Collingridge 1993.
102   Long-term potentiation: Bliss and Lømo 1973.
102   Memory formation: Schwärzel and Müller 2006.
104   Of the twenty-four subjects: Loftus and Pickrell 1995; Loftus 1993.
104   A research group in Israel: Mendelson et al. 2009.
105   group of neuroscientists at Duke University: Botzung et al. 2010.
106   medial prefrontal cortex lit up: Craik et al. 1999; Kelley et al. 2002.
107   "I'd be *happy* to do it": Rankin 2009.
109   participants recalling 9/11: Kvavilashvili et al. 2010.
110   Members of the midtown group: Sharot et al. 2007.
110   more emotionally affected people: Schmidt 2004.
110   In a 2013 study: Cunningham et al. 2013.
111   "I know in my heart": Anderson 1990.
114   George Franklin was found guilty: *Franklin v. Duncan,* 1995.
115   memory for negative feelings: Ritchie et al. 2006.
115   more likely to neglect them: Sedikides and Green 2004.
116   "Doctor, do you know": Gazzaniga 2000.
118   study in London: Kopelman 1987.
119   exclusively the result of brain damage: Schnider, von Däniken, and Gutbrod 1996.
119   Some researchers believe: Metcalf, Langdon, and Coltheart 2007.
120   Confabulation usually results: Dalla and Boisse 2010.

120   it's a defense mechanism: The counterargument to this view, as expertly expressed
       by Dr. Morris Moscovitch (Moscovitch 1995) goes as follows: If confabulation were
       truly an attempt to reconcile discrepancies in beliefs to protect the ego, then shouldn't
       it happen to everyone regardless of whether they have any brain damage? Perhaps the
       psychodynamic explanation we discussed doesn't account for the entire syndrome.
       Then again, maybe the capacity for confabulation does exist in everyone, but in
       those with brain damage the threshold to confabulate is lower than it is in those with
       healthy brains.
121   In one experiment: Schnider 2003.
121   set of correct answers: Images from Schnider 2013.
122   classic fairy tales or Bible stories: Asaf Gilboa et al. 2006.
123   A patient in a related study: Turner et al. 2008.
123   Confabulating patients were no more likely: Schnider, von Däniken, and Gutbrod
       1996; Mercer et al. 1977.
123   In a similar study: Moscovitch 1989.


5.
WHY DO PEOPLE BELIEVE IN ALIEN ABDUCTIONS?

127   "Most visions of extraterrestrial life": Myhrvold 1996.
128   One in four people: Gallup and Newport 1991.
128   Nine percent said: "Poll: U.S. Hiding Knowledge of Aliens," 1997.
128   Psychological assessments demonstrate: Chequers, Joseph, and Diduca 1997.
129   "The subject awakes to consciousness": Mitchell 1876.
129   feeling of suffocation: Simons and Hughes 1985.
130   8 percent of the population: Sharpless and Barber 2011.
130   Studies show that people who struggle: Solomonova 2008.
131   "Where is this shadow person?": Arzy 2006.
132   "God loves me": Carrazana and Cheng 2011.
132   "I saw an angel close": Teresa of Ávila 1565.
133   the neurologist determines: Carrazana and Cheng 2011.
133   Gazzaniga, at least, suspects as much: Gazzaniga 2005, 156–57.
134   induced these mystical encounters: Hill and Persinger 2003.
136   man who developed the delusion after a motorcycle accident: Young et al. 1992.
136   failure to connect perceptions with emotions: Ramirez-Bermudez et al. 2010.
136   without having any emotional reaction: Gerrans 2002.
137   "Every time you left the room": Corlett, D'Souza, and Krystal 2010.
137   he assumed he was getting away with it: Thomas-Antérion et al. 2008.
137   syndromes were two sides of a coin: McKay and Cipolotti 2007.
137   paranoid explanation of his symptoms: Kinderman and Bentall 1997.
137   depressive, nihilistic approach: Peterson et al. 1982.
138   "I was spending my summer": Facco and Agrillo 2012.
138   table below shows the breakdown: van Lommel et al. 2001.
139   welcomed as part of the natural order: Facco and Agrillo 2012.

140  "the next thing I knew": Fulgham 2006.

140  About 10 percent of pilots: Rickards and Newman 2005.

141  Many pilots reported feelings: Carter 2010; Whinnery 1997.

141  The periphery of their vision: Lambert and Wood 1946.

141  Studies suggest that impaired: Nelson et al. 2007; Blackmore and Troscianko 1989.

141  Studies of near-death experience: Nelson et al. 2006.

142  counteraction by the nervous system: Ibid.

142  people who suffer from sleep paralysis: Ibid.

143  A twenty-five-year-old soldier: Siegel 1984.

143  study of those two people: Ibid.

144  "I'm totally pissed": Clancy 2005, 50.

146  "I can feel it comin' on": Quotations all taken from Ness 1978.

146  *kokma:* Ibid.

147  *subirse el muerto:* Jiménez-Genchi et al. 2009.

147  stand-stills: Dahlitz and Parkes 1993.

147  In West Africa: De Jong 2005.

147  "The tall man with the white hat": Ibid.

6.

## WHY DO SCHIZOPHRENICS HEAR VOICES?

149  "If you talk to God": Szasz 1973, 101.

152  electrical signaling pathway continues: Guenther, Ghosh, and Tourville 2006; Simonyan and Horwitz 2011.

153  a form of subvocal speech: Watson 1913.

153  disproven after an experiment: Smith et al. 1947.

153  speech muscles were contracting: Garrity 1977.

154  Gould compared the EMG: Gould 1948.

154  emerged as a soft whisper: Gould 1949.

155  *"If you're in his mind":* Green and Preston 1981.

156  nearly 60 percent: Green and Kinsbourne 1990.

156  counting aloud: Nelson, Thrasher, and Barnes 1991.

158  someone other than themselves: Johns et al. 2006.

158  "Someone else is speaking": Frith 1995.

158  mormyrid nervous system: Feulner et al. 2009b.

159  mormyrid females are attracted: Feulner et al. 2009a.

160  Here's what happened: Adapted from Russell and Bell 1978.

161  the receptors detected nothing: Ibid.

161  Bell showed: Bell 1981; Bell and Grant 1989.

162  known as the corollary discharge: Caputi and Nogueira 2012; Bell and Grant 1989.

163  Songbirds like the finch: Crapse and Sommer 2008.

163  subjects lifted a container: Nowak and Hermsdörfer 2003.

164  vestibulo-ocular reflex: Herdman, Schubert, and Tusa 2001; Davidson and Wolpert 2005.

164 catch a ball at just the right moment: Zago et al. 2004.

165 internal system of prediction: Gentili et al. 2004.

166 N100: Ford et al. 2001.

167 patients incorrectly identified the voice: Heinks-Maldonado et al. 2007; Shergill et al. 2000.

168 deaf population at the same rate: Altshuler and Rainer 1958; Evans and Elliott 1981.

168 few such patients: du Feu and McKenna 1999; Critchley et al. 1981.

169 "How do I know, I'm deaf": Thacker 1994.

170 neuroimaging studies of language: MacSweeney et al. 2002.

170 deaf participants underwent a PET scan: McGuire et al. 1997.

171 Syd Barrett: Schaffner 2005, 106.

171 locked his girlfriend in a room: Ibid., 77.

171 likely that Barrett suffered from schizophrenia: Greene 2006.

172 "possibly the ultimate self-diagnosis": Schaffner 2005, 99.

172 "I look out the window": Mellor 1970.

172 "One man said": Spence and Frith 1997.

172 "When I reach my hand": Mellor 1970.

173 "I cry, tears roll": Ibid. (emphasis added).

173 "The sudden impulse": Ibid. (emphasis added).

174 tickling machine: Blakemore, Frith, and Wolpert 1999.

175 The defenses are down: Something similar probably goes on in the brain when we talk on a phone with a bad connection and hear an echo of our voice after a delay. It must be a bit confusing for the brain, just like having the feeling of tickling after a delay. Perhaps that's why echoes on the phone are so annoying.

175 When a group of schizophrenic patients: Blakemore et al. 2000.

176 déjà vu: Lisman and Sternberg 2013.

7.

CAN SOMEONE BE HYPNOTIZED TO COMMIT MURDER?

178 "The conscious mind": Freud 1913.

178 Palle Hardrup: Streatfeild 2007, 135–39.

180 study of thirty burn victims: Patterson, Goldberg, and Ehde 1996.

181 pain in cancer patients: Syrjala, Cummings, and Donaldson 1992.

181 Ellen DeGeneres: You can watch it for yourself on YouTube.

181 Debra Messing: "Messing Calls on Hypnosis to Help Her with Underwater Scenes," 2005.

181 "Company B will leave at 2100 tonight": Watkins 1947.

182 "The real origin and essence": Braid 1843.

184 did not notice the gorilla: Chabris and Simons 2009, 6–8.

184 continued to provide the directions: Simons and Levin 1998.

185 Research on the neurobiology of attention: Haykin and Chen 2005.

186 zebra finch: Narayan et al. 2007.

188 Stroop effect: Stroop 1935.

188   Present in more than 99 percent: MacLeod 1991.

188   hypnotized subjects attempt the Stroop: Raz et al. 2002.

188   Neuroimaging studies of the brain: Botvinick et al. 2001; Kerns, Cohen, and Mac-Donald 2004.

188   anterior cingulate has many functions: Lane et al. 1998; Posner and Petersen 1990.

189   anterior cingulate is hard at work: Botvinick, Cohen, and Carter 2004; Barch et al. 2000. There are some, however, who contend that its role is even more prominent. A German research group conducted a study in which it monitored subjects' brain activity while the subjects experienced pain in three different situations. In the first situation, the subjects used a heated probe to zap one of their hands. In the second scenario, someone else zapped their hands for them. In the third trial, the subjects used a device designed so that when they pulled on a rope with one hand, the probe would zap their other hand. The first two trials represented self-initiated and externally initiated pain, while the third trial represented something in between, what we might call indirectly self-initiated pain. The fMRI data the group collected revealed that a different region of the anterior cingulate was activated during each of the three trials. The researchers concluded that the anterior cingulate is used not only for conflict monitoring but also for distinguishing between self-generated and externally generated stimuli (Mohr et al. 2005).

189   John Gruzelier: Egner, Jamieson, and Gruzelier 2005.

190   Gruzelier says: As quoted in Gosline 2004.

191   "EAT POPCORN": Pratkanis 1992.

191   "the most alarming invention": Streatfeild 2007, 185.

191   "If the device is successful": Cousins 1957.

191   "abolish the free will almost completely": Aldous Huxley to Humphry Osmond, April 8, 1957, in Huxley 1970.

192   hidden in the album cover: Streatfeild 2007, 181.

192   "You have seen 'SEX' embedded": Ibid., 204, quoting cross-examination by Bill Peterson, March 29, 1990.

193   Canadian Broadcasting Corporation: Pratkanis 1992.

193   It was even discovered: Streatfeild 2007, 194.

193   known as backward masking: Higgins and Bargh 1987; Kihlstrom, 1987.

194   graduate students underwent: Baldwin, Carrell, and Lopez 1990.

195   twenty-six people were primed: Lee et al. 2011.

195   primed with angry or sad faces: Yang and Tong 2010.

195   Studies using fMRI show: Fahrenfort et al. 2008.

196   amygdala lights up: Whalen et al. 1998.

196   two groups of undergraduates: Mayer and Merckelbach 1999.

197    "I am honest, I will not steal": Paraskevas-Thadani 1997.

197   incidence of shoplifting fell: Arrington 1982.

198   1984 commercial for British Airways: Heath 2012, 92–93.

199   "Advertisers begin": Yapko 1995, 38.

200   Here are some examples: Kaplan 2007.

201   In a 2007 study: Ibid.

201   A 2007 neuroimaging study: Schaefer and Rotte 2007.

202   Pepsi paradox: Koenigs and Tranel 2008.

202  Coca-Cola sells nearly twice: D'Altorio 2012.
202  The experimenters concluded: Koenigs and Tranel 2008.
204  "Germany": Searle 2004, 157.
205  "It's just my luck": Dalrymple 2001, 6.


8.
WHY CAN'T SPLIT PERSONALITIES SHARE PRESCRIPTION GLASSES?

210  "I learned to recognize": Stevenson 1991, 43.
210  Evelyn was in bad shape: Evelyn's case was taken from Bhuvaneswar and Spiegel 2013.
211  "I have noticed": This quotation was taken from an interview of the patient before a medical school class. The interview was led by Dr. David Spiegel of Stanford University.
211  "When I come to": Ibid.
212  excerpt of a conversation: Ibid.
214  a gynecologist named Peter: Pachalska et al. 2011.
216  right frontotemporal lobe damage: Feinberg and Shapiro 1989; Moscovitch 1995.
216  recorded the following exchange: Feinberg 2001, 18.
217  Asomatognosia results from damage: Feinberg et al. 2010.
217  Experiments using fMRI: Herwig et al. 2012; Keenan et al. 2000.
217  consensus seems to be: Keenan, Gallup, and Falk 2003, 204.
218  Just ask Vicki: Wolman 2012.
219  alien hand syndrome: Verleger et al. 2011.
219  if Vicki's left hemisphere: Baynes et al. 1998.
219  Gazzaniga thought so: Gazzaniga 1972.
219  showed the word "walk": Gazzaniga 2005, 148–49.
220  flashed a picture of apples: Gazzaniga 1970, 106.
220  displayed the word "smile": Wolman 2012.
220  "left-hemisphere interpreter": Gazzaniga 1989; Turk et al. 2003.
221  It was a day the Ackermans: Lanius, Hopper, and Menon 2003.
222  short fMRI study: Ibid.
223  Dissociative conditions: Armstrong 1991.
223  victims of long-standing abuse: Watkins and Watkins 1998.
224  "emotional parts": Reis 1993.
224  "apparently normal parts": Nijenhuis, Van der Hart, and Steele, 2002; Reis 1993.
224  personality may respond: Miller and Triggiano 1992; Putnam, Zahn, and Post 1990.
225  When Evelyn arrived: Stankiewicz and Golczyńska 2006.
225  researchers in the Netherlands: Reinders et al. 2006.
225  stress is a trigger: Barlow and Chu 2014.
226  neutral personalities: Simeon et al. 2000.
227  2013 experiment: Schlumpf et al. 2013.
227  recalling autobiographical memories: Fink et al. 1996.
228  hippocampus is 19.2 percent smaller: Vermetten et al. 2006.

228  memories may be repressed: Though, as discussed in chapter 4, this is controversial.
228  studies we've seen: Also see Van der Kolk and Fisler 1995.
228  several isolated cases: Tsai et al. 1999; Saxe et al. 1992; Savoy et al. 2012.
228  reduced activity in the orbitofrontal cortex: Sar, Unal, and Ozturk 2007.
229  Evelyn and her alter egos: Bhuvaneswar and Spiegel 2013.
230  defining characteristics: Howell 2011, 148.
230  Hypnosis helps soothe: Smith 1993; Howland 1975.
230  "I feel better": This quotation was taken from an actual hospital progress note from Stanford University Medical Center. Used with permission of the patient's physician, Dr. David Spiegel. Notes were sent via password-protected files with names and dates removed.
230  some psychiatrists subscribe: Gleaves 1996.
230  Studies using fMRI: Kas et al. 2014.
231  same neurological pattern: Thomaes et al. 2013; Bremner 2007.
231  "auto-suggestive": Oakley 1999; Bell et al. 2011.
232  An Eye for an I: This section title was borrowed from Bhuvaneswar and Spiegel 2013.
233  Compared with the healthy controls: Werring et al. 2004.
233  neuroscientists have also noticed: Becker et al. 2013; Bell et al. 2011.
234  French neurologist Jean-Martin Charcot: Bogousslavsky, Walusinski, and Veyrunes 2009.
234  public demonstrations: Goetz, Bonduelle, and Gelfand 1995, 203.
234  hypnosis can *induce* the symptoms: Vaudreuil and Trieu 2013; Bell et al. 2011; Pyka et al. 2011.
234  induce left leg paralysis: Halligan et al. 2000.
235  case of Brett: Patterson 1980.
235  guided hypnotic sessions: Stonnington, Barry, and Fisher 2006; Bühler and Heim 2011.
235  The evidence points: Lane et al. 1998; Posner and Petersen 1990.
236  emotional trauma can divert: Vuilleumier 2005.
236  autosuggestion, or self-hypnosis: Oakley 1999; Halligan, Bass, and Wade 2000.
238  brain's process of creating vision: Manning and Manning 2009.
239  Some neuroscientists theorize: Staunton 2001.

# Bibliography

Ackerman, J. M., C. C. Nocera, and J. A. Bargh. "Incidental Haptic Sensations Influence Social Judgments and Decisions." *Science* 328, no. 5986 (2010): 1712–15.

Ackman, D. "How Big Is Porn?" Forbes.com, May 25, 2001. http://www.forbes.com/2001/05/25/0524porn.html.

Altshuler, K. Z., and M. B. Rainer. "Patterns and Course of Schizophrenia in the Deaf." *Journal of Nervous and Mental Disease* 127, no. 1 (1958): 77–83.

Anderson, D. "Recollections." *New York Times,* April 14, 1990, B9.

Anderson, J. R., M. Myowa-Yamakoshi, and T. Matsuzawa. "Contagious Yawning in Chimpanzees." *Proceedings of the Royal Society Biological Sciences* 271, no. 6 (2004): 68–70.

Armstrong, J. "The Psychological Organization of Multiple Personality Disordered Patients." *Psychiatric Clinics of North America* 14, no. 3 (1991): 533–46.

Arnott, S. R., A. Singhal, and M. A. Goodale. "An Investigation of Auditory Contagious Yawning." *Cognitive, Affective, and Behavioral Neuroscience* 9, no. 3 (2009): 335–42.

Arrington, R. L. "Advertising and Behavior Control." *Journal of Business Ethics* 1 (1982): 3–12.

Arzy, S., et al. "Induction of an Illusory Shadow Person." *Nature* 443, no. 7109 (2006): 287.

Asaf Gilboa, C. A., et al. "Mechanisms of Spontaneous Confabulations: A Strategic Retrieval Account." *Brain* 129 (2006): 1399–414.

Atkinson, J. R. "The Perceptual Characteristics of Voice-Hallucinations in Deaf People: Insights into the Nature of Subvocal Thought and Sensory Feedback Loops." *Schizophrenia Bulletin* 32, no. 4 (2006): 701–8.

Avenanti, A., et al. "Transcranial Magnetic Stimulation Highlights the Sensorimotor Side of Empathy for Pain." *Nature Neuroscience* 8, no. 7 (2005): 955–60.

Avillac, M., et al. "Reference Frames for Representing Visual and Tactile Locations in Parietal Cortex." *Nature Neuroscience* 8, no. 7 (2005): 941–49.

Baker, C. L., R. F. Hess, and J. Zihl. "Residual Motion Perception in a 'Motion-Blind' Patient, Assessed with Limited-Lifetime Random Dot Stimuli." *Journal of Neuroscience* 11, no. 2 (1991): 454–61.

Baldwin, M. W., S. E. Carrell, and D. F. Lopez. "Priming Relationship Schemas: My Advisor and the Pope Are Watching Me from the Back of My Mind." *Journal of Experimental Social Psychology* 26, no. 5 (1990): 435–54.

Balleine, B. W., and A. Dickinson. "Goal-Directed Instrumental Action: Contingency and Incentive Learning and Their Cortical Substrates." *Neuropharmacology* 37, no. 4–5 (1998): 407–19.

Barch, D. M., et al. "Anterior Cingulate and the Monitoring of Response Conflict: Evidence from an fMRI Study of Overt Verb Generation." *Journal of Cognitive Neuroscience* 12, no. 2 (2000): 298–309.

Barlow, M. R., and J. A. Chu. "Measuring Fragmentation in Dissociative Identity Disorder: The Integration Measure and Relationship to Switching and Time in Therapy." *European Journal of Psychotraumatology* 5 (2014): 22250.

Baron-Cohen, S. "Empathizing, Systemizing, and the Extreme Male Brain Theory of Autism." *Progress in Brain Research* 186 (2010): 167–75.

Baron-Cohen, S., and S. Wheelwright. "The Empathy Quotient: An Investigation of Adults with Asperger Syndrome or High Functioning Autism, and Normal Sex Differences." *Journal of Autism and Developmental Disorders* 34, no. 2 (2004): 163–75.

Barr, K., and C. Hall. "The Use of Imagery by Rowers." *International Journal of Sport Psychology* 23, no. 3 (1992): 243–61.

Barrett, J., and H. Ehrlichman. "Bilateral Hemispheric Alpha Activity During Visual Imagery." *Neuropsychologia* 20, no. 6 (1982): 703–8.

Bartholomew, A. J., and E. T. Cirulli. "Individual Variation in Contagious Yawning Susceptibility Is Highly Stable and Largely Unexplained by Empathy or Other Known Factors." *PLOS ONE* 9, no. 3 (2014).

Baynes, K., et al. "Modular Organization of Cognitive Systems Masked by Interhemispheric Integration." *Science* 280 (1998): 902–5.

Bechara, A., H. Damasio, and A. R. Damasio. "Emotion, Decision Making, and the Orbitofrontal Cortex." *Cerebral Cortex* 10, no. 3 (2000): 295–307.

Bechara A., et al. "Insensitivity to Future Consequences Following Damage to Human Prefrontal Cortex." *Cognition* 50, no. 1–3 (1994): 7–15.

Becker, B., et al. "Deciphering the Neural Signature of Conversion Blindness." *American Journal of Psychiatry* 170, no. 1 (2013): 121–22.

Beilock, S. L., et al. "Haste Does Not Always Make Waste: Expertise, Direction of Attention, and Speed Versus Accuracy in Performing Sensorimotor Skills." *Psychonomic Bulletin and Review* 11 (2004): 373–79.

Béjot, Y., et al. "Sexsomnia: An Uncommon Variety of Parasomnia." *Clinical Neurology and Neurosurgery* 112, no. 1 (2010): 72–75.

Bell, C. C. "An Efference Copy Which Is Modified by Reafferent Input." *Science* 214, no. 23 (1981): 50–53.

Bell, C. C., and K. Grant. "Corollary Discharge Inhibition and Preservation of Temporal Information in a Sensory Nucleus of Mormyrid Electric Fish." *Journal of Neuroscience* 9, no. 3 (1989): 1029–44.

Bell, V., et al. "Dissociation in Hysteria and Hypnosis: Evidence from Cognitive Neuroscience." *Journal of Neurology, Neurosurgery, and Psychiatry* 82, no. 3 (2011): 332–39.

Berkowitz, A. L., and D. Ansari. "Generation of Novel Motor Sequences: The Neural Correlates of Musical Improvisation." *NeuroImage* 41, no. 2 (2008): 535–43.

Bernardi, N. F., et al. "Mental Practice Promotes Motor Anticipation: Evidence from Skilled Music Performance." *Frontiers in Human Neuroscience* 7, no. 451 (2013): 1–14.

Bértolo, H., et al. "Visual Dream Content, Graphical Representation, and EEG Alpha Activity in Congenitally Blind Subjects." *Cognitive Brain Research* 15, no. 3 (2003): 277–84.

Bhuvaneswar, C., and D. Spiegel. "An Eye for an I: A 35-Year-Old Woman with Fluctuating Oculomotor Deficits and Dissociative Identity Disorder." *International Journal of Clinical and Experimental Hypnosis* 61, no. 3 (2013): 351–70.

Bischof, M., and C. L. Bassetti. "Total Dream Loss: A Distinct Neuropsychological Dysfunction After Bilateral PCA Stroke." *Annals of Neurology* 56, no. 4 (2004): 583–86.

Blakemore, S. J., C. D. Frith, and D. M. Wolpert. "Spatio-temporal Prediction Modulates the Perception of Self-Produced Stimuli." *Journal of Cognitive Neuroscience* 11, no. 5 (1999): 551–59.

Blackmore, S. J., and T. S. Troscianko. "The Physiology of the Tunnel." *Journal of Near-Death Studies* 8, no. 1 (1989): 15–28.

Blakemore, S. J., et al. "The Perception of Self-Produced Sensory Stimuli in Patients with Auditory Hallucinations and Passivity Experiences: Evidence for a Breakdown in Self-Monitoring." *Psychological Medicine* 30, no. 5 (2000): 1131–39.

Bliss, T. V., and G. L. Collingridge. "A Synaptic Model of Memory: Long-Term Potentiation in the Hippocampus." *Nature* 361 (1993): 31–39.

Bliss, T. V., and T. Lømo. "Long-Lasting Potentiation of Synaptic Transmission in the Dentate Area of the Anaesthetized Rabbit Following Stimulation of the Perforant Path." *Journal of Physiology* 232, no. 2 (1973): 331–56.

Blythe, W. *To Hate Like This Is to Be Happy Forever: A Thoroughly Obsessive, Intermittently Uplifting, and Occasionally Unbiased Account of the Duke–North Carolina Basketball Rivalry*. New York: HarperCollins, 2006.

Bogousslavsky, J., O. Walusinski, and D. Veyrunes. "Crime, Hysteria, and Belle Epoque Hypnotism: The Path Traced by Jean-Martin Charcot and Georges Gilles de la Tourette." *European Neurology* 62, no. 4 (2009): 193–99.

Botvinick, M. M., J. D. Cohen, and C. S. Carter. "Conflict Monitoring and Anterior Cingulate Cortex: An Update." *Trends in Cognitive Sciences* 8, no. 12 (2004): 539–46.

Botvinick, M. M., et al. "Conflict Monitoring and Cognitive Control." *Psychological Review* 108, no. 3 (2001): 624–52.

Botzung, A., et al. "Mental Hoop Diaries: Emotional Memories of a College Basketball Game in Rival Fans." *Journal of Neuroscience* 30, no. 6 (2010): 2130–37.

Braid, J. *Neurypnology; or, The Rationale of Nervous Sleep Considered in Relation to Animal Magnetism*. London: John Churchill, 1843.

Bremner, J. D. "Neuroimaging in Posttraumatic Stress Disorder and Other Stress-Related Disorders." *Neuroimaging Clinics of North America* 17, no. 4 (2007): 523–43.

Brooks, S. J., et al. "Exposure to Subliminal Arousing Stimuli Induces Robust Activation in the Amygdala, Hippocampus, Anterior Cingulate, Insular Cortex, and Primary Visual Cortex: A Systematic Meta-analysis of fMRI Studies." *NeuroImage* 59, no. 3 (2012): 2962–73.

Broughton, R., et al. "Homicidal Somnambulism: A Case Report." *Sleep* 17, no. 3 (1994): 253–64.

Brown, R. M., and C. Palmer. "Auditory and Motor Imagery Modulate Learning in Music Performance." *Frontiers in Human Neuroscience* 7, no. 320 (2013): 1–13.

Brumm, K., et al. "Functional MRI of a Child with Alice in Wonderland Syndrome During an Episode of Micropsia." *Journal of American Association for Pediatric Ophthalmology* 14, no. 4 (2010): 317–22.

Buccino, G., et al. "Action Observation Activates Premotor and Parietal Areas in a Somatotopic Manner: An fMRI Study." *European Journal of Neuroscience* 13, no. 2 (2001): 400–404.

Bühler, K. E., and G. Heim. "Etiology, Pathogenesis, and Therapy According to Pierre Janet Concerning Conversion Disorders and Dissociative Disorders." *American Journal of Psychotherapy* 65, no. 4 (2011): 281–309.

Burke, W. "The Neural Basis of Charles Bonnet Hallucinations: A Hypothesis." *Journal of Neurology, Neurosurgery, and Psychiatry* 73, no. 5 (2002): 535–41.

Butler, A. J., and S. J. Page. "Mental Practice with Motor Imagery: Evidence for Motor Recovery and Cortical Reorganization After Stroke." *Archives of Physical Medicine and Rehabilitation* 87, no. 12, S2 (2006): S2–S11.


Cahill, C. "Psychotic Experiences Induced in Deluded Patients Using Distorted Auditory Feedback." *Cognitive Neuropsychiatry* 1, no. 3 (1996): 201–11.

Cantero, J. L., et al. "Alpha Power Modulation During Periods with Rapid Oculomotor Activity in Human REM Sleep." *Neuroreport* 10, no. 9 (1999): 1817–20.

Caputi, A. A., and J. Nogueira. "Identifying Self- and Nonself-Generated Signals: Lessons from Electrosensory Systems." In *Sensing in Nature,* edited by C. López-Larrea, 1–19. New York: Landes Bioscience and Springer Science and Business Media, 2012.

Carrazana, E., and J. Cheng. "St. Theresa's Dart and a Case of Religious Ecstatic Epilepsy." *Cognitive and Behavioral Neurology* 24, no. 3 (2011): 152–55.

Carroll, L. *Alice in Wonderland.* New York: Tribeca Books, 2013.

Carter, C. *Science and the Near-Death Experience: How Consciousness Survives Death.* Rochester, Vt.: Inner Traditions, 2010.

Chabris, C., and D. Simons. *The Invisible Gorilla: How Our Intuitions Deceive Us.* New York: Random House, 2009.

Chalmers, D. *The Conscious Mind: In Search of a Fundamental Theory.* Oxford: Oxford University Press, 1995.

Chang, Y., et al. "Neural Correlates of Motor Imagery for Elite Archers." *NMR in Biomedicine* 24, no. 4 (2011): 366–72.

Chartrand, T. L., and J. A. Bargh. "The Chameleon Effect: The Perception-Behavior Link and Social Interaction." *Journal of Personality and Social Psychology* 76, no. 6 (1999): 893–910.

Chellappa, S. L., et al. "Cortical Activation Patterns Herald Successful Dream Recall After NREM and REM Sleep." *Biological Psychology* 87, no. 2 (2011): 251–56.

Chequers, J., S. Joseph, and D. Diduca. "Belief in Extraterrestrial Life, UFO-Related Beliefs, and Schizotypal Personality." *Personality and Individual Differences* 23, no. 3 (1997): 519–52.

Choi, W., and P. C. Gordon. "Word Skipping During Sentence Reading: Effects of Lexicality on Parafoveal Processing." *Attention, Perception, and Psychophysics* 76, no. 1 (2004): 201–13.

Cicogna, P., et al. "Slow-Wave and REM Sleep Mentation." *Sleep Research Online* 3 (2000): 67–72.

Clancy, S. A. *Abducted: How People Come to Believe They Were Kidnapped by Aliens.* Cambridge, Mass.: Harvard University Press, 2005.

Cohen, L., et al. "Selective Deficit of Visual Size Perception: Two Cases of Hemimicropsia." *Journal of Neurology, Neurosurgery, and Psychiatry* 57, no. 1 (1994): 73–78.

Cole, J. "Empathy Needs a Face." *Journal of Consciousness Studies* 8, no. 5–7 (2001): 51–68.

Colon-Rivera, H. A., and M. A. Oldham. "The Mind with a Radio of Its Own: A Case Report and Review of the Literature on the Treatment of Musical Hallucinations." *General Hospital Psychiatry* 36, no. 2 (2013): 220–24.

Corlett, P. R., D. C. D'Souza, and J. H. Krystal. "Capgras Syndrome Induced by Ketamine in a Healthy Subject." *Biological Psychiatry* 68, no. 1 (2010): e1–e2.

Corradini, A., and A. Antonietti. "Mirror Neurons and Their Function in Cognitively Understood Empathy." *Consciousness and Cognition* 22, no. 3 (2013): 1152–61.

Cousins, N. "Smudging the Subconscious." *Saturday Review,* Oct. 5, 1957.

Cowey, A. "The Blindsight Saga." *Experimental Brain Research* 200 (2010): 3–24.

Craik, F. I. M., et al. "In Search of the Self: A Positron Emission Tomography Study." *Psychological Science* 10, no. 1 (1999): 26–34.

Crapse, T. B., and M. A. Sommer. "Corollary Discharge Across the Animal Kingdom." *Nature Reviews Neuroscience* 9 (2008): 587–600.

Creutzfeldt, O., G. Ojeman, and E. Lettich. "Neuronal Activity in the Human Lateral Temporal Lobe: II. Responses to the Subject's Own Voice." *Experimental Brain Research* 77 (1989): 476–89.

Critchley, E. M., et al. "Hallucinatory Experiences of Prelingually Profoundly Deaf Schizophrenics." *British Journal of Psychiatry* 138 (1981): 30–32.

Cunningham, S., et al. "Survival of the Selfish: Contrasting Self-Referential and Survival-Based Encoding." *Consciousness and Cognition* 22, no. 1 (2013): 237–44.

Dahlitz, M., and J. D. Parkes. "Sleep Paralysis." *Lancet* 341, no. 8842 (1993): 406–7.

Dalí, S. *The Secret Life of Salvador Dalí.* New York: Dover, 1993.

Dalla, B. G., and M. F. Boisse. "Temporal Consciousness and Confabulation: Is the Medial Temporal Lobe 'Temporal'?" *Cognitive Neuropsychiatry* 15, no. 1 (2010): 95–117.

Dalrymple, T. *Life at the Bottom: The Worldview That Makes the Underclass.* Chicago: Ivan R. Dee, 2001.

D'Altorio, T. "Coke vs. Pepsi . . . Are the Cola Wars Finally Over?" Accessed July 3, 2012. http://www.investmentu.com/2012/February/are-the-coke-vs-pepsi-cola-wars-over .html.

Damasio, A. *Descartes' Error: Emotion, Reason, and the Human Brain.* New York: Avon Books, 1994.

Davidson, P. R., and D. M. Wolpert. "Widespread Access to Predictive Models in the Motor System: A Short Review." *Journal of Neural Engineering* 2, no. 3 (2005): S313–S19.

Davis, M. H., F. Meunier, and W. D. Marslen-Wilson. "Neural Responses to Morphological, Syntactic, and Semantic Properties of Single Words: An fMRI Study." *Brain and Language* 89, no. 3 (2004): 439–49.

Decety, J., J. Jeannerod, and C. Prablanc. "The Timing of Mentally Represented Actions." *Behavioural Brain Research* 34, no. 1–2 (1989): 35–42.

Decety, J., and F. Michel. "Comparative Analysis of Actual and Mental Movement Times in Two Graphic Tasks." *Brain and Cognition* 11, no. 1 (1989): 87–97.

de Gelder, B., et al. "Intact Navigation Skills After Bilateral Loss of Striate Cortex." *Current Biology* 18, no. 24 (2008): R1128–R29.

De Jong, J. T. V. "Cultural Variation in the Clinical Presentation of Sleep Paralysis." *Transcultural Psychiatry* 42, no. 1 (2005): 78–92.

Dement, W., and E. A. Wolpert. "The Relation of Eye Movements, Body Motility, and External Stimuli to Dream Content." *Journal of Experimental Psychology* 55, no. 6 (1958): 543–53.

D'Esposito, M., et al. "A Functional MRI Study of Mental Imagery Generation." *Neuropsychologia* 35, no. 5 (1997): 724–30.

Diaz, J. "Masters Plan." *Sports Illustrated,* April 13, 1998. http://sportsillustrated.cnn.com/vault/article/magazine/MAG1012553/2/index.htm.

Dimberg, U., M. Thunberg, and K. Elmehed. "Unconscious Facial Reactions to Emotional Facial Expressions." *Psychological Science* 11, no. 1 (2000): 86–89.

Dinstein, I., et al. "Normal Movement Selectivity in Autism." *Neuron* 66, no. 3 (2010): 461–69.

Di Pellegrino, G., et al. "Understanding Motor Events: A Neurophysiological Study." *Experimental Brain Research* 91, no. 1 (1992): 176–80.

Domhoff, G. W. "The Dreams of Men and Women: Patterns of Gender Similarity and Difference" (2005). Accessed Dec. 31, 2013. http://dreamresearch.net/Library/domhoff_2005c.html.

Donnay, G. F., et al. "Neural Substrates of Interactive Musical Improvisation: An fMRI Study of 'Trading Fours' in Jazz." *PLOS ONE* 9, no. 2 (2014): e88665.

Downing, S. *On Course: Study Skills Plus Edition.* Boston: Wadsworth, 2011.

Dresler, M., et al. "Neural Correlates of Dream Lucidity Obtained from Contrasting Lucid Versus Non-Lucid REM Sleep: A Combined EEG/fMRI Case Study." *Sleep* 35, no. 7 (2012): 1017–20.

Driediger, M., C. Hall, and N. Callow. "Imagery Use by Injured Athletes: A Qualitative Analysis." *Journal of Sports Sciences* 24, no. 3 (2006): 261–71.

"Driving You Crazy." WHNT News 19, Huntsville, Ala. Accessed Dec. 10, 2012. http://www.dailymotion.com/video/xfz183_driving-out-of-habit-becoming-dangerous_news#.UOCNQW_edJ6.

Drysdale, G. "Kaethe Kollwitz (1867–1945): The Artist Who May Have Suffered from Alice in Wonderland Syndrome." *Journal of Medical Biography* 17, no. 2 (2009): 106–10.

Duchenne, G.-B. *The Mechanism of Human Facial Expression.* New York: Cambridge University Press, 1990.

du Feu, M., and P. J. McKenna. "Prelingually, Profoundly Deaf Schizophrenic Patients Who Hear Voices: A Phenomenological Analysis." *Acta Psychiatrica Scandinavica* 99, no. 6 (1999): 453–59.


Egner, T., G. Jamieson, and J. Gruzelier. "Hypnosis Decouples Cognitive Control from Conflict Monitoring Processes of the Frontal Lobe." *NeuroImage* 27, no. 4 (2005): 969–78.

Eiser, A. S. "Physiology and Psychology of Dreams." *Seminars in Neurology* 25, no. 1 (2005): 97–105.

Erickson, T. D., and M. E. Mattson. "From Words to Meaning: A Semantic Illusion." *Journal of Verbal Learning and Verbal Behavior* 20, no. 5 (1981): 540–51.

Evans, J., and H. Elliott. "Screening Criteria for the Diagnosis of Schizophrenia in Deaf Patients." *Archives of General Psychiatry* 38, no. 7 (1981): 787–90.

Eysel, U. T., et al. "Reorganization in the Visual Cortex After Retinal and Cortical Damage." *Restorative Neurology and Neuroscience* 15, no. 2–3 (1999): 153–64.

Facco, E., and C. Agrillo. "Near-Death-Like Experiences Without Life-Threatening Conditions or Brain Disorders: A Hypothesis from a Case Report." *Frontiers in Psychology* 3, no. 490 (2012): 1–6.

Fahrenfort, J. J., et al. "The Spatiotemporal Profile of Cortical Processing Leading Up to Visual Perception." *Journal of Vision* 8, no. 1 (2008): 11–12.

Feinberg, T. E. *Altered Egos: How the Brain Creates the Self.* New York: Oxford University Press, 2001.

Feinberg, T. E., and R. M. Shapiro. "Misidentification-Reduplication and the Right Hemisphere." *Cognitive and Behavioral Neurology* 2, no. 1 (1989): 39–48.

Feinberg, T. E., et al. "The Neuroanatomy of Asomatognosia and Somatoparaphrenia." *Journal of Neurology, Neurosurgery, and Psychiatry* 81, no. 3 (2010): 276–81.

Feulner, P. G., et al. "Electrifying Love: Electric Fish Use Species-Specific Discharge for Mate Recognition." *Biology Letters* 5, no. 2 (2009a): 225–28.

Feulner, P. G., et al. "Magic Trait Electric Organ Discharge (EOD): Dual Function of Electric Signals Promotes Speciation in African Weakly Electric Fish." *Communicative and Integrative Biology* 2, no. 4 (2009b): 329–31.

Ffytche, D. H., et al. "The Anatomy of Conscious Vision: An fMRI Study of Visual Hallucinations." *Nature Neuroscience* 1, no. 8 (1998): 738–42.

Filimon, F., et al. "Human Cortical Representations for Reaching: Mirror Neurons for Execution, Observation, and Imagery." *NeuroImage* 37, no. 4 (2007): 1315–28.

Fink, G. R., et al. "Cerebral Representation of One's Own Past: Neural Networks Involved in Autobiographical Memory." *Journal of Neuroscience* 16, no. 13 (1996): 4275–82.

Flanagan, J. R., and A. M. Wing. "The Role of Internal Models in Motion Planning and Control: Evidence from Grip Force Adjustments During Movements of Hand-Held Loads." *Journal of Neuroscience* 17, no. 4 (1997): 1519–28.

Ford, J. M., and D. H. Mathalon. "Electrophysiological Evidence of Corollary Discharge Dysfunction in Schizophrenia During Talking and Thinking." *Journal of Psychiatric Research* 38, no. 1 (2004): 37–46.

Ford, J. M., et al. "Neurophysiological Evidence of Corollary Discharge Dysfunction in Schizophrenia." *American Journal of Psychiatry* 158, no. 12 (2001): 2069–71.

Fosse, M. J., et al. "Dreaming and Episodic Memory: A Functional Dissociation?" *Journal of Cognitive Neuroscience* 15, no. 1 (2003): 1–9.

*Franklin v. Duncan,* 884 F. Supp. 1435 (N.D. Cal. 1995).

Franklin, M., and M. Zyphur. "The Role of Dreams in the Evolution of the Human Mind." *Evolutionary Psychology* 3 (2005): 59–78.

Freud, S. *The Interpretation of Dreams.* London: Macmillan, 1913.

Frith, C. D. "The Cognitive Abnormalities Underlying the Symptomatology and the Disability of Patients with Schizophrenia." *International Clinical Psychopharmacology* 10, no. 3 (1995): 87–98.

Fulgham, D. Interview with Jad Abumrad. "Out of Body, Roger." *Radiolab,* May 5, 2006.

Gallese, V., et al. "Action Recognition in the Premotor Cortex." *Brain* 119, no. 2 (1996): 593–609.

Gallup, G. H., and F. Newport Jr. "Belief in Paranormal Phenomena Among Adult Americans." *Skeptical Inquirer* 15, no. 2 (1991): 137–46.

Gangitano, M., F. M. Mottaghy, and A. Pascual-Leone. "Phase-Specific Modulation of

Cortical Motor Output During Movement Observation." *Neuroreport* 12, no. 7 (2001): 1489–92.

García Márquez, G. *Love in the Time of Cholera*. New York: Alfred A. Knopf, 1985.

Garrity, L. I. "Electromyography: A Review of the Current Status of Subvocal Speech Research." *Memory and Cognition* 5, no. 6 (1977): 615–22.

Gazzaniga, M. S. *The Bisected Brain*. New York: Appleton-Century-Crofts, 1970.

———. "Cerebral Specialization and Interhemispheric Communication: Does the Corpus Callosum Enable the Human Condition?" *Brain* 123 (2000): 1293–326.

———. *The Ethical Brain*. New York: Dana Press, 2005.

———. "One Brain—Two Minds?" *American Scientist* 60 (1972): 311–17.

———. "Organization of the Human Brain." *Science* 245, no. 4921 (1989): 947–52.

Gazzaniga, M. S., R. Ivry, and G. R. Mangun. *Cognitive Neuroscience: The Biology of the Mind*. New York: W. W. Norton, 2002.

Gentili, R., C. Papaxanthis, and T. Pozzo. "Improvement and Generalization of Arm Motor Performance Through Motor Imagery Practice." *Neuroscience* 137, no. 3 (2006): 761–72.

Gentili, R., et al. "Inertial Properties of the Arm Are Accurately Predicted During Motor Imagery." *Behavioural Brain Research* 155, no. 2 (2004): 231–39.

Gerrans, P. "A One-Stage Explanation of the Cotard Delusion." *Philosophy, Psychiatry, and Psychology* 9, no. 1 (2002): 47–53.

Gleaves, D. H. "The Sociocognitive Model of Dissociative Identity Disorder: A Reexamination of the Evidence." *Psychological Bulletin* 120, no. 1 (1996): 42–59.

Goetz, C. G., M. Bonduelle, and T. Gelfand. *Charcot: Constructing Neurology*. New York: Oxford University Press, 1995.

Goldberg, E. *The Executive Brain: The Frontal Lobes and the Civilized Mind*. Oxford: Oxford University Press, 2001.

Goller, A. I., et al. "Mirror-Touch Synaesthesia in the Phantom Limbs of Amputees." *Cortex* 49, no. 1 (2013): 243–51.

Gosline, A. "Hypnosis Really Changes Your Mind." *New Scientist*, Sept. 10, 2004.

Gould, L. N. "Auditory Hallucinations and Subvocal Speech." *Journal of Nervous and Mental Disease* 109, no. 5 (1949): 418–27.

———. "Verbal Hallucinations and the Activity of the Vocal Musculature." *American Journal of Psychiatry* 105, no. 5 (1948): 367–72.

Grant, K., et al. "Neural Command of Electromotor Output in Mormyrids." *Journal of Experimental Biology* 202 (1999): 1399–407.

Green, M. F., and M. Kinsbourne. "Subvocal Activity and Auditory Hallucinations: Clues for Behavioral Treatments?" *Psychological Bulletin* 16, no. 4 (1990): 617–25.

Green, P., and M. Preston. "Reinforcement of Vocal Correlate of Auditory Hallucinations by Auditory Feedback: A Case Study." *British Journal of Psychiatry* 139 (1981): 204–8.

Greene, A. "Syd Barrett (1946–2006): Founding Frontman and Songwriter for Pink Floyd Dead at 60." *Rolling Stone*, July 11, 2006. http://www.rollingstone.com/music/news/syd-barrett-1946-2006-20060711.

Guenther, F. H., S. S. Ghosh, and J. A. Tourville. "Neural Modeling and Imaging of the Cortical Interactions Underlying Syllable Production." *Brain and Language* 96, no. 3 (2006): 280–301.

Guillot, A., et al. "Motor Imagery and Tennis Serve Performance: The External Focus Efficacy." *Journal of Sports Science Medicine* 12, no. 2 (2013): 332–38.

Haker, H., et al. "Mirror Neuron Activity During Contagious Yawning—an fMRI Study." *Brain Imaging and Behavior* 7, no. 1 (2013): 28–34.

Halligan, P. W., C. Bass, and D. T. Wade. "New Approaches to Conversion Hysteria." *British Medical Journal* 320, no. 7248 (2000): 1488–89.

Halligan, P. W., et al. "Imaging Hypnotic Paralysis: Implications for Conversion Hysteria." *Lancet* 355, no. 9208 (2000): 986–87.

Hamson-Utley, J. J., S. Martin, and J. Walters. "Athletic Trainers' and Physical Therapists' Perceptions of the Effectiveness of Psychological Skills Within Sport Injury Rehabilitation Programs." *Journal of Athletic Training* 43, no. 3 (2008): 258–64.

Hanson-Vaux, G., A. S. Crisinel, and C. Spence. "Smelling Shapes: Crossmodal Correspondences Between Odors and Shapes." *Chemical Senses* 38, no. 2 (2013): 161–66.

Haykin, S., and Z. Chen. "The Cocktail Party Problem." *Neural Computation* 17, no. 9 (2005): 1875–902.

Head, P. D. "Synaesthesia: Pitch-Color Isomorphism in RGB-Space?" *Cortex* 42, no. 2 (2006): 164–74.

Heath, R. *Seducing the Subconscious: The Psychology of Emotional Influence in Advertising.* West Sussex, U.K.: Wiley-Blackwell, 2012.

Heilman, K. M. "Anosognosia: Possible Neuropsychological Mechanisms." In *Awareness of Deficit After Brain Injury: Clinical and Theoretical Issues,* edited by G. P. Prigatano and D. L. Schacter. New York: Oxford University Press, 1991.

Heinks-Maldonado, T. H., et al. "Relationship of Imprecise Corollary Discharge in Schizophrenia to Auditory Hallucinations." *Archives of General Psychiatry* 64, no. 3 (2007): 286–96.

Helt, M. S., et al. "Contagious Yawning in Autistic and Typical Development." *Child Development* 81, no. 5 (2010): 1620–31.

Hemayattalab, R., and A. Movahedi. "Effects of Different Variations of Mental and Physical Practice on Sport Skill Learning in Adolescents with Mental Retardation." *Research in Developmental Disabilities* 31, no. 1 (2010): 81–86.

Henderson, W. R., and G. E. Smyth. "Phantom Limbs." *Journal of Neurology, Neurosurgery, and Psychiatry* 11, no. 2 (1948): 88–112.

Herdman, S. J., M. C. Schubert, and R. J. Tusa. "Role of Central Preprogramming in Dynamic Visual Acuity with Vestibular Loss." *Archives of Otolaryngology—Head and Neck Surgery* 127, no. 10 (2001): 1205–10.

Herwig, U., et al. "Neural Activity Associated with Self-Reflection." *BMC Neuroscience* 13, no. 52 (2012): 1–12.

Higgins, E. T., and J. A. Bargh. "Social Cognition and Social Perception." *Annual Review of Psychology* 38 (1987): 369–425.

Hill, D. R., and M. A. Persinger. "Application of Transcerebral, Weak (1 microT) Complex Magnetic Fields and Mystical Experiences: Are They Generated by Field-Induced Dimethyltryptamine Release from the Pineal Organ?" *Perceptual and Motor Skills* 97 (2003): 1049–50.

Hobson, J. A. "REM Sleep and Dreaming: Towards a Theory of Protoconsciousness." *Nature Reviews Neuroscience* 10 (2009): 803–13.

———. "Sleep and Dream Suppression Following a Lateral Medullary Infarct: A First-Person Account." *Consciousness and Cognition* 11, no. 3 (2002): 377–90.

Hobson, J. A., and K. J. Friston. "Waking and Dreaming Consciousness: Neurobiological and Functional Considerations." *Progress in Neurobiology* 98, no. 1 (2012): 82–98.

Hobson, J. A., and R. W. McCarley. "The Brain as a Dream State Generator: An Activation-Synthesis Hypothesis of the Dream Process." *American Journal of Psychiatry* 134, no. 12 (1977): 1335–48.

Hobson, J. A., E. F. Pace-Schott, and R. Stickgold. "Dreaming and the Brain: Toward a Cognitive Neuroscience of Conscious States." *Behavioral and Brain Sciences* 23, no. 6 (2000): 793–842.

Hofle, N., et al. "Regional Cerebral Blood Flow Changes as a Function of Delta and Spindle Activity During Slow Wave Sleep in Humans." *Journal of Neuroscience* 17, no. 12 (1997): 4800–4808.

Holmes, P. S., and D. J. Collins. "The PETTLEP Approach to Motor Imagery: A Functional Equivalence Model for Sport Psychologists." *Journal of Applied Sport Psychology* 13, no. 1 (2001): 60–83.

Hong, C. C., et al. "fMRI Evidence for Multisensory Recruitment Associated with Rapid Eye Movements During Sleep." *Human Brain Mapping* 30, no. 5 (2008): 1705–22.

Howell, E. *Understanding and Treating Dissociative Identity Disorder.* New York: Routledge, 2011.

Howland, J. S. "The Use of Hypnosis in the Treatment of a Case of Multiple Personality." *Journal of Nervous and Mental Disease* 161, no. 2 (1975): 138–42.

Huber, R., et al. "Arm Immobilization Causes Cortical Plastic Changes and Locally Decreases Sleep Slow Wave Activity." *Nature Neuroscience* 9, no. 9 (2006): 1169–76.

Hurovitz, C., et al. "The Dreams of Blind Men and Women: A Replication and Extension of Previous Findings." *Dreaming* 9, no. 2–3 (1999): 183–93.

Hutchison, W., et al. "Pain-Related Neurons in the Human Cingulate Cortex." *Nature Neuroscience* 2 (1999): 403–5.

Huxley, A. *Letters of Aldous Huxley.* Ed. Grover Smith. New York: Harper & Row, 1970.

Ibáñez, A., et al. "Subliminal Presentation of Other Faces (but Not Own Face) Primes Behavioral and Evoked Cortical Processing of Empathy for Pain." *Brain Research* 1398 (2011): 72–85.

Ietswaart, M., et al. "Mental Practice with Motor Imagery in Stroke Recovery: Randomized Controlled Trial of Efficacy." *Brain* 134, no. 5 (2011): 1373–86.

*The International Classification of Sleep Disorders: Diagnostic and Coding Manual.* 2nd ed. Westchester, Ill.: American Academy of Sleep Medicine, 2005.

Jackson, P. L., A. N. Meltzoff, and J. Decety. "How Do We Perceive the Pain of Others? A Window into the Neural Processes Involved in Empathy." *NeuroImage* 24, no. 3 (2005): 771–79.

Jacob, A., et al. "Charles Bonnet Syndrome—Elderly People and Visual Hallucinations." *British Medical Journal* 328, no. 7455 (2004): 1552–54.

Jacome, D. "Phantom Itching Relieved by Scratching Phantom Feet." *Journal of the American Medical Association* 240, no. 22 (1978): 2432.

Jarrett, C. "A Calm Look at the Most Hyped Concept in Neuroscience—Mirror Neurons." Wired.com. Accessed Dec. 13, 2013. http://www.wired.com/wiredscience/2013/12/a-calm-look-at-the-most-hyped-concept-in-neuroscience-mirror-neurons/.

Jiménez-Genchi, A., et al. "Sleep Paralysis in Adolescents: The 'A Dead Body Climbed on Top of Me' Phenomenon in Mexico." *Psychiatry and Clinical Neurosciences* 63, no. 4 (2009): 546–49.

Joel, B. Interview with Alec Baldwin. *Here's the Thing*. Produced by Emily Botein and Kathie Russo. New York: WNYC. July 30, 2012.

Johns, L. C., et al. "Impaired Verbal Self-Monitoring in Psychosis: Effects of State, Trait, and Diagnosis." *Psychological Medicine* 36, no. 4 (2006): 465–74.

Johnson, A., and A. D. Redish. "Neural Ensembles in CA3 Transiently Encode Paths Forward of the Animal at a Decision Point." *Journal of Neuroscience* 27, no. 45 (2007): 12176–89.

Joly-Mascheroni, R. M., A. Senju, and A. J. Shepherd. "Dogs Catch Human Yawns." *Biology Letters* 4, no. 5 (2008): 446–48.

Jung, C. G. *The Archetypes and the Collective Unconscious*. Princeton, NJ: Princeton University Press, 1959.


Kan, I. P., et al. "Memory Monitoring Failure in Confabulation: Evidence from the Semantic Illusion Paradigm." *Journal of the International Neuropsychological Society* 16, no. 6 (2010): 1006–17.

Kanner, L. "Autistic Disturbances of Affective Contact." *Nervous Child* 2 (1943): 217–50.

Kaplan, O. "The Effect of the Hypnotic-Suggestive Communication Level of Advertisements on Their Effectiveness." *Contemporary Hypnosis* 24, no. 2 (2007): 53–63.

Kas, A., et al. "Feeling Unreal: A Functional Imaging Study in Patients with Kleine-Levin Syndrome." *Brain* 37, pt. 7 (2014): 2077–87.

Kaski, D. "Revision: Is Visual Perception a Requisite for Visual Imagery?" *Perception* 31, no. 6 (2002): 717–31.

Keenan, J. P., G. Gallup Jr., and D. Falk. *The Face in the Mirror: How We Know Who We Are*. New York: Ecco, 2003.

Keenan, J. P., et al. "Self-Recognition and the Right Prefrontal Cortex." *Trends in Cognitive Sciences* 4, no. 9 (2000): 338–44.

Kelley, W. M., et al. "Finding the Self? An Event-Related fMRI Study." *Journal of Cognitive Neuroscience* 15, no. 5 (2002): 785–94.

Kerns, J. G., J. D. Cohen, and A. W. MacDonald. "Anterior Cingulate Conflict Monitoring and Adjustments in Control." *Science* 303, no. 5660 (2004): 1023–26.

Kerr, N. H., and G. W. Domhoff. "Do the Blind Literally 'See' in Their Dreams? A Critique of a Recent Claim That They Do." *Dreaming* 14, no. 4 (2004): 230–33.

Kerr, N. H., et al. "The Structure of Laboratory Dream Reports in Blind and Sighted Subjects." *Journal of Nervous and Mental Disease* 170, no. 5 (1982): 247–64.

Kew, J., A. Wright, and P. W. Halligan. "Somesthetic Aura: The Experience of 'Alice in Wonderland.'" *Lancet* 351, no. 9120 (1998): 1934.

Kihlstrom, J. F. "The Cognitive Unconscious." *Science* 237, no. 4821 (1987): 1445–52.

Kilner, J. M., Y. Paulignan, and S. J. Blakemore. "An Interference Effect of Observed Biological Movement on Action." *Current Biology* 13, no. 6 (2003): 522–25.

Kim, Y. T., et al. "Neural Correlates Related to Action Observation in Expert Archers." *Behavioural Brain Research* 223, no. 2 (2011): 342–47.

Kinderman, P., and R. P. Bentall. "Causal Attributions in Paranoia and Depression: Internal, Personal, and Situational Attributions for Negative Events." *Journal of Abnormal Psychology* 106, no. 2 (1997): 341–45.

Kleiter, I., et al. "A Lightning Strike to the Head Causing a Visual Cortex Defect with Simple and Complex Visual Hallucinations." *Journal of Neurology, Neurosurgery, and Psychiatry* 78, no. 4 (2007): 423–26.

Koelsch, S. "Towards a Neural Basis of Music-Evoked Emotions." *Trends in Cognitive Sciences* 14, no. 3 (2010): 131–37.

Koenigs, M., and D. Tranel. "Prefrontal Cortex Damage Abolishes Brand-Cued Changes in Cola Preference." *Social, Cognitive, and Affective Neuroscience* 3, no. 1 (2008): 1–6.

Kondziella, D., and S. Frahm-Falkenberg. "Anton's Syndrome and Eugenics." *Journal of Clinical Neurology* 7, no. 2 (2011): 96–98.

Kopelman, M. D. "Two Types of Confabulation." *Journal of Neurology, Neurosurgery, and Psychiatry* 50, no. 11 (1987): 1482–87.

Kosslyn, S. M., et al. "Neural Systems Shared by Visual Imagery and Visual Perception: A Positron Emission Tomography Study." *NeuroImage* 6, no. 4 (1997): 320–34.

Kosslyn, S. M., et al. "Visual Mental Imagery Activates Topographically Organized Visual Cortex: PET Investigations." *Journal of Cognitive Neuroscience* 5, no. 3 (1993): 263–87.

Kreiman, G., C. Koch, and I. Fried. "Category-Specific Visual Responses of Single Neurons in the Human Medial Temporal Lobe." *Nature Neuroscience* 3 (2000): 946–53.

Kremer, W. "Human Echolocation: Using Tongue-Clicks to Navigate the World." *BBC World Service,* Sept. 12, 2012. http://www.bbc.co.uk/news/magazine-19524962.

Krieger, R. A. *Civilization's Quotations: Life's Ideal.* New York: Algora, 2002.

Krosnick, J. A., et al. "Subliminal Conditioning of Attitudes." *Personality and Social Psychology Bulletin* 18, no. 2 (1992): 152.

Kumar, B. "Complex Visual Hallucinations in a Patient with Macular Degeneration: A Case of the Charles Bonnet Syndrome." *Age and Ageing* 42, no. 3 (2013): 411.

Kupers, R., et al. "Neural Correlates of Virtual Route Recognition in Congenital Blindness." *Proceedings of the National Academy of Sciences* 107, no. 28 (2010): 12716–21.

Kvavilashvili, L., et al. "Effects of Age on Phenomenology and Consistency of Flashbulb Memories of September 11 and a Staged Control Event." *Psychology and Aging* 25, no. 2 (2010): 391–404.

Lacourse, M. G., et al. "Brain Activation During Execution and Motor Imagery of Novel and Skilled Sequential Hand Movements." *NeuroImage* 27, no. 3 (2005): 505–19.

Lambert, E. H., and E. H. Wood. "Direct Determination of Man's Blood Pressure on the Human Centrifuge During Positive Acceleration." *Federation Proceedings* 5, no. 1, pt. 2 (1946): 59.

Lane, R. D., et al. "Neural Correlates of Levels of Emotional Awareness: Evidence of an Interaction Between Emotion and Attention in the Anterior Cingulate Cortex." *Journal of Cognitive Neuroscience* 10, no. 4 (1998): 525–35.

Lanius, R. A., J. W. Hopper, and R. S. Menon. "Individual Differences in a Husband and Wife Who Developed PTSD After a Motor Vehicle Accident: A Functional MRI Case Study." *American Journal of Psychiatry* 160, no. 4 (2003): 667–69.

"Leading Causes of Blindness in the U.S." National Eye Institute. Accessed Dec. 30, 2013. http://www.nei.nih.gov/health/fact_sheet.asp.

Lee, S. Y., et al. "Differential Priming Effect for Subliminal Fear and Disgust Facial Expressions." *Attention, Perception, and Psychophysics* 2, no. 73 (2011): 473–81.

Lessard, N., et al. "Early-Blind Human Subjects Localize Sound Sources Better Than Sighted Subjects." *Nature* 395, no. 6699 (1998): 278–80.

Lewis, M. "Obama's Way." *Vanity Fair,* Oct. 2012.

Lhermitte, F., et al. "Human Autonomy and the Frontal Lobes. Part I: Imitation and Utilization Behavior: A Neuropsychological Study of 75 Patients." *Annals of Neurology* 19, no. 4 (1986): 326–34.

———. "'Utilization Behavior' and Its Relation to Lesions of the Frontal Lobes." *Brain* 106, no. 2 (1983): 237–55.

Lhermitte, J. "Syndrome de la calotte du pédoncule cérébral: Les troubles psychosensoriels dans les lésions du mésocéphale." *Revue Neurologique* 38 (1922): 1359–65.

Lippman, C. W. "Certain Hallucinations Peculiar to Migraine." *Journal of Nervous and Mental Disease* 116, no. 4 (1952): 346–51.

Lisman, J., and E. J. Sternberg. "Habit and Nonhabit Systems for Unconscious and Conscious Behavior: Implications for Multitasking." *Journal of Cognitive Neuroscience* 25, no. 2 (2013): 273–83.

Litke, J. "If Duke Played the Taliban, I'd Pull for Taliban." Associated Press, *Yahoo! News,* March 23, 2012. sports.yahoo.com/blogs/ncaab-the-dagger/us-rep-brad-miller-duke -playing-taliban-d-191910616.html.

Lockhart, J. G., trans. and ed. *Ancient Spanish Ballads: Historical and Romantic.* New York: Wiley and Putnam, 1842.

Loftus, E. F. "The Reality of Repressed Memories." *American Psychologist* 48, no. 5 (1993): 518–37.

Loftus, E. F., and J. E. Pickrell. "The Formation of False Memories." *Psychiatric Annals* 15, no. 12 (1995): 720–25.

Lui, F., et al. "Neural Substrates for Observing and Imagining Non-Object-Directed Actions." *Society for Neuroscience* 3, no. 3–4 (2008): 261– 75.

MacDonald, K., and T. MacDonald. "Peas, Please: A Case Report and Neuroscientific Review of Dissociative Amnesia and Fugue." *Journal of Trauma and Dissociation* 10, no. 4 (2009): 420–35.

MacIntyre, T., and A. Moran. "Imagery Use Among Canoeists: A Worldwide Survey of Novice, Intermediate, and Elite Slalomists." *Journal of Applied Sport Psychology* 8 (1996): S132.

MacLeod, C. M. "Half a Century of Research on the Stroop Effect: An Integrative Review." *Psychological Bulletin* 109, no. 2 (1991): 163–203.

Maclin, E. L., K. E. Mathewson, and K. A. Low. "Learning to Multitask: Effects of Video Game Practice on Electrophysiological Indices of Attention and Resource Allocation." *Psychophysiology* 48, no. 9 (2011): 1173–83.

MacSweeney, M., et al. "Neural Systems Underlying British Sign Language and Audio-Visual English Processing in Native Users." *Brain* 125 (2002): 1583–93.

Maggin, D. L. *Stan Getz: A Life in Jazz.* New York: William Morrow, 1996.

Manford, M., and F. Andermann. "Complex Visual Hallucinations: Clinical and Neuro-biological Insights." *Brain* 121, no. 10 (1998): 1819–40.

Manning, M. L., and R. L. Manning. "Convergent Paradigms for Visual Neuroscience and Dissociative Identity Disorder." *Journal of Trauma and Dissociation* 10, no. 4 (2009): 405–19.

Mark, V. W., C. A. Kooistra, and K. M. Heilman. "Hemispatial Neglect Affected by Non-Neglected Stimuli." *Neurology* 38, no. 8 (1988): 1207–11.

Martineau, J., et al. "Atypical Activation of the Mirror Neuron System During Perception of Hand Motion in Autism." *Brain Research* 1320 (2010): 168–75.

Massen, J. J., D. A. Vermunt, and E. H. Sterck. "Male Yawning Is More Contagious Than Female Yawning Among Chimpanzees (*Pan troglodytes*)." *PLoS ONE* 7, no. 7 (2012).

Mast, F. W., D. M. Merfeld, and S. M. Kosslyn. "Visual Mental Imagery During Caloric Vestibular Stimulation." *Neuropsychologia* 44, no. 1 (2006): 101–19.

Mathalon, D. H., and J. M. Ford. "Corollary Discharge Dysfunction in Schizophrenia: Evidence for an Elemental Deficit." *Clinical EEG and Neuroscience* 39, no. 2 (2008): 82–86.

Mathersul, D., S. McDonald, and J. A. Rushby. "Automatic Facial Responses to Affective Stimuli in High-Functioning Adults with Autism Spectrum Disorder." *Physiology and Behavior* 109 (2013): 14–22.

Mayer, B., and H. Merckelbach. "Do Subliminal Priming Effects on Emotion Have Clinical Potential?" *Anxiety, Stress, and Coping* 12, no. 2 (1999): 217–29.

McCarley, R. W., O. Benoit, and G. Barrionuevo. "Lateral Geniculate Nucleus Unitary Discharge in Sleep and Waking: State- and Rate-Specific Aspects." *Journal of Neurophysiology* 50, no. 4 (1983): 798–818.

McGuire, P. K., et al. "Neural Correlates of Thinking in Sign Language." *Neuroreport* 8, no. 3 (1997): 695–98.

McGurk, H., and J. MacDonald. "Hearing Lips and Seeing Voices." *Nature* 264, no. 5588 (1976): 746–48.

McKay, R., and L. Cipolotti. "Attributional Style in a Case of Cotard Delusion." *Consciousness and Cognition* 16, no. 2 (2007): 349–59.

Mellor, C. S. "First Rank Symptoms of Schizophrenia. I. The Frequency in Schizophrenics on Admission to Hospital. II. Differences Between Individual First Rank Symptoms." *British Journal of Psychiatry* 117, no. 536 (1970): 15–23.

Mendelsohn, A., et al. "Subjective vs. Documented Reality: A Case Study of Long-Term Real-Life Autobiographical Memory." *Learning and Memory* 16, no. 2 (2009): 142–46.

Mercer, B., et al. "A Study of Confabulation." *Archives of Neurology* 34, no. 7 (1977): 429–33.

Mercer, J. "Hidden Persuaders." *Ode,* May/June 2012.

"Messing Calls on Hypnosis to Help Her with Underwater Scenes." ContactMusic.com, Oct. 21, 2005. Accessed Oct. 28, 2012. http://www.contactmusic.com/news-article/messing-calls-on-hypnosis-to-help-her-with-underwater-scenes.

Metcalf, K., R. Langdon, and M. Coltheart. "Models of Confabulation: A Critical Review and a New Framework." *Cognitive Neuropsychology* 24, no. 1 (2007): 23–47.

Miller, G. "Hunting for Meaning After Midnight." *Science* 315, no. 5817 (2007): 1360–63.

Miller, S. D., and P. J. Triggiano. "The Psychophysiological Investigation of Multiple Personality Disorder: Review and Update Review." *American Journal of Clinical Hypnosis* 35, no. 1 (1992): 47–61.

Minio-Paluello, I., et al. "Absence of Embodied Empathy During Pain Observation in Asperger Syndrome." *Biological Psychiatry* 65, no. 1 (2009): 55–62.

Mitchell, S. W. "On Some of the Disorders of Sleep." *Virginia Medical Monthly* 2 (1876): 769–81. In *Handbook of Clinical Neurology*. Vol. 15. Edited by D. D. Daly et al. Amsterdam: North Holland Publishing Company, 1974.

Mohr, C., et al., "The Anterior Cingulate Cortex Contains Distinct Areas Disassociating External from Self-Administered Painful Stimulation: A Parametric fMRI Study." *Pain* 114, no. 3 (2005): 347–57.

Morrison, I., et al. "Vicarious Responses to Pain in Anterior Cingulate Cortex: Is Empathy a Multisensory Issue?" *Cognitive, Affective, and Behavioral Neuroscience* 4, no. 2 (2004): 270–78.

Moscovitch, M. "Confabulation." In *Memory Distortion,* edited by D. L. Schacter, J. T. Coyle, G. D. Fischbach, M. M. Mesulam, and L. E. Sullivan, 226–51. Cambridge, Mass.: Harvard University Press, 1995.

———. "Confabulation and the Frontal Systems: Strategic Versus Associative Retrieval in Neuropsychological Theories of Memory." In *Varieties of Memory and Consciousness: Essays in Honour of Endel Tulving,* edited by H. L. Roediger and F. I. M. Craik, 133–60. Hillsdale, N.J.: Erlbaum, 1989.

Mouras, H., et al. "Activation of Mirror-Neuron System by Erotic Video Clips Predicts Degree of Induced Erection: An fMRI Study." *NeuroImage* 42, no. 3 (2008): 1142–50.

Mullins, S., and S. A. Spence. "Re-examining Thought Insertion: Semi-Structured Literature Review and Conceptual Analysis." *British Journal of Psychiatry* 182 (2003): 293–98.

Murphy, M., et al. "The Cortical Topography of Local Sleep." *Current Topics in Medical Chemistry* 11, no. 19 (2011): 2438–46.

Myhrvold, N. "Mars to Humanity: Get Over Yourself." Slate.com, Aug. 15, 1996. http://www.slate.com/articles/briefing/articles/1996/08/mars_to_humanity_get_over_your self.html.

Narayan, R., et al. "Cortical Interference Effects in the Cocktail Party Problem." *Nature Neuroscience* 10, no. 12 (2007): 1601–7.

Nelson, H. E., S. Thrasher, and T. R. Barnes. "Practical Ways of Alleviating Auditory Hallucinations." *British Medical Journal* 302, no. 6772 (1991): 327.

Nelson, K. R., et al. "Does the Arousal System Contribute to Near Death Experience?" *Neurology* 66, no. 7 (2006): 1003–9.

Nelson, K. R., et al. "Out-of-Body Experience and Arousal." *Neurology* 68, no. 10 (2007): 794–95.

Ness, R. C. "The Old Hag Phenomenon as Sleep Paralysis: A Biocultural Interpretation." *Culture, Medicine, and Psychiatry* 2, no. 1 (1978): 15–39.

Nicklaus, Jack. *Play Better Golf.* New York: King Features, 1976.

Niedenthal, P. M., et al. "Embodiment in Attitudes, Social Perception, and Emotion." *Personality and Social Psychology Review* 9, no. 3 (2005): 184–211.

Nijenhuis, E. R. S., O. Van der Hart, and K. Steele. "The Emerging Psychobiology of Trauma-Related Dissociation and Dissociative Disorders." In *Biological Psychiatry,* edited by H. D'Haenen, J. A. den Boer, and P. Willner, 1079–80. London: Wiley, 2002.

Nowak, D. A., and J. Hermsdörfer. "Sensorimotor Memory and Grip Force Control: Does Grip Force Anticipate a Self-Produced Weight Change When Drinking with a Straw from a Cup?" *European Journal of Neuroscience* 18, no. 10 (2003): 2883–92.

Oakley, D. A. "Hypnosis and Conversion Hysteria: A Unifying Model." *Cognitive Neuropsychiatry* 4, no. 3 (1999): 243–65.

Oishi, K., T. Kasai, and T. Maeshima. "Autonomic Response Specificity During Motor Imagery." *Journal of Physiology and Anthropology of Applied Human Sciences* 19, no. 6 (2000): 255–61.

O'Keefe, J. "A Review of the Hippocampal Place Cells." *Progress in Neurobiology* 13, no. 4 (1979): 419–39.

Oudiette, D., et al. "Dreamlike Mentations During Sleepwalking and Sleep Terrors in Adults." *Sleep* 32, no. 12 (2009): 1621–27.

Pachalska, M., et al. "A Case of 'Borrowed Identity Syndrome' After Severe Traumatic Brain Injury." *Medical Science Monitor* 17, no. 2 (2011): 18–28.

Packard, M. G., and J. L. McGaugh. "Inactivation of Hippocampus or Caudate Nucleus with Lidocaine Differentially Affects Expression of Place and Response Learning." *Neurobiology of Learning and Memory* 65, no. 1 (1996): 65–72.

Palagi, E., et al. "Contagious Yawning in Gelada Baboons as a Possible Expression of Empathy." *Proceedings of the National Academy of Sciences* 106, no. 46 (2009): 19262–67.

Paraskevas-Thadani, E. "Banning the Thought: Saving the Lungs of Children by Banning Subliminal Messages in Tobacco Advertisements." *Syracuse Journal of Legislation and Policy* 2 (1997): 133–63.

Park, M., et al. "Differences Between Musicians and Non-Musicians in Neuro-Affective Processing of Sadness and Fear Expressed in Music." *Neuroscience Letters* 566 (2014): 120–24.

Park, Y. W., et al. "Alien Hand Syndrome in Stroke—Case Report and Neurophysiologic Study." *Annals of Rehabilitation Medicine* 36, no. 4 (2012): 556–60.

Parton, A., P. Malhotra, and M. Husain. "Hemispatial Neglect." *Journal of Neurology, Neurosurgery, and Psychiatry* 75 (2004): 13–21.

Pascual-Leone, A., et al. "Modulation of Muscle Responses Evoked by Transcranial Magnetic Stimulation During the Acquisition of New Fine Motor Skills." *Journal of Neurophysiology* 74, no. 3 (1995): 1037–45.

Patterson, D. R., M. L. Goldberg, and D. M. Ehde. "Hypnosis in the Treatment of Patients with Severe Burns." *American Journal of Clinical Hypnosis* 38, no. 3 (1996): 200–212.

Patterson, R. B. "Hypnotherapy of Hysterical Monocular Blindness: A Case Report." *American Journal of Clinical Hypnosis* 23, no. 2 (1980): 119–21.

Pavlides, C., and J. Winson. "Influences of Hippocampal Place Cell Firing in the Awake State on the Activity of These Cells During Subsequent Sleep Episodes." *Journal of Neuroscience* 9, no. 8 (1989): 2907–18.

Pehrs, C., et al. "How Music Alters a Kiss: Superior Temporal Gyrus Controls Fusiform-Amygdalar Effective Connectivity." *Social Cognitive and Affective Neuroscience* 9, no. 11 (2014): 1–9.

Peigneux, P., et al. "Are Spatial Memories Strengthened in the Human Hippocampus During Slow Wave Sleep?" *Neuron* 44, no. 3 (2004): 535–45.

Peterson, C., et al. "The Attributional Style Questionnaire." *Cognitive Therapy and Research* 6, no. 3 (1982): 287–300.

Pfeiffer, J. H., et al. "Mirroring Others' Emotions Relates to Empathy and Interpersonal Competence in Children." *NeuroImage* 39, no. 4 (2008): 2076–85.

Platek, S. M. "Yawn, Yawn, Yawn, Yawn; Yawn, Yawn, Yawn! The Social, Evolutionary, and Neuroscientific Facets of Contagious Yawning." *Frontiers of Neurology and Neuroscience* 28 (2010): 107–12.

Podoll, K., and D. Robinson. "Lewis Carroll's Migraine Experiences." *Lancet* 353, no. 9161 (1999): 1366.

"Poll: U.S. Hiding Knowledge of Aliens." CNN.com, June 15, 1997. http://articles.cnn .com/1997-06-15/us/9706_15_ufo.poll.

Poppel, E., et al. "Residual Visual Function After Brain Wounds Involving the Central Visual Pathways in Man." *Nature* 243, no. 5405 (1973): 295–96.

Posner, M. I., and S. E. Petersen. "The Attention System of the Human Brain." *Annual Review of Neuroscience* 13 (1990): 25–42.

Powell, L. J., et al. "Dissociable Neural Substrates for Agentic Versus Conceptual Representations of Self." *Journal of Cognitive Neuroscience* 22, no. 10 (2010): 2186–97.

Prasad, S., and A. L. Berkowitz. "Modified Target Cancellation in Hemispatial Neglect." *Practical Neurology* 14, no. 4 (2014): 277.

Pratkanis, A. R. "The Cargo-Cult Science of Subliminal Persuasion." *Skeptical Inquirer* 16, no. 3 (1992).

Price, A., and D. Price. *Introducing Psychology of Success: A Practical Guide.* London: Icon Books, 2011.

Prigatano, G. P., and D. L. Schacter. *Awareness of Deficit After Brain Injury: Clinical and Theoretical Issues.* Oxford: Oxford University Press, 1991.

Proust, M. *Remembrance of Things Past: Swann's Way.* New York: Vintage Books, 1982.

Provine, R. R. "Yawning." *American Science* 93, no. 6 (2005): 532–39.

Putnam, F. W., T. P. Zahn, and R. M. Post. "Differential Autonomic Nervous System Activity in Multiple Personality Disorder." *Physical Review* 31, no. 3 (1990): 251–60.

Pyka, M., et al. "Brain Correlates of Hypnotic Paralysis—a Resting-State fMRI Study." *NeuroImage* 56, no. 4 (2011): 2173–82.

Quian Quiroga, R. "Concept Cells: The Building Blocks of Declarative Memory Functions." *Nature Reviews Neuroscience* 13, no. 8 (2012): 587–97.

Quian Quiroga, R., et al. "Explicit Encoding of Multimodal Percepts by Single Neurons in the Human Brain." *Current Biology* 19, no. 15 (2009): 1308–13.

Quian Quiroga, R., et al. "Invariant Visual Representation by Single Neurons in the Human Brain." *Nature* 435 (2005): 1102–7.

*Rabey v. R.*, [1980] 2 S.C.R. 513 (Can.) (Dickson, J. dissenting).

Ramachandran, V. S., and D. Brang. "Sensations Evoked in Patients with Amputation from Watching an Individual Whose Corresponding Intact Limb Is Being Touched." *Archives of Neurology* 66, no. 10 (2009): 1281–84.

Ramachandran, V. S., and L. M. Oberman. "Broken Mirrors: A Theory of Autism." *Scientific American* 295, no. 5 (2006): 62–69.

Ramachandran, V. S., and D. Rogers-Ramachandran. "Synaesthesia in Phantom Limbs Induced with Mirrors." *Proceedings of the Royal Society B: Biological Sciences* 263, no. 1369 (1996): 377–86.

Ramakonar, H., E. A. Franz, and C. R. Lind. "The Rubber Hand Illusion and Its Application to Clinical Neuroscience." *Journal of Clinical Neuroscience* 18, no. 12 (2011): 1596–601.

Ramirez-Bermudez, J., et al. "Cotard Syndrome in Neurological and Psychiatric Patients." *Journal of Neuropsychiatry and Clinical Neurosciences* 22, no. 4 (2010): 409–16.

Ranganathan, V. K., et al. "From Mental Power to Muscle Power—Gaining Strength by Using the Mind." *Neuropsychologia* 42, no. 7 (2004): 944–56.

Rankin, K. P. "Detecting Sarcasm from Paralinguistic Cues: Anatomic and Cognitive Correlates in Neurodegenerative Disease." *NeuroImage* 47, no. 4 (2009): 2005–15.

Raposo, A., and J. F. Marques. "The Contribution of Fronto-parietal Regions to Sentence Comprehension: Insights from the Moses Illusion." *NeuroImage* 83 (2013): 431–37.

Raz, A., et al. "Hypnotic Suggestion and the Modulation of Stroop Interference." *Archives of General Psychiatry* 59, no. 12 (2002): 1155–61.

Reder, L. M., and G. W. Kusbit. "Locus of the Moses Illusion: Imperfect Encoding, Retrieval, or Match?" *Journal of Memory and Language* 30 (1991): 385–406.

Reinders, A. A., et al. "Psychobiological Characteristics of Dissociative Identity Disorder: A Symptom Provocation Study." *Biological Psychiatry* 60, no. 7 (2006): 730–40.

Reis, B. E. "Toward a Psychoanalytic Understanding of Multiple Personality Disorder." *Bulletin of the Menninger Clinic* 57, no. 3 (1993): 309–18.

Ricard, P. "Vision Loss and Visual Hallucinations: The Charles Bonnet Syndrome." *Community Eye Health* 22, no. 69 (2009): 14.

Rickards, C. A., and D. G. Newman. "G-induced Visual and Cognitive Disturbances in a Survey of 65 Operational Fighter Pilots." *Aviation, Space, and Environmental Medicine* 76, no. 5 (2005): 496–500.

Riddoch, G. "Dissociation of Visual Perceptions due to Occipital Injuries, with Especial Reference to Appreciation of Movement." *Brain* 40, no. 1 (1917a): 15–57.

———. "On the Relative Perceptions of Movement and a Stationary Object in Certain Visual Disturbances due to Occipital Injuries." *Proceedings of the Royal Society of Medicine* 10 (1917b): 13–34.

Ritchie, T. D., et al. "Event Self-Importance, Event Rehearsal, and the Fading Affect Bias in Autobiographical Memory." *Self and Identity* 5 (2006): 172–95.

Roland, P. E., and B. Gulyas. "Visual Memory, Visual Imagery, and Visual Recognition of Large Field Patterns by the Human Brain: Functional Anatomy by Positron Emission Tomography." *Cerebral Cortex* 5, no. 1 (1995): 79–93.

Ross, S. *Higher, Further, Faster: Is Technology Improving Sport?* Chichester, U.K.: John Wiley and Sons, 2008.

Rudolph, K., and T. Pasternak. "Transient and Permanent Deficits in Motion Perception After Lesions of Cortical Areas MT and MST in the Macaque Monkey." *Cerebral Cortex* 9, no. 1 (1999): 90–100.

Russell, C. J., and C. C. Bell. "Neuronal Responses to Electrosensory Input in Mormyrid Valvula Cerebelli." *Journal of Neurophysiology* 41, no. 6 (1978): 1495–510.

Sakamaki, T. "Social Grooming Among Wild Bonobos (*Pan paniscus*) at Wamba in the Luo Scientific Reserve, DR Congo, with Special Reference to the Formation of Grooming Gatherings." *Primates* 54, no. 4 (2013): 349–59.

Sakreida, K., et al. "Motion Class Dependency in Observers' Motor Areas Revealed by Functional Magnetic Resonance Imaging." *Journal of Neuroscience* 25, no. 6 (2005): 1335–42.

Saleem, K. S., and K. Tanaka. "Divergent Projections from the Anterior Inferotemporal Area TE to the Perirhinal and Entorhinal Cortices in the Macaque Monkey." *Journal of Neuroscience* 16, no. 15 (1996): 4757–75.

Sar, V., S. N. Unal, and E. Ozturk. "Frontal and Occipital Perfusion Changes in Dissociative Identity Disorder." *Psychiatry Research* 156, no. 3 (2007): 217–23.

Savoy, R. L., et al. "Voluntary Switching Between Identities in Dissociative Identity Disorder: A Functional MRI Case Study." *Cognitive Neuroscience* 3, no. 2 (2012): 112–19.

Saxe, G. N., et al. "SPECT Imaging and Multiple Personality Disorder." *Journal of Nervous and Mental Disease* 180, no. 10 (1992): 662–63.

Schaefer, M., and M. Rotte. "Thinking on Luxury or Pragmatic Brand Products: Brain Responses to Different Categories of Culturally Based Brands." *Brain Research* 1165 (2007): 98–104.

Schaffner, N. *Saucerful of Secrets: The Pink Floyd Odyssey.* London: Helter Skelter, 2005.

Schlumpf, Y. R., et al. "Dissociative Part-Dependent Biopsychosocial Reactions to Backward Masked Angry and Neutral Faces: An fMRI Study of Dissociative Identity Disorder." *NeuroImage: Clinical* 3 (2013): 54–64.

Schmidt, S. R. "Autobiographical Memories for the September 11th Attacks: Reconstructive Errors and Emotional Impairment of Memory." *Memory and Cognition* 32, no. 3 (2004): 443–54.

Schnider, A. "Orbitofrontal Reality Filtering." *Frontiers in Behavioral Neuroscience* 7, no. 67 (2013): 1–8.

———. "Spontaneous Confabulation and the Adaptation of Thought to Ongoing Reality." *Nature Reviews Neuroscience* 4, no. 8 (2003): 662–71.

Schnider, A., C. von Däniken, and K. Gutbrod. "The Mechanisms of Spontaneous and Provoked Confabulations." *Brain* 119 (1996): 1365–75.

Schulte-Rüther, M., et al. "Mirror Neuron and Theory of Mind Mechanisms Involved in Face-to-Face Interactions: A Functional Magnetic Resonance Imaging Approach to Empathy." *Journal of Cognitive Neuroscience* 19, no. 8 (2007): 1354–72.

Schuster, C., et al. "Best Practice for Motor Imagery: A Systematic Literature Review on Motor Imagery Training Elements in Five Different Disciplines." *BMC Medicine* 9, no. 75 (2011): 1–35.

Schwärzel, M., and U. Müller. "Dynamic Memory Networks: Dissecting Molecular Mechanisms Underlying Associative Memory in the Temporal Domain." *Cellular and Molecular Life Sciences* 63, no. 9 (2006): 989–98.

Searle, J. R. *Mind: A Brief Introduction.* New York: Oxford University Press, 2004.

Sedikides, C., and J. D. Green. "What I Don't Recall Can't Hurt Me: Information Negativity Versus Information Inconsistency as Determinants of Memorial Self-Defense." *Social Cognition* 22, no. 1 (2004): 4–29.

Seif-Barghi, T., et al. "The Effect of an Ecological Imagery Program on Soccer Performance of Elite Players." *Asian Journal of Sports Medicine* 3, no. 2 (2012): 81–89.

Senju, A., et al. "Brief Report: Does Eye Contact Induce Contagious Yawning in Children with Autism Spectrum Disorder?" *Journal of Autism and Developmental Disorders* 39, no. 11 (2009): 1598–602.

Shahar, A., et al. "Induction of an Illusory Shadow Person." *Nature* 443 (2006): 287.

Sharot, T., et al. "How Personal Experience Modulates the Neural Circuitry of Memories of September 11." *Proceedings of the National Academy of Sciences* 104, no. 1 (2007): 389–94.

Sharpless, B. A., and J. P. Barber. "Lifetime Prevalence Rates of Sleep Paralysis: A Systematic Review." *Sleep Medicine Reviews* 15, no. 5 (2011): 311–15.

Shergill, S. S., et al. "Mapping Auditory Hallucinations in Schizophrenia Using Functional Magnetic Resonance Imaging." *Archives of General Psychiatry* 57, no. 11 (2000): 1033–38.

Sherman, R. A., C. J. Sherman, and L. Parker. "Chronic Phantom and Stump Pain Among American Veterans: Results of a Survey." *Pain* 18, no. 1 (1984): 83–95.

Shmuelof, L., and E. Zohary. "Mirror-Image Representation of Action in the Anterior Parietal Cortex." *Nature Neuroscience* 11, no. 11 (2008): 1267–69.

Siegel, R. K. "Hostage Hallucinations: Visual Imagery Induced by Isolation and Life-Threatening Stress." *Journal of Nervous and Mental Disease* 172, no. 5 (1984): 264–72.

Sigman, M., S. J. Spence, and A. T. Wang. "Autism from Developmental and Neuropsychological Perspectives." *Annual Review of Clinical Psychology* 2 (2006): 327–55.

Silk, J., D. Cheney, and R. Seyfarth. "A Practical Guide to the Study of Social Relationships." *Evolutionary Anthropology* 22, no. 5 (2013): 213–25.

Simeon, D., et al. "Feeling Unreal: A PET Study of Depersonalization Disorder." *American Journal of Psychiatry* 157, no. 11 (2000): 1782–88.

Simons, D. J., and D. T. Levin. "Failure to Detect Changes to People During a Real-World Interaction." *Psychonomic Bulletin and Review* 5, no. 4 (1998): 644–49.

Simons, R. C., and C. C. Hughes. *The Culture-Bound Syndromes: Folk Illnesses of Psychiatric and Anthropological Interest (Culture, Illness, and Healing)*. Dordrecht: Reidel, 1985.

Simonyan, K., and B. Horwitz. "Laryngeal Motor Cortex and Control of Speech in Humans." *Neuroscientist* 17, no. 2 (2011): 197–208.

Singer, T., et al. "Empathy for Pain Involves the Affective but Not Sensory Components of Pain." *Science* 303, no. 5661 (2004): 1157–62.

Smith, D., C. J. Wright, and C. Cantwell. "Beating the Bunker: The Effect of PETTLEP Imagery on Golf Bunker Shot Performance." *Research Quarterly for Exercise and Sport* 79, no. 3 (2008): 385–91.

Smith, S. M., et al. "The Lack of Cerebral Effects of *d*-Tubocurarine." *Anesthesiology* 8, no. 1 (1947): 1–14.

Smith, W. H. "Incorporating Hypnosis into the Psychotherapy of Patients with Multiple Personality Disorder." *Bulletin of the Menninger Clinic* 57, no. 3 (1993): 344–54.

Solomonova, E., et al. "Sensed Presence as a Correlate of Sleep Paralysis Distress, Social Anxiety, and Waking State Social Imagery." *Consciousness and Cognition* 17, no. 1 (2008): 49–63.

Spence, C., and O. Deroy. "Hearing Mouth Shapes: Sound Symbolism and the Reverse McGurk Effect." *Iperception* 3, no. 8 (2012): 550–52.

Spence, S. A., and C. Frith. "A PET Study of Voluntary Movement in Schizophrenic Patients Experiencing Passivity Phenomena." *Brain* 120, no. 11 (1997): 1997–2011.

Spoormaker, V., and J. van den Bout. "Lucid Dreaming Treatment for Nightmares: A Pilot Study." *Psychotherapy and Psychosomatics* 75, no. 6 (2006): 389–94.

Stankiewicz, S., and M. Golczyńska. "Dispute over the Multiple Personality Disorder: Theoretical or Practical Dilemma?" *Psychiatria Polska* 40, no. 2 (2006): 233–43.

Staunton, H. "The Function of Dreaming." *Reviews in the Neurosciences* 12, no. 4 (2001): 365–71.

Stephan, K. E., et al. "Dysconnection in Schizophrenia: From Abnormal Synaptic Plasticity to Failures of Self-Monitoring." *Schizophrenia Bulletin* 35, no. 3 (2009): 509–27.

Stevenson, R. L. *The Strange Case of Dr. Jekyll and Mr. Hyde*. New York: Dover, 1991.

Stinson, B., and D. Arthur. "A Novel EEG for Alpha Brain State Training, Neurobiofeedback and Behavior Change." *Complementary Therapies in Clinical Practice* 19, no. 3 (2013): 114–18.

Stone, S. P., P. W. Halligan, and R. J. Greenwood. "The Incidence of Neglect Phenomena and Related Disorders in Patients with an Acute Right or Left Hemisphere Stroke." *Age and Ageing* 22, no. 1 (1993): 46–52.

Stonnington, C. M., J. J. Barry, and R. S. Fisher. "Conversion Disorder." *American Journal of Psychiatry* 163, no. 9 (2006): 1510–17.

Strayer, D. L., et al. "Cell Phone–Induced Failures of Visual Attention During Simulated Driving." *Journal of Experimental Psychology: Applied* 9, no. 1 (2003): 23–32.

Streatfeild, D. *Brainwash: The Secret History of Mind Control.* New York: St. Martin's Press, 2007.

Stroop, J. R. "Studies of Interference in Serial Verbal Reactions." *Journal of Experimental Psychology* 18, no. 16 (1935): 643–62.

Suzuki, W. A. "Neuroanatomy of the Monkey Entorhinal, Perirhinal, and Parahippocampal Cortices: Organization of Cortical Inputs and Interconnections with Amygdala and Striatum." *Seminars in Neuroscience* 8, no. 1 (1996): 3–12.

Syrjala, K. L., C. Cummings, and G. W. Donaldson. "Hypnosis or Cognitive Behavioral Training for the Reduction of Pain and Nausea During Cancer Treatment: A Controlled Clinical Trial." *Pain* 48, no. 2 (1992): 137–46.

Szasz, T. *The Second Sin.* New York: Doubleday, 1973.

Tataranni, P. A., J.-F. Gautier, and K. Chen. "Neuroanatomical Correlates of Hunger and Satiation in Humans Using Positron Emission Tomography." *Proceedings of the National Academy of Sciences* 96, no. 8 (1999): 4569–74.

Taylor, J. *Prime Golf: Triumph of the Mental Game.* Lincoln, Neb.: Writers Club Press, 2001.

Taylor, J. B. *My Stroke of Insight: A Brain Scientist's Personal Journey.* New York: Viking, 2006.

"The 10 Most Interesting Rituals in Sports." ExactSports.com, Oct. 6, 2011. http://exactsports.com/blog/the-10-most-interesting-rituals-in-sports/2011/10/06/.

Teresa of Ávila. *The Life of St. Teresa of Jesus, of the Order of Our Lady of Carmel* (ca. 1565). Translated by David Lewis (1904), chap. 29. Reproduced by BiblioLife, 2007.

Teunisse, R. J., et al. "The Charles Bonnet Syndrome: A Large Prospective Study in the Netherlands: A Study of the Prevalence of the Charles Bonnet Syndrome and Associated Factors in 500 Patients Attending the University Department of Ophthalmology at Nijmegen." *British Journal of Psychiatry* 166, no. 2 (1995): 254–57.

Thacker, A. J. "Formal Communication Disorder: Sign Language in Deaf People with Schizophrenia." *British Journal of Psychiatry* 165, no. 6 (1994): 818–23.

Thaler, L., S. R. Arnott, and M. A. Goodale. "Neural Correlates of Natural Human Echolocation in Early and Late Blind Echolocation Experts." *PLoS ONE* 6, no. 5 (2011): e20162.

Thomaes, K., et al. "Increased Anterior Cingulate Cortex and Hippocampus Activation in Complex PTSD During Encoding of Negative Words." *Social Cognitive and Affective Neuroscience* 8, no. 2 (2013): 190–200.

Thomas-Antérion, C., et al. "An Odd Manifestation of the Capgras Syndrome: Loss of Familiarity Even with the Sexual Partner." *Clinical Neurophysiology* 38, no. 3 (2008): 177–82.

"Tiger's Daily Routine." Accessed Feb. 6, 2014. http://www.tigerwoods.com/fitness/tiger
DailyRoutine.

Toiviainen, P., et al. "Capturing the Musical Brain with Lasso: Dynamic Decoding of
Musical Features from fMRI Data." *NeuroImage* 88C (2013): 170–80.

Travis, K. E., et al. "Spatiotemporal Neural Dynamics of Word Understanding in 12- to
18-Month-Old-Infants." *Cerebral Cortex* 21, no. 8 (2011): 1832–39.

Tricomi, E., B. W. Balleine, et al. "A Specific Role for Posterior Dorsolateral Striatum
in Human Habit Learning." *European Journal of Neuroscience* 29, no. 11 (2009):
2225–32.

Tsai, Guochuan, E., et al. "Functional Magnetic Resonance Imaging of Personality Switches
in a Woman with Dissociative Identity Disorder." *Harvard Review of Psychiatry* 7, no. 2
(1999): 119–22.

Turk, D. J., et al. "Mike or Me? Self-Recognition in a Split-Brain Patient." *Nature Neuroscience* 5, no. 9 (2002): 841–42.

Turk, D. J., et al. "Out of Contact, out of Mind: The Distributed Nature of the Self." *Annals
of the New York Academy of Sciences* 1001 (2003): 65–78.

Turner, M. S., et al. "Confabulation: Damage to a Specific Inferior Medial Prefrontal System." *Cortex* 44 (2008): 637–48.

Twersky, T. "Ray Allen Q + A." *Slam* Online. Feb. 10, 2011. http://www.slamonline.com/
online/nba/2011/02/ray-allen-qa/.

Usui, S., et al. "Presence of Contagious Yawning in Children with Autism Spectrum Disorder." *Autism Research and Treatment* 2013 (2013).

Van der Kolk, B. A., and R. Fisler. "Dissociation and the Fragmentary Nature of Traumatic
Memories: Overview and Exploratory Study." *Journal of Traumatic Stress* 8, no. 4 (1995):
505–25.

van Elk, M., et al. "Neural Evidence for Compromised Motor Imagery in Right Hemiparetic Cerebral Palsy." *Frontiers in Neurology* 1, no. 150 (2010): 1–7.

van Lommel, P., et al. "Near-Death Experiences in Survivors of Cardiac Arrest: A Prospective Study in the Netherlands." *Lancet* 358, no. 9298 (2001): 2039–45.

van Veluw, S. J., and S. A. Chance. "Differentiating Between Self and Others: An ALE
Meta-analysis of fMRI Studies of Self-Recognition and Theory of Mind." *Brain Imaging
in Behavioral Medicine and Clinical Neuroscience* 8, no. 1 (2014): 24–38.

Vaudreuil, C., and M. Trieu. "Symptom-Inducibility in a Case of Conversion Disorder."
*Psychosomatics* 54, no. 5 (2013): 505–6.

Verleger, R., et al. "Anarchic-Hand Syndrome: ERP Reflections of Lost Control over the
Right Hemisphere." *Brain and Cognition* 77, no. 1 (2011): 138–50.

Vermetten, E., et al. "Hippocampal and Amygdalar Volumes in Dissociative Identity Disorder." *American Journal of Psychiatry* 163, no. 4 (2006): 630–36.

Vignal, J. P., et al. "The Dreamy State: Hallucinations of Autobiographic Memory Evoked
by Temporal Lobe Stimulations and Seizures." *Brain* 130, no. 1 (2007): 88–99.

Vita, M. G., et al. "Visual Hallucinations and Pontine Demyelination in a Child: Possible
REM Dissociation?" *Journal of Clinical Sleep Medicine* 4, no. 6 (2008): 588–90.

Vuilleumier, P. "Hysterical Conversion and Brain Function." *Progress in Brain Research* 150
(2005): 309–29.

Wagner, U., et al. "Sleep Inspires Insight." *Nature* 427 (2004): 352–55.

Watkins, J. G. "Antisocial Compulsions Induced Under Hypnotic Trance." *Journal of Abnormal and Social Psychology* 42, no. 2 (1947): 256–59.

Watkins, J. G., and H. H. Watkins. "The Management of Malevolent Ego States in Multiple Personality Disorder." *Dissociation* 1, no. 1 (1998): 67–71.

Watson, J. B. "Psychology as the Behaviorist Views It." *Psychological Review* 20 (1913): 158–77.

Weiskrantz, L., J. L. Barbur, and A. Sahraie. "Parameters Affecting Conscious Versus Unconscious Visual Discrimination with Damage to the Visual Cortex (V1)." *Proceedings of the National Academy of Science* 92, no. 13 (1995): 6122–26.

Weiskrantz, L., et al. "Visual Capacity in the Hemianopic Field Following a Restricted Occipital Ablation." *Brain* 97, no. 4 (1974): 709–28.

Werring, D. J., et al. "Functional Magnetic Resonance Imaging of the Cerebral Response to Visual Stimulation in Medically Unexplained Visual Loss." *Psychological Medicine* 34, no. 4 (2004): 583–89.

Whalen, P. J., et al. "Masked Presentations of Emotional Facial Expressions Modulate Amygdala Activity Without Explicit Knowledge." *Journal of Neuroscience* 18, no. 1 (1998): 411–18.

Whinnery, J. E. "Psychophysiologic Correlates of Unconsciousness and Near-Death Experiences." *Journal of Near-Death Studies* 15, no. 4 (1997): 231–58.

Williams, L. M., et al. "Amygdala-Prefrontal Dissociation of Subliminal and Supraliminal Fear." *Human Brain Mapping* 27, no. 8 (2006): 652–61.

Wolman, D. "The Split Brain: A Tale of Two Halves." *Nature* 483, no. 7389 (2012): 260–63.

Wright, M. J., et al. "Brain Regions Concerned with the Identification of Deceptive Soccer Moves by Higher-Skilled and Lower-Skilled Players." *Frontiers in Human Neuroscience* 7 (2013): 851.

Yang, Z., and E. M. Tong. "The Effects of Subliminal Anger and Sadness Primes on Agency Appraisals." *Emotion* 10, no. 6 (2010): 915–22.

Yapko, M. D. *Essentials of Hypnosis*. New York: Brunner/Mazel, 1995.

Yin, H. H., and B. J. Knowlton. "The Role of the Basal Ganglia in Habit Formation." *Nature Reviews Neuroscience* 7, no. 6 (2006): 464–76.

Yin, H. H., et al. "Lesions of Dorsolateral Striatum Preserve Outcome Expectancy but Disrupt Habit Formation in Instrumental Learning." *European Journal of Neuroscience* 19, no. 1 (2004): 181–89.

Young, A. W., et al. "Cotard Delusion After Brain Injury." *Psychological Medicine* 22, no. 3 (1992): 799–804.

Zago, M., et al. "Internal Models of Target Motion: Expected Dynamics Overrides Measured Kinematics in Timing Manual Interceptions." *Journal of Neurophysiology* 91, no. 4 (2004): 1620–34.

Zeki, S., and D. H. Ffytche. "The Riddoch Syndrome: Insights into the Neurobiology of Conscious Vision." *Brain* 121 (1998): 25–45.

Zimmermann-Schlatter, A., et al. "Efficacy of Motor Imagery in Post-Stroke Rehabilitation: A Systematic Review." *Journal of Neuroengineering and Rehabilitation* 5 (2008): 1–10.

# Index

Page numbers in *italics* refer to illustrations.

ILLUSTRATION CREDITS

PAGE 6: Copyright © OpenStax College, Anatomy & Physiology. OpenStax CNX. Jul 30, 2014. Used under terms of Creative Commons Attribution License.

PAGE 11: *Dream Caused by the Flight of a Bee Around a Pomegranate a Second Before Waking Up,* 1944, by Salvador Dalí. Oil on panel. Copyright © 2014, Museo Thyssen-Bornemisza/ Scala, Florence.

PAGE 17: *Seeds for Sowing Must Not be Ground,* 1941, by Käthe Kollowitz (Knesebeck 274). Copyright © 2014 Artists Rights Society (ARS), New York/VG Bild-Kunst, Bonn. Photo courtesy of Galerie St. Etienne, New York.

PAGE 21: From "Complex Visual Hallucinations in a Patient with Macular Degeneration: A Case of the Charles Bonnet Syndrome," by B. Kumar, in *Age and Ageing* 42, no. 3 (2013): 411. By permission of Oxford University Press.

PAGE 31: From "Neural Correlates of Natural Human Echolocation in Early and Late Blind Echolocation Experts," by L. Thaler, S. R. Arnott, and M. A. Goodale, *PLoS ONE* 6, no. 5. Used under terms of Creative Common License.

PAGES 33 (left and right) and 34: From "Visual Dream Content, Graphical Representation, and EEG Alpha Activity in Congenitally Blind Subjects," by H. Bértolo et al., in *Cognitive Brain Research* 15, no. 3: 277–84. Copyright © 2003. Used with permission from Elsevier.

PAGE 43: From "Hemispatial Neglect," by A. Parton, P. Malhotra, and M. Husain, in *Journal of Neurology, Neurosurgery, and Psychiatry* 75: 13–21. Copyright © 2004. Used with permission from BMJ Publishing Group Ltd.

PAGE 44: From "Modified Target Cancellation in Hemispatial Neglect," by S. Prasad and A. L. Berkowitz, in *Practical Neurology* 14, no. 4 (2014): 277. Used with permission from Modern Neurology LLC.

PAGES 47 and 48: From "The Role of Basal Ganglia in Habit Formation," by H. H. Yin and B. J. Knowlton, in *Nature Reviews Neuroscience* 7, no. 6: 464–76. Copyright © 2006. Reprinted by permission from Macmillian Publishers Ltd.

PAGE 52 (top and bottom): From *The Mechanism of Human Facial Expression,* by B. Duchenne, R. A. Cuthbertson, trans. New York: Cambridge University Press, 1990.

PAGE 74: From "Improvement and Generalization of Arm Motor Performance Through Motor Imagery Practice," by R. Gentili, C. Papaxanthis, and T. Pozzo, in *Neuroscience* 137, no. 3: 761–72. Copyright © 2006. Used with permission from Elsevier.

PAGE 77: From "Beating the Bunker: The Effect of PETTLEP Imagery on Golf Bunker Shot Performance," by D. Smith, C. J. Wright, and C. Cantwell, in *Research Quarterly for Exercise and Sport* 79, no. 3 (2008): 385–91. Reprinted by permission of Taylor & Francis Ltd.

PAGES 121 and 122: From "Spontaneous Confabulation and the Adaptation of Thought to Ongoing Reality," by A. Schnider, in *Nature Reviews Neuroscience* 4, no. 8: 662–72. Copyright © 2003. Reprinted by permission from Macmillan Publishers Ltd.

PAGE 157: Adapted from"Subvocal Activity and Auditory Hallucinations: Clues for Behavioral Treatments," by M. F. Green and M. Kinsbourne, in *Psychological Bulletin* 16, no. 4 (1990): 617–25.

PAGE 159: Photo by Daiju Azuma.

PAGE 160 (top and bottom): From "Neuronal Responses to Electrosensory Input in Mormyrid Valvula Cerebelli," by C. J. Russell and C. C. Bell, in *Journal of Neurophysiology* 41, no. 6 (1978): 1495–1510. Copyright © The American Physiological Society (APS).